RHEUMATIC DISEASE:

OCCUPATIONAL THERAPY
AND REHABILITATION

RHEUMATIC DISEASE:

OCCUPATIONAL THERAPY AND REHABILITATION

Edition 2

**JEANNE LYNN MELVIN,
O.T.R., M.S. Ed., F.A.O.T.A.**

**Director, Arthritis and Health Resource Center,
Wellesley, Massachusetts. Formerly Director of
Occupational Therapy at the Brigham and Women's
Hospital and the Robert B. Brigham Hospital,
Boston, Massachusetts.**

Illustrated by Lois R. Barnes

 F. A. DAVIS COMPANY • Philadelphia

Library of Congress Cataloging in Publication Data

Melvin, Jeanne L.
    Rheumatic disease.

    Includes bibliographies and index.
    1. Rheumatism—Patients—Rehabilitation.   2. Occupational therapy.   I. Title.   [DNLM:
1. Arthritis—Rehabilitation.   2. Occupational   therapy.   3. Rheumatism—Rehabilitation.
WE 344 M531r]
RC927.M43   1982   616.7'2306   81-19596
ISBN 0-8036-6136-3   AACR2

CONSULTANTS

HAND SURGERY CONSULTANT

Edward A. Nalebuff, M.D.

Professor of Orthopaedic Surgery, Tufts University School of Medicine; Chief, Hand Surgical Service, New England Baptist Hospital; Orthopaedic Staff, Brigham and Women's Hospital. Formerly, Chief, Hand Service, Robert B. Brigham Hospital, Boston.

MEDICAL CONSULTANT

Kenneth M. Nies, M.D.

Associate Professor of Medicine, and Associate Chief, Division of Rheumatology, Harbor-UCLA Medical Center, Torrance, California.

ORTHOPAEDIC SURGERY CONSULTANT

Clement B. Sledge, M.D.

John B. and Buckminster Brown Professor of Orthopaedic Surgery, Harvard Medical School; Chairman, Department of Orthopaedic Surgery, Brigham and Women's Hospital, Boston.

PREFACE

The treatment of chronic diseases such as arthritis is rapidly undergoing change in this country. It has become clear in the field of rheumatology that optimal care is obtained for the person with joint disease when several specialized personnel interact as a team to achieve the common goal of physical and functional independence for the client. The physician, occupational therapist, physical therapist, nurse, social worker, and other health professionals must have a common understanding of the disease, of the available treatment methods, and of each other's role in order to effectively share their expertise in enhancing the client's well being.

It is hoped that this text will further the development of the team approach to patient care by presenting the medical and surgical information from an allied health frame of reference and by communicating to other professionals the role of occupational therapy in the treatment of rheumatic disease.

This book is designed as a clinical reference guide, with material organized according to how problems or issues present themselves in the clinic. The introductory chapter provides an overview of therapy for joint involvement common to all the rheumatic diseases. It is brief to provide a gestalt of treatment. The reader is then referred to subsequent chapters for detailed information.

The topics of psychology and patient education are combined in Part 1 to alert the reader to some of the basic psychological issues that need to be dealt with before effective patient instruction can take place. This part has been expanded to include guidelines for patient education programs.

Nine major rheumatic diseases are reviewed in Part 2, including a new chapter on psoriatic arthritis. This addition reflects the recent research that makes this disease and its classification more comprehensible. Treatment for the diseases discussed in Part 2 is listed according to the common clinical symptoms or by the body areas affected, thereby allowing easy reference for treatment of specific symptoms.

Part 3 (Chapter 12) on drug therapy is brief and focuses on how medications can affect allied health effectiveness in administering quantitative measurements and patient education.

In Part 4, seven chapters have been added on surgical rehabilitation to cover the advances in hand surgery and joint replacement surgery over the past several years. These advances have created many new options for improving functional ability. These new chapters discuss the theory or rationale for selecting a surgical procedure as well as guidelines for postoperative management. It is important that therapists and rheumatologists understand the limitations of conservative measures and the indications for surgical intervention in order to provide the most effective options to a patient.

Part 5 concerns evaluation and relates standard evaluation methods specifically to patients with joint disease. Other texts that define the standard range of motion and strength assessments, for example, relate the procedure only to normal joint anatomy. Assessment of damaged joints requires special considerations.

The chapter on hand pathodynamics and assessment has been expanded and reorganized to reflect the growing knowledge about these processes. Systematic comprehensive hand assessments, conducted by therapists knowledgeable in both arthritis pathodynamics and therapeutic intervention, can result in the early detection and prevention of many deformities. The comprehensive hand assessment process described in this chapter is the result of eight years of development and refinement.

Part 6 covers five basic occupational therapy modalities as they apply to joint involvement: splinting, joint protection and energy conservation techniques, assistive equipment, functional activities, and a general discussion of range of motion and strengthening. The text is not intended to teach basic occupational therapy methods but is intended to review the unique aspects of these activities as they apply to joint disease.

In addition to the major changes listed previously, the second edition includes 32 new clinical photographs and drawings. The text throughout the book has been updated and revised to include recent research and clinical trends, including the changes in therapeutic management over the past seven years that involved changes in attitude and philosophy rather than the development of new treatments. There is more openness and flexibility in the delivery of therapy, as well as a greater appreciation of the patient's individual needs. For example, the teaching of joint protection techniques has evolved from handing patients a list of absolute do's and don'ts to teaching them how to monitor the signs of inflammation so they can evaluate the appropriateness and consequences of their own daily activities. This trend of teaching self-management is now being reflected in all areas of arthritis management.

A glossary of common rheumatologic terms is included as a resource for terms not found in medical dictionaries.

Occupational therapy for rheumatic diseases is in a state of evolution and varies considerably across the country. In some facilities the occupational therapist carries out training only in activities of daily living and does not do any splinting or exercises. In other centers the occupational therapist carries out all treatment for the upper extremities. The treatment procedures that are a part of current occupational therapy regimens have been included to accommodate the needs of various clinics.

ACKNOWLEDGMENTS
FOR THE FIRST EDITION

In 1973 the Arthritis Foundation provided the first Allied Health Professions Fellowship. This book is a result of the research portion of that two year Fellowship. I am indebted to the Arthritis Foundation and the Allied Health Professions Section for their support.

As I review the work involved in producing this book, appreciative thoughts are reflected to physician and therapist friends who helped through manuscript critiques and personal support. One person, in particular, holds a special place in this project for he has been a major influence in its completion. Throughout our five year working liaison Dr. Kenneth Nies has continually challenged my professional skills. His clear, pragmatic approach to rheumatology has guided the medical philosophy put forth in this text. I hope that this book will, in part, acknowledge my gratitude for his support over the years and for his supervision of the second year of the Fellowship.

Thanks is given to the following people for the cooperation and work they put into this endeavor. Consultants Patricia MacBain, Hanna Gruen, and Dena Shapiro provided the necessary feedback to make material applicable to a wide variety of clinical settings. Patricia MacBain was particularly helpful in supplying references and sources of information. Dr. James London provided guidance with the surgery and hand sections. Working with him can best be described as an unique and enjoyable educational experience. Dr. Robert Swezey supervised the first year of the Fellowship and the Rehabilitation section. Linda Olt, Medical Editor at the University of California at Los Angeles, and Eleanor Mora, Production Editor with the F. A. Davis Company, provided excellent editorial assistance. The concern and research Lois Barnes put into the project is reflected in the high quality of her illustrations.

I am also indebted to Robert Craven, President of the F. A. Davis Company, for his guidance and friendship throughout the publishing process.

Finally I extend my appreciation to Max Weiner and Bob Richardson, Past Presidents of the Allied Health Professions Section of the Arthritis Foundation, and Dr. James Louie, Chief of Rheumatology at Harbor General Hospital, for their support and encouragement during the Fellowship program.

ACKNOWLEDGMENTS FOR THE SECOND EDITION

Several individuals have played an important role in creating this Second Edition. I am very grateful for their assistance, support, and friendship.

Long before my move to the East Coast, Dr. Edward Nalebuff, through his writings, was a teacher and a guide in hand management. Working with him these past four years has been a memorable experience. His skill as a surgeon is matched only by his keen ability to review, analyze, and organize complex processes into comprehensible functional forms. The chapter on hand surgery was possible in part because of his previous work in classifying rheumatic hand disorders. He is also responsible for the length of the hand chapter, by continually challenging me with such questions as: "Is this *all* you are going to write?" After each such question the chapter would lengthen considerably. I am also indebted to Dr. Nalebuff for his generous loan of clinical and surgical hand photographs that helped immeasurably to illustrate teaching points.

In a similar vein, Dr. Clement Sledge is responsible for the remaining five chapters on rheumatologic surgery. His writings on joint replacement surgery along with the surgical reviews he encouraged as co-editor of the new *Textbook of Rheumatology* have filled a major gap in the rheumatologic literature. This new literature base made writing the chapters on surgery in this edition a feasible and manageable task. His critical editing of these chapters was invaluable for insuring the accuracy of this technical material. Dr. Sledge's support and encouragement over the past four years have been greatly appreciated.

Dr. Kenneth Nies made a special contribution to the continuity between the First and Second Editions by reminding me of the original purpose of the book. He coaxed additions to the medical section into a consistent style and because of this process can be credited with the brevity of several sections. He also kept me in touch with my California rheumatologic roots which helped create an East Coast-West Coast balance in the presentation of material. I am indebted to Dr. Nies for his teachings, encouragement, and friendship throughout the writing of both editions of this book.

I am also very grateful to the talented publishing staff at F. A. Davis, who literally created this Edition—Robert Martone, Allied Health Editor, who coordinated this endeavor; Sally Burke, for her gentle, patient, and thorough editing; and Lenoire Brown, for overseeing the design and production.

CONTENTS

ABBREVIATIONS

ADL	Activities of daily living
AS	Ankylosing spondylitis
CARS	Canadian Arthritis and Rheumatism Society
CMC	Carpometacarpal
DIP	Distal interphalangeal
DJD	Degenerative joint disease
IP	Interphalangeal
JCPA	Juvenile chronic polyarthritis
MCP	Metacarpophalangeal
MTP	Metatarsophalangeal
NSAID	Nonsteroidal anti-inflammatory drug
PA	Psoriatic arthritis
PIP	Proximal interphalangeal
PSS	Progressive systemic sclerosis
RA	Rheumatoid arthritis
RID	Remission-inducing drug
ROM	Range of Motion
SLE	Systemic lupus erythematosus

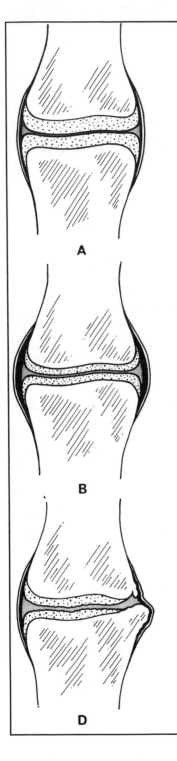

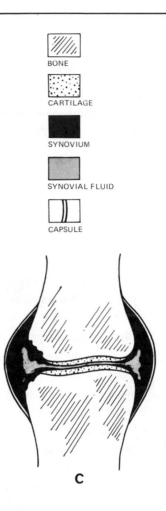

BONE

CARTILAGE

SYNOVIUM

SYNOVIAL FLUID

CAPSULE

A

B

C

D

FIGURE 1. Types of joint disease. (*A*), Normal joint with synovial lining one to three cells thick. (*B*), Early inflammatory disease with symmetric cartilage reduction, including thickened synovium, increased synovial fluid, and fusiform swelling. (*C*), Advanced inflammatory disease showing marked synovial hypertrophy with pannus formation, bone and cartilage erosions, and severely diminished cartilage. (*D*), Noninflammatory disease with characteristic asymmetric cartilage destruction and osteophyte formation without synovial involvement.

1

INTRODUCTION AND OVERVIEW OF THERAPY FOR JOINT DISEASE

There are over one hundred conditions in which joint disease can be a significant feature. The common denominator of joint involvement characterizes these conditions as the rheumatic diseases. Joint involvement, be it localized to a single joint or in combination with a systemic disease, universally interferes with a person's functional ability. Thus effective patient care involves treating both the disease and the person.

Treatment for joint disease is accomplished through control of inflammation, removal of irritating causal factors, and protection of joint structures during periods of exacerbation. From this point treatment must be directed towards the person and towards relief or control of pain, improvement of functional ability, psychological adjustment to functional loss, and development of health behaviors with regard to nutrition, rest, and exercise.

The physical, personal, familial, social, and vocational consequences of chronic joint disease are so extensive that skilled assistance is beyond the scope of any one professional. Consultation and cooperation among various health care workers become an integral part of treatment.

The rehabilitative approaches described and advocated in this book are based on the premise that effective treatment of joint disease is *experimental* in all phases. There are no absolute answers in therapy; no treatment can be applied with complete certainty as to outcome. There is no treatment without disadvantages as well as advantages and no treatment that cannot be improved. There are many successful treatment methods to be developed by therapists.

THERAPY FOR JOINT DISEASE

The goals of therapy vary depending on the chronicity of the disease and the responsiveness of the patient to medication. In the beginning stages of rheumatoid arthritis (RA), particulary the first two years, there is a high incidence of sustained remission. It is estimated that 20 to 40 percent of all people diagnosed with RA have only one or two episodes of arthritis and then go into "spontaneous" remission. Spontaneous is the term used when the reason for the remission is not understood. Some clinicians report that the incidence of spontaneous remission may be as high as 80 percent when the diagnosis is made early (within the first two months of the disease).[1] It is unclear whether these patients actually develop RA and then, through some unknown process, are able to mobilize their immune system to control the inflammation or whether they have developed an unidentified short-term, more benign inflammatory condition. It is likely that both of these factors, as well as several other unknown factors, play a role in the development of sustained remissions.[1] In this discussion, RA is used as an example because it is the most common condition treated by therapists and because there is the most information available about the natural course of the disease. However, it is possible to have spontaneous remissions in all of the major rheumatic diseases.

The remissions seen in patients diagnosed with RA may last for several years or may be indefinite. The initial episodes vary in intensity and duration. They may be mild, lasting several weeks with no residual limitation, or they may be quite severe, lasting as long as a year. If proper therapy is not received, these patients may, despite complete remission of the disease, have to live with deformities incurred during the initial episodes.

Other patients—an estimated 20 to 30 percent—have a variable or intermittent course of RA, with alternating periods of remission and exacerbation. For others, the condition is slowly or rapidly progressive. Fortunately, most of these patients are responsive to antirheumatic medications. It is really a small percentage of patients (3 to 5 percent) with RA that have a severe progressive disease that is not responsive to medications.[1]

In addition to spontaneous remissions it is possible for some of the stronger antirheumatic medications, such as gold, hydroxychloroquine (Plaquenil), and penicillamine, to induce a complete or nearly complete remission of symptoms. So in the early stages of the disease there is considerable opportunity for the patient to experience sustained remissions. (See Chapter 12, Drug Therapy.)

When a therapist is working with a patient early in the course of the disease (within the first two years), *the overriding goal of therapy should be to preserve the integrity of the musculoskeletal system during periods of exacerbation, so the patient will have optimal functioning during periods of remission or throughout his or her life, in the event of a spontaneous remission.*

Occupational and physical therapy should be initiated early in the course of the disease (during the first six months), so that treatment can be preventive rather than salvage in nature.

Many therapists work in facilities in which physicians do not refer patients to rehabilitation until the patient develops significant limitations. In these facilities it is the responsibility of the therapist to make physicians aware of the preventive role of therapy and the value of early patient education. Many of the deformities that occur in arthritis can be avoided, as they are the result of the patient having inadequate information about the disease and lacking instruction regarding appropriate or effective exercise technique. Throughout this text there will be an emphasis on early treatment and the procedures that are most effective for preventing deformity or limitations. Preventive therapy is one of the most rewarding and satisfying aspects of rheumatologic rehabilitation, for the therapist as well as the patient.

Joint disease can take two forms: inflammatory or noninflammatory (which includes osteoarthritis and traumatic arthritis). Figure 1 compares these two forms of joint involvement with a normal joint. Inflammatory joint disease is described as having phases. It may start as acute and then diminish to subacute. If it persists over time it is referred to as chronic-active.[2]

Rehabilitative therapy for each phase of joint disease is symptomatic and preventive in nature; that is, it is directed towards reducing the signs and symptoms of arthritis and preventing limitations related to specific joints. The principles of rehabilitation are the same whether the disease occurs in a single joint or in association with a major rheumatic disease. For example, rehabilitative therapy for synovitis of the wrist is the same if it is the only joint involved or if it occurs in conjunction with rheumatoid arthritis, psoriatic arthritis, juvenile polyarthritis, or any other rheumatic disease. In many instances, it is not possible to ascribe a specific diagnostic label until a clear pattern of joint involvement is established. This may take as long as 6 months. But when medical or rehabilitative treatment is symptomatic, the lack of a definite diagnosis does not alter the course of therapy. However, critical to the treatment process is an understanding of how to reduce the symptoms of arthritis and how to preserve the specific joint structures from the effects of chronic arthritis.

To understand the consequences of chronic arthritis in specific joints it is necessary to be familiar with only three rheumatic diseases. These diseases have characteristic patterns of joint involvement and therefore provide a prototype or model for understanding the consequences of chronic arthritis in specific joints. These diseases are *rheumatoid arthritis,* a chronic inflammatory joint disease of the peripheral joints and the cervical spine; *ankylosing spondylitis* (AS), a chronic inflammatory joint disease of the axial joints; and *degenerative joint disease* (DJD) (osteoarthritis), a noninflammatory joint disease of any joint. This means, for example, that the rehabilitative treatment for chronic synovitis of the peripheral joints in any disease is the same as for rheumatoid arthritis. A case in point is psoriatic arthritis, a condition that may result in inflammatory arthritis of both the peripheral and axial joints. Consequently, rehabilitative treatment for the peripheral joints is the same as for RA, and the treatment of the axial joints is the same as for AS.

Since the treatment for arthritis is symptomatic and common to all of the rheumatic diseases, it is reviewed separately in this chapter. The following overview is purposely brief to provide a gestalt of treatment for easy reference. The specific application of treatment of a person with a major rheumatic disease is discussed in Part II.

INFLAMMATORY JOINT DISEASE

The site of inflammation is in the synovial membrane, which lines the joint capsules, tendon sheaths, and bursae throughout the body. It is theorized that the synovial lining (or membrane) performs two functions. First, it contributes to the production of synovial fluid, which coats the articular surfaces and aids lubrication by synthesizing a major component of the fluid, hyaluronic acid.[3] Second, it provides for removal of the synovial fluid from the joint. When the synovial lining becomes inflamed, these two functions become impaired.[3] An excess of joint fluid is produced, the drainage mechanism becomes inadequate, and the fluid becomes trapped within the capsule (an effusion), resulting in characteristic fusiform-shaped swelling.

If the inflammation is prolonged the synovial cells begin to proliferate, increasing the thickness of the membrane from the normal one to four cells to possibly twenty or more.[3] The inflammatory process directly infiltrates and damages the capsule, supporting ligaments, cartilage, and subchondral bone.[1,4]

Both the effusion and thickened synovium result in an increase in intra-articular pressure that places the joint capsule and supporting structures on tension or stretch. This mechanical stress, in addition to the tissue damage caused by direct inflammatory infiltration, makes the joint structures extremely vulnerable to overstretching during functional use.[3] (All forms of exercise should take into account the tension to which joint structures are subjected during active synovitis.)

If the synovitis is severe, chronic synovial granulation tissue (pannus) can develop in the joint, furthering the inflammatory process and causing erosive changes in the cartilage and subchondral bone. All deformities, joint destruction, and pathologic anatomy encountered in severe inflammatory arthritis are the result of the way in which hypertrophied synovial tissue affects its surroundings.[3] A single (limited) acute bout of synovitis usually does not result in residual deformity.

Pain appears to result from the force exerted by increased intra-articular pressure on the innervated capsule and on the attachment of the capsule to the sensitive bone and possible pressure on small areas of exposed bone within the confines of the capsule. Evidence for this theory is often demonstrated by patients with mild synovitis who perceive pain only when compression or motion further increases the intra-articular pressure. Patients with severe synovitis often feel pain at rest.[3]

Pain and stretch of the joint capsule are also believed to be responsible for secondary changes such as protective muscle spasm. The natural protective response of the body, in the presence of pain, is excitation of the flexors and inhibition of the extensors. Protective spasm is most frequently seen in the flexor and adductor muscles and in the spinal muscles.[4,5,6,7]

The terminology for describing the various phases of inflammation varies considerably across the country. The Manual for Allied Health Professionals published by the Arthritis Foundation lists four phases of arthritis: acute, subacute, chronic-active, and chronic-inactive, the last referring to the end stage or "burned-out" phase of arthritis.[2,8] These terms can be helpful in describing joint status or relating therapy to severity of inflammation. However, most physicians do not recognize these categories and instead refer to synovitis as acute, chronic, active, or inactive. (Inactive is used but technically it is a misnomer, since synovitis by definition is active.) Sometimes the term controlled is used to describe a low-grade synovitis kept in check by medication. Probably no single classification prevails because the terminology can not be applied equally to all patients. Acute inflammation for one patient may be considered moderate or subacute for another. Some patients never develop hot, red, exquisitely tender joints even at the height of an exacerbation.

The symptoms are the same in the three phases of inflammatory joint disease (acute, subacute, and chronic-active); that is, the classic pattern of joint inflammation (pain, tenderness, swelling, warmth, and limited range of motion) is present. The symptoms are the most severe in the *acute phase*. When the symptoms diminish, the patient is entering the *subacute phase* of the disease. If the symptoms continue at a low-grade inflammatory level for an extended period, the disease is in the *chronic-active phase*.[2]

The subacute and chronic-active phases seem very similar. The main difference is that the chronic-active phase is a stable condition. In this phase individuals usually feel better than in the acute or subacute phases, have adjusted somewhat to the pain, and are more active. Thus therapy can be more vigorous in the chronic-active phase.[2]

Clients who have systemic diseases may demonstrate also the classic symptoms of systemic illness (fever, chills, malaise, weakness, and anorexia) and in addition have stiffness. As with articular involvement, these symptoms are more severe in the acute phase and less so in the subacute period. In the chronic-active phase, these symptoms may be reduced to fatigue, morning stiffness, and malaise.[1] When there is systemic involvement, all the joints may be involved during an exacerbation.

Primary Occupational Therapy Goals and Suggested Modalities

The following is an outline of basic treatment for both isolated and multiple joint involvement. The reader is referred to specific chapters for a detailed discussion and references.

I. Acute and subacute phases
A. Reduce pain and inflammation
   1. Splinting or positioning to rest specific joints: wrist/hand resting splints (see Chapter 25); posterior leg or ankle splints; soft neck collars; proper support for back and neck while sitting in bed. (See Chapter 30.)
   2. Elimination of unnecessary joint stress by adequate systemic rest during the day. For inpatients it is essential that the medical, nursing, and rehabilitation programs be coordinated so the patient can get adequate rest: bed or chair rest for inflamed joints of lower extremities and instruction in joint protection methods relevant to involved joints and daily activities of the client. For hospitalized patients instruction may be limited to appropriate transfer and ambulation methods. (See Chapter 26.) When there is severe synovitis, joint protection instruction is minimal because the patient is in too much pain to participate in activities. As the inflammation becomes less acute and the patient starts feeling better and more active, joint protection methods and use of assistive equipment play a more important role in reducing pain and stress to involved joints.
   3. Application of ice compresses, heating pads, or hot packs to relieve pain secondary to joint inflammation and to reduce protective muscle spasm. For acute joint inflammation and tenosynovitis, ice compresses are usually the most beneficial. As the swelling decreases, ice becomes less effective and heat may help the most. Generally, the hotter the joint, the more responsive it is to ice. Acute tenosynovitis may present with neither heat nor pain; the only symptoms may be swelling and decreased tendon excursion. Ice is the most effective modality for reducing swelling.[9-11] For children with severe muscle spasm, contrast hot-cold compresses or baths may be the most effective intervention for reducing swelling or spasm.[12]
B. Maintain range of motion (ROM) and joint integrity
   1. Gentle passive or active ROM to the point of discomfort (without stretch) two times per day. (Stretch is *not* recommended when there is severe intra articular swelling since this in itself causes the supportive joint structures to be on stretch. See Chapter 29, Exercise Treatment.) The client may be able to do effective active self-ranging of the neck, elbows, hands, knees, and ankles but may require gentle passive ranging of the shoulders and hips (passive ranging allows maximal muscle relaxation). The flexor, adductor, internal rotators, and supinator muscles are the most prone to developing contractures and therefore need emphasis in the ROM program.
   2. Proper positioning for lying or sitting. This includes a firm mattress, small head pillow or cervical pillow, no knee pillows, and the hospital bed *not elevated* at the patient's knees. (See Chapter 30.) For subacute involvement, proper positioning during leisure activities becomes more important, for example, while reading (especially reading in bed), watching television, or doing homework. Proper positioning includes back and neck support to achieve straight alignment,[10] elevation of the feet with knees extended and supported (for knee or ankle involvement) and an open or extended position for fingers at rest. (See Chapter 30.) For clients with hip involvement or on prolonged bed rest, lying prone to tolerance is an important adjunct to maintaining hip ROM.[10] (See Chapter 30.)
   3. Use of resting hand, ankle, or leg splints. Posterior ankle splints are the most effective method for preventing ankle plantar-flexion contractures. Footboards are

helpful in keeping bedcovers elevated so they don't pull the feet into plantar flexion, but they are not sufficient for preventing foot drop contractures.

    4. Deep breathing and postural exercises to maintain thoracic and scapular joint mobility.

    5. Exercises to maintain jaw mobility are indicated for clients with temporomandibular joint movement.

  C. Maintain strength and endurance

    1. Performance of activities of daily living to tolerance.

    2. Isometric exercises: one to three full contractions per muscle group once a day may be sufficient for maintaining strength. (See Exercise for Muscle Strength and Endurance, for rationale.) *Note*: Philosophy regarding exercises to maintain strength during the acute phase is controversial. It is also important to consider the effect of exercises on protective muscle spasm. Strengthening usually is delayed when the client has acute systemic illness.

    3. An appropriate amount of rest is critical during all phases of active disease. At least 10 to 12 hours of sleep are recommended in a 24-hour period. This concept needs more reinforcement in the subacute and chronic phases when the patient is more active than in the acute phase.

    4. Initiation of work simplification and energy conservation as the inflammation decreases.

II. Chronic-active phase

    The treatment protocol is the same as outlined for the subacute phase, but the emphasis is different because clients are able to perform more activities than in the acute or subacute phases. However, they still have synovitis, thus making the supporting joint structures vulnerable to deformity.

    In this phase *joint protection techniques, assistive equipment,* and *splinting* are the most important treatment modalities for maintaining joint integrity. (See Chapters 25, 26, and 27.)

    In addition to an exercise maintenance program, exercises to *improve* muscle strength and *increase* ROM can be started. (The type and amount of exercise recommended are discussed in detail in Chapter 29.)

    Other valuable interventions that are growing in availability across the country include:

    1. Relaxation and stress management training (with or without biofeedback instrumentation). This type of training can be particularly valuable for helping patients to develop a sense of control over their lives (and bodies), reducing fatigue, pain and depression, as well as improving ability for sleeping. [13,14,15,16]

    2. Foot orthotics to reduce stress, pain, and inflammation in the affected joints. These should be incorporated into the patient's program, *before* subluxation occurs, as a measure to reduce or prevent deforming forces. (Foot orthotics are described in Chapter 26, Joint Protection and Energy Conservation Instruction.)

    3. Foot ROM exercise program to reduce the effects of chronic protective spasm of the toe flexors that may result in muscle and joint contractures.

    4. Vocational counseling. All of the concepts of joint protection and energy conservation need to be applied in the work setting as well as in the home.

NONINFLAMMATORY JOINT DISEASE

Noninflammatory joint disease primarily refers to degenerative arthritis (osteoarthritis) and traumatic arthritis. It is characterized by (1) the absence of inflammatory signs; (2) pain on motion or weight bearing rather than pain at rest; (3) joint stiffness, particularly after prolonged static positioning; (4) residual deformity; (5) residual muscle weakness and disuse atrophy; and (6) muscle spasm secondary to pain.[17] The client with DJD may also have poor endurance secondary to inactivity or to coexistent systemic condition.

Although DJD is classified as a noninflammatory condition, some patients have periods of localized inflammation. The exact mechanism for this type of inflammation is not clear.[16] Sometimes it appears to be related to mucoidal cyst formation (in the digits) and often disappears after the cyst solidifies. In other cases it appears to be a "wear and tear" phenomenon, causing irritation to the joint capsule. When patients with DJD have pain at rest, they are usually experiencing a localized synovitis associated with DJD.

Primary Occupational Therapy Goals and Suggested Modalities

The following is an outline of treatment for both isolated and multiple joint involvement. For treatment of degenerative joint disease of specific joints see Chapter 10.

I. Improve functional independence
   A. Utilization of assistive equipment. (See Chapter 27 for detailed treatment methods and rationale.) Instruction in adapted methods to compensate for physical limitations.
   B. Improvement of functional endurance through instruction in work simplification and energy conservation methods. (See Chapter 26.)
   C. Reduction of pain through use of joint protection techniques (Chapter 26) and assistive equipment (Chapter 27). For pain secondary to muscle spasm, heat applications or ice massage can be beneficial.[9]
II. Maintain and/or increase muscle strength and ROM
   A. To maintain muscle strength, have the client perform one to three isometric exercises, once a day. (See Chapter 29.) To increase muscle strength, increase the number of contractions sufficiently to elicit fatigue but not pain.
   B. To maintain ROM, move the joint through a complete arc of motion once per day. To increase ROM, position the joint to allow gentle sustained passive stretch. (See Chapter 29.) For DJD of the upper extremities, increasing ROM is hardly ever possible, since most limitations are due to bony blocks.

REFERENCES

1. Harris, E. D.: *Rheumatoid arthritis: The clinical spectrum.* In Kelley, W. M., et al. (eds.): *Textbook of Rheumatology.* W. B. Saunders, Philadelphia, 1981.
2. Kendall, P. H.: *Exercise for arthritis.* In Licht, S. (ed.): *Therapeutic Exercise,* ed. 2. Elizabeth Licht Pub., New Haven, Conn., 1965.
3. Harris, E. D.: *Biology of the joint.* In Kelley, W. M., et al. (eds.): *Textbook of Rheumatology.* W. B. Saunders, Philadelphia, 1981.

4. Vasey, J. R., and Crozier, L. W.: *Neuromuscular approach to knee joint problems.* Physiotherapy 66(6):193, 1980.

5. Sherrington, C. S.: *The Integrative Action of the Nervous System.* Yale University Press, New Haven, Conn., 1906. (This is the original source on pain reflex inhibition and excitation.)

6. deAndrade, J. R. et al.: *Joint distension and reflex muscle inhibition in the knee.* J. Bone Joint Surg. 47A:313, 1965.

7. Cohen, L. A., and Cohen, M. L.: Arthrokinetic reflex of the knee. Am. J. Physiol. 184:433, 1956.

8. *Manual for Allied Health Professionals.* Arthritis Foundation, New York, 1973.

9. Lehmann, J. F., Warren, C. G., and Scham, S. M.: *Therapeutic heat and cold.* Clin. Orthop. 99:207, 1974. (Review article)

10. Kabet, H.: *Proprioceptive facilitation in therapeutic exercise.* In Licht, S. (ed.): *Therapeutic Exercise,* ed. 2. Elizabeth Licht Pub., New Haven, Conn., 1965.

11. Mead, S., and Knott, M.: *Ice therapy in joint restriction, spasticity and certain types of pain.* Gen. Pract. Feb. 1961, p. 16.

12. Knox, S.: Director of Occupational Therapy, Children's Hospital of Los Angeles. Personal communication, June, 1978.

13. Goldwag, E. M. (ed.): *Inner Balance: The Power of Holistic Healing.* Prentice-Hall, Englewood Cliffs, N.J., 1979.

14. Grezesiak, R. C.: *Relaxation techniques in treatment of chronic pain.* Arch. Phys. Med. Rehab. 58:270, June, 1977.

15. Olton, D. S., and Noonber, A. R.: *Biofeedback: Clinical Applications in Behavioral Medicine.* Prentice-Hall, Englewood Cliffs, N.J., 1980. (Contains a chapter on the treatment of Raynaud's disease.)

16. Achterberg, J., McGraw, and Lawlis, G. F.: *Rheumatoid arthritis: A study of relaxation and temperature biofeedback training as an adjunctive therapy.* Biofeedback and Self Reg. 6(2):207, 1981.

17. Bland, J. H., and Stulberg, S. D.: *Osteoarthritis: Pathology and clinical patterns.* In Kelley, W. M., et al. (eds.): Textbook of Rheumatology. W. B. Saunders, Philadelphia, 1981.

ADDITIONAL SOURCES

Ice and Heat Therapy

Fisher, E., and Solomon, S.: *Physiological response to heat and cold.* In Licht, S. (ed.): *Therapeutic Heat and Cold,* ed. 5. Elizabeth Licht Pub., New Haven, Conn., 1965.

McMaster, W. C.: *A literary review on ice therapy.* Am. J. Sports Med. 5(3):124, 1977.

Mennell, J. M.: *The therapeutic use of cold.* J. Am. Osteopath. Assoc. 74(12):1146, 1975.

Pegg, S. M. H., Littler, T. R., and Littler, E. W.: *A trial of ice therapy and exercise in chronic arthritis.* Physiotherapy 55:51, 1969.

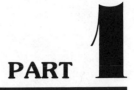

PART **1**

PSYCHOLOGY, EDUCATION, AND PATIENT CARE

2

PSYCHOLOGICAL CONSIDERATIONS IN PATIENT EDUCATION AND TREATMENT

The greater percentage of an effective treatment program for chronic arthritis involves patient instruction. Treatment issues such as when to take medication, how to use hand splints or assistive devices, joint protection methods, or basic disease information involve a definite learning-teaching process. The education component is even greater for patients with arthritis as compared with other diseases, because of the need to counteract the extensive folklore and quackery regarding arthritis.

Over the past five years, patient education has gained increasing importance in rheumatologic rehabilitation. Several major publications and audio-visual resources have been produced to help the clinician develop effective patient education programs. These resources are listed at the end of the chapter.

An effective instructional program includes three components: specific educational goals, clear presentation of the material, and assessment of the learning process. But, before any of these processes can be effective, the patient has to be willing and psychologically ready to learn the material. This chapter explores the basic psychological and medical factors that need to be dealt with before an effective teaching program can be initiated.

PATIENT-PROFESSIONAL RELATIONSHIP

The relationship between a patient and the health professional is an extremely sensitive one. The stakes are high: for the former it is an issue of health and of life at a basic survival level; for the latter it is personal satisfaction and good job performance. In spite of these contingencies, it is hoped that, with each encounter, optimal patient care will result and the patient will emerge with a greater sense of well being.

These goals can be achieved only if both parties have a clear understanding of their responsibilities and if the health professional is aware of the effect of his or her behavior on the achievement of these goals.

In general, the optimal treatment situation occurs when the patient takes responsibility for his or her own health care by (a) actively seeking skilled advice, (b) understanding the illness and treatment rationale, and (c) following through with prescribed therapy; and when the health professional takes responsibility by (a) providing competent treatment and (b) providing the appropriate environment and sufficient information for the patient to carry out his or her responsibilities.

The health professional's philosophy and approach is the keystone to the method of patient care described above. Some of the processes essential to sharing responsibility are:

Education. Many patients believe that a person goes to a hospital or to therapy to be taken care of. They are not aware of the active role they need to play in order to make the system work. In other words, patients need to have their role and responsibilities clearly defined.

Modeling the process. The professional's role in the relationship needs to be defined and he or she must carry out the appropriate responsibilities.

Un-mothering. The professional should not assume the patient's responsibilities; once a professional does that, there is no reason for the patient to assume those responsibilities.

In the patient-professional relationship only one person can comply with the treatment instructions, and that is the patient. No one can do it for him or her. The odds on the patient carrying out that responsibility appear to be increased if the patient is assuming responsibility for his or her health care throughout the treatment process.

PSYCHOLOGICAL FACTORS RELATED TO RHEUMATIC DISEASES

The search to discover a unique etiologic or reactive link between a specific psychological variable and joint diseases has been extensive, but a *definite association has not been found.*[1,2] Many investigators have reported certain predominant personality patterns in the arthritis patients studied; however, it is evident by reviewing their research methodology that a conclusive study with controls for all of the important variables has not been carried out.[3-26] Furthermore, greater psychosocial variance has been found within a single disease entity than is evident in a variety of diseases.[28] The personality typically described for patients with rheumatoid arthritis can also be found in other chronic diseases and among people without disease.[1,24,28] The most promising work in this area has been in discovering the relationship of emotions to immunologic response, but again, a unique or definite association cannot be established for patients with arthritis.[29-32]

A discussion on the psychological aspects of the rheumatic diseases is essentially a discussion on the psychological aspects of chronic disease. *The natures of the diseases vary but the patient response is to illness and chronic disability.*[33,34,35,36] Therefore the psychological and educational factors relevant to treating patients with rheumatic diseases can be generalized to treatment of patients with other chronic conditions.

The psychological responses necessary to cope with the trauma of arthritis can be compared with those necessary to cope with personal death, as identified by leading theorists and researchers in the field of thanatology (study of death and dying).[37] Encountering a life-threatening disease such as cancer or sustaining a limb amputation involves a very obvious and absolute personal loss. Psychologists and other theorists have carried out a great deal of research in order to understand patient response to amputations and terminal disease and to develop approaches for helping patients cope with the trauma of loss.[38,39] The results of this research can also be applied to patients with rheumatic diseases for, although the loss involved with the rheumatic diseases is not as obvious as in the above conditions, its effect on the patient can be equally traumatic. For instance, the loss involved in arthritis can be conceptualized in two ways. First, it is a loss of a joint or body part. Second, it is the loss or death of "a self," of the ability to carry out a personal, family, or societal role (since we consist of many "selves" in many roles). The permanent loss of the ability to fulfill one or more of these roles is an emotional trauma equal to that of losing a limb.

From a practical viewpoint, the emphasis in therapy needs to be placed on the psychological reaction of the individual to the disability rather than to the etiologic or predispositional factors involved.

PSYCHOLOGICAL FACTORS RELATED TO PATIENT EDUCATION AND COMPLIANCE

The psychological issues relevant to patient instruction and compliance cluster around two processes: the patient's response to the disability and the interaction of, or relationship between, the patient and the health professional. The patient's response follows in this section. The patient-professional relationship is discussed at the beginning of this chapter.

Patient Response to Disability

Disability carries a distinct meaning for each person and each person's method of coping is unique. It is important to identify each patient's response, to find out how he or she perceives the disease, to determine what is most important to him or her, and then to relate the method and content of the instruction to the individual's needs.

Although individual response patterns are unique, certain responses occur more frequently and have a stronger influence on patient-professional interaction. These responses are denial, depression, need for control, dependency, and acceptance.[37,38] Denial and depression are the two most common specific responses that have the potential for inhibiting therapy. The need for control and dependency issues are two fundamental concerns that are always present and, therefore, continually need to be considered. Acceptance, as defined later in this section, has a strong positive influence on therapy and allows maximal utilization of health resources to take place. There are many other responses such as family, cultural, and societal contingencies that influence the patient's response to disability, but a thorough discussion of patient psychology is beyond the scope of this text.

DENIAL

Denial is an amazing defense mechanism. Very few processes will allow one to wipe out bad events so neatly. If a denial mechanism is in good working order, a person can be told he has rheumatoid arthritis or cancer and it will not affect his outlook on life in the least. Denial, like other defense mechanisms, comes into existence when an issue becomes a threat to a person's reality. Therefore, it is a very valuable and necessary process for that person.

However, while denial can be a positive mechanism for the patient, it can at the same time be a negative mechanism for the therapist or physician who believes the patient needs to understand the disease and appropriate treatment for optimal care. If a person does not believe that he or she has a serious disease, or a painful wrist, there is no reason to learn the treatment procedures.

This brings up the question of how to determine if denial is present. This is done simply by talking to the patient, by finding out how the patient perceives the disease and disability, and his or her expectations and attitudes about complying with the instructions and by determining the source of discrepancies between the patient's and therapist's perspective.

It may or may not be possible to reconcile the needs of the patient and the professional concerning denial, but certain measures can help. If the health professional's goal is to do what is best for the patient, it is important to recognize the positive value of denial for the patient. The patient needs the denial or it would not be there. When denial is present, the major concern is to protect the patient from self-harm through actions he or she may take such as not taking medication or discarding splints. Therefore, it is not necessary to eliminate the denial but to work around it. In fact, it is impossible for the professional to alter the denial; only the patient can do that. Any attempts to eliminate it by "making him or her face reality" probably will be in vain or only increase the patient's stress. The patient is doing the right thing, i.e., taking care of himself or herself by using denial to avoid overwhelming issues.

It is possible to work around the denial by acknowledging the patient's beliefs and designing the treatment regimen to accommodate them. This is somewhat easy to do with the rheumatic diseases because the course is variable and the definite prognosis is not known in the early stages. So one can honestly give patients the hope of remission while asking them to comply with the current physical problems.

Before dealing with the issue of denial it is extremely important to make sure the patient has accurate information about the disease. It is not enough to describe the disease or give the patient literature to read. No matter how the patient obtains information it is absolutely essential to have him or her explain the information to you. For example in a personal experience, I asked a patient to read a pamphlet about rheumatoid arthritis prepared by the Arthritis Foundation. When she had finished I answered her questions. About three months later I learned that she had interpreted the passage which read "RA *can* cause disease in the lungs, skin, blood vessels, muscles . . . ," to mean "RA *will* cause disease. . . ." We cannot protect patients from all misinterpretations but the only way we can find out what they actually understand is by asking. Had the woman's misinterpretation not been corrected, she might have expected all of her organs to become seriously damaged. This is not a specific example of denial, but misconceptions about the severity of the disease may needlessly elicit defense mechanisms such as denial.

A point of crisis often causes a person to interpret information literally or to amplify the meaning, thus making a casual statement into something definite and absolute. This often stems from an acute need for structure and definition at a time of emotional chaos when nothing, not even the individual's body, seems to be stable.

The patient's accurate understanding of both the positive and negative aspects of his or her condition is important in helping him or her deal honestly with the condition.

DEPRESSION

Psychological depression is probably the most difficult response to identify and work with, especially in patients with systemic diseases, because the symptoms of depression are identical to those of systemic illness, e.g., fatigue, loss of appetite, malaise, decreased motivation, and diminished sexual drive.[40] The identification of depression becomes further complicated by several issues:

1. There are many medications that cause depression.
2. There are two forms of depression, i.e., *reactive* or *exogenous*, in which the depression is linked with a specific cause; or *endogenous*, in which the severe depression occurs without a discernible cause. This category includes depression related to physiologic changes.[37]
3. Sadness over loss (grief) appears similar to depression.
4. Patients with medical problems often attribute the symptoms of mild depression to the physical ailment, thus deferring diagnosis and treatment of the real problem.

The following methods are often helpful in identifying depression:

1. The nature of the fatigue can be a key to distinguishing depression from systemic symptoms. Systemic fatigue is related to activity level and commonly occurs after four to six hours of activity, whereas fatigue associated with depression is usually constant.
2. Question the patient regarding depressed behavior. When asked, many patients can clearly identify their depression. Patients who initially attribute their depressed behavior to a physical ailment without considering a psychological source often gain insight simply from discussion about possible sources. Depression can result from a variety of causes with the most common being suppression of anger.
3. It is important to distinguish true depression from sadness. When a person encounters loss in any form, it is vital that he or she fully experience the associated grief or sorrow to get beyond it.
4. There are psychological assessments available to help identify depression. These tests are not recommended for routine use in occupational or physical therapy clinics; however, they are helpful in learning what to look for when evaluating for depression. (There are several depression inventories. Their availability changes yearly. A listing of current tests and their reliability and validity scores can be found in Buros, O.V. (ed.): *The Eighth Mental Measurements Yearbook*. Gryphon Press, Highland Park, N.J., 1979.)

The symptoms of depression can pose a real threat to the therapy program. Patients experiencing a sense of hopelessness and futility are not likely to participate in programs designed to make the future brighter. When treatment procedures require rigorous compliance, assessment of depression should be part of the pre-evaluation and the depression should be resolved before treatment is started. For instance, marked depression has become such an obvious deterrent to rehabilitation of total knee arthroplasties that it is now considered a contraindication at some centers.

It is easy to talk about resolving a depression but significantly harder to do. It is difficult even to discuss methods of working with depression, since the method of choice depends upon the patient—why he or she is depressed, the need to be depressed, and how the depression is interfering with the treatment.

Once a person develops strong feelings about something, he or she has difficulty seeing or avoids seeing the opposite viewpoint. This can happen with a health problem. To the patient, the disease is a bad event and the patient focuses on the negative aspects, which can feed a depressive cycle. The health professional can best help the patient and himself or herself by acknowledging the negative aspects, by acknowledging the person's need to relate those aspects, and by giving the patient positive issues to respond to. Patients who need to be depressed will stay depressed no matter what is said, but patients in a depressive cycle who are ready to break out of it will pick up on the positive issues mentioned.

Along this line, two specific approaches are often helpful. First, whenever doing an evaluation that focuses on what the patient *cannot do*, such as an ADL assessment or hand function test, end the procedure on items that the patient can do successfully. This reinforces the patient's awareness of function rather than dysfunction. Second, have the patient clarify the meaning of his or her negative generalities. For example: (1) When a patient says he "has arthritis all over," asking him to be specific will probably turn up several uninvolved joints. (2) Statements like "I can't cook anymore," upon being clarified may really mean the person can no longer lift heavy pots or open cans. (3) Almost all statements like "I'm no good," "I'm a terrible mother," or "I'm a failure," can become less overwhelming and more realistic and positive by having the patient be more specific.

NEED FOR CONTROL

Basic to life, sanity, and happiness is the need for sensing control over one's body, actions, and environment. Most people who are afflicted with an illness of unknown cause, especially if it strikes suddenly, have a prevailing feeling of incredible helplessness. There is no reason for, or control of, the situation. "Why me?" becomes a repetitive forever-unanswered question.

Society, through the health profession, has devised an incredible answer to this problem. When people become ill and sense no control over their bodies, they are placed in a hospital in which they have no control over their environment. Even a healthy person in the hospital for a routine physical examination becomes acutely aware of a lack of control in the hospital environment.

There are many ways for the patient to gain or restore control. Some people do it by being cooperative and agreeable during clinic interaction, then follow their own wishes when authority figures are not around. This is commonly referred to as a passive-aggressive approach. Other people may overtly establish control by refusing to comply and by managing their own treatment.

Everyone needs to sense control over his or her environment. The professional's awareness of how patients maintain a sense of control when they are ill and in a structured environment allows for more effective treatment planning. For example, if the patient's method of gaining control is to resist treatment then the health professional can reduce the resistance and increase the patient's sense of control by telling the patient the treatment methods available, the alternative to treatment (a consequence of no treatment) and letting the patient choose the option he or she prefers.

DEPENDENCY

Another psychological factor that often comes to the forefront when illness strikes is dependency.[38] The conflict between autonomy and dependency is with us from the first year of life. Unresolved conflicts in this area become dominant factors when a person is placed in a position of dependency (becoming disabled) or independency (taking care of someone disabled). A person with strong unresolved dependency needs may assume an independent posture in defense of being overpowered by the desire to be taken care of. Examples of behavior patterns that allow symbolic or unconscious satisfaction for dependency but maintain control of the situation are: (1) demanding behavior, for example, constant requests for attention, water, pills, equipment; (2) super-cooperative behavior that manipulates others into caring for them without directly requesting care; (3) indecisive behavior in which there is difficulty making or carrying out decisions. The last is a more overt dependent behavior, especially when it consistently results in people other than the patient making the final decisions.[38,41]

Any of these behaviors can negatively affect a treatment program. When the above behaviors are serving dependency needs, cognizance of that fact can allow the professional to respond to the patient's needs rather than getting caught up in the patient's demands or manipulations, for the latter will only perpetuate a cyclic process. For example, responding to a demanding patient by retaliation and not giving attention to the patient only increases the dependency conflict, whereas increasing the attention often helps reduce the need and demand.

Treatment programs and discharge planning should also take dependency issues into consideration. A patient with strong dependency needs is not likely to follow through on a program that requires independent action or perseverance.

ACCEPTANCE

The ideal situation exists when the patient can experience and deal with the emotional trauma of disability and arrive at some point of acceptance.

Acceptance of a disability is a difficult concept to define because it is a process unique for each person. However, in general terms, acceptance can describe *an honest* relationship with the disability—one in which the person acknowledges and experiences the anger, rage, fear, sadness, and helplessness associated with having to live with a miserable disease but at the same time acknowledges those aspects of life not affected by the disease. For example, arthritis of the knees may stop a man from playing basketball with his son but it does not need to interfere with his ability to be a loving husband, father, and competent provider for his family. Nonacceptance may be indicated when the man does not acknowledge the limitations of the arthritis and continues to play ball, possibly causing unnecessary joint damage and greater debility. On the other hand, if he becomes depressed over the inability to play with his son, he will allow the depression to interfere with his role as a husband and provider. In this case, acceptance means anger at the limitations imposed by the arthritis but also recognition of what the true limitations are.

This example is a simplified version of a complex process and acceptance or nonacceptance is never the sole issue because it is extremely difficult for people to deal openly with issues that threaten their physical existence. However, it *is* possible, and it is a process that can be facilitated by health professionals who are oriented to helping patients deal honestly with all health issues.

MEDICAL FACTORS RELATED TO PATIENT EDUCATION AND COMPLIANCE

In addition to the basic psychological factors related to patient responses and client-professional interaction it is important to consider the effects of the disability on the learning process.

Three medical contingencies that can influence learning for people with joint disease are invariably present in the clinic: pain or discomfort, concern about illness (or health), and the effect of medication. The patient with systemic lupus erythematosus may additionally have central nervous system involvement that can interfere with learning.

Pain or Discomfort

Pain and the influence it can have on the therapeutic relationship is an extremely complex issue. The significance of experiencing pain is unique for each patient and the significance of being with someone in pain is unique for each professional. Pain presents competing stimuli for attention and in general is an inhibitor to learning. However, it does not have to stop the learning process and when motivation or desire is strong enough a person can learn even when pain is present. The amount of instruction should be adjusted to the amount of patient participation, this being influenced by the severity of pain.

Concern About Health

Concern over one's health status with such reactions as anxiety or fear may not only limit learning in a given session but also prohibit it altogether. This reference to the client's day-to-day concern over health differs from the general psychological response to the disease. It is often more contingent upon sudden changes in his or her health status or upon misinformation obtained from such sources as friends or the news media. Along this line arthritis creates a double problem. It is a common but extremely misunderstood condition and it is the only chronic disease that carries extensive folklore. Consequently, patients are often inundated with misinformation about their specific type of arthritis, a fact which can be extremely disconcerting. For example: (1) a patient with mild degenerative joint disease of the hands may believe his or her hands will become deformed like the patient with rheumatoid arthritis on the other side of the clinic, (2) a patient with a misconception that the rheumatoid nodule on his or her forearm is cancerous may be scared to mention it to anyone and his or her anxiety may severely interfere with learning, or (3) a patient may have a remission of certain symptoms and believe the disease is cured and therefore believe that he or she does not need to learn a certain necessary procedure.

Many patients are very open about such concerns and seek correct information but others have been conditioned to listen to the health professional rather than to talk or disclose their own concerns. However, most patients will respond to encouragement to discuss such issues.

Effect of Medication

The effect of medication on learning ability has both positive and negative features. If the medication relieves pain, it removes a block from learning and thus can facilitate the process. This is often the case with medications taken for a specific or focal problem. However, common rheumatic disease medications can have side effects. Sometimes a side effect such as nausea can be an obvious distraction to learning. More often the side effects are so subtle, such as very slight lightheadedness or vague uneasiness, that the patient might not mention it or may not even be able to define the feeling. These mild effects can also compete with the learning process. Steroid therapy in particular can produce a wide range of emotional side effects. Euphoric responses create such emotional detachment that the patient is not able to attend to instructions. Health professionals need to be well versed on the effects of medication. (See Drug Therapy, Chapter 12, for a review of the side effects.) When patients are on medication that can affect learning or retention, *all* instructions should be written out and should be reviewed at a later date if possible.

Instructing the Patient

Methods of instructing patients in the presence of pain, anxiety, or drug side effects are the same for all factors. First, it is important to find out what factors are competing for attention with the information you want to get across. This can be done only by asking the patient; that is, finding out how he or she feels, or if anything about the arthritis is particularly worrisome to the patient, or if he or she is aware of any side effects from medication.

The competing factors must be acknowledged if their influence on the teaching process is to be dealt with. Many professionals believe that if they don't talk about the patient's pain the patient will ignore it and pay attention to the instruction. Nevertheless, it is impossible to ignore pain or other conflicting stimuli. It is just a matter of overt or covert attention to it.

Conversely, this raises the issue of what to do with the patient who wants to talk incessantly about his or her pain or concerns. When this occurs it is usually the patient's talking that becomes the hindrance to teaching rather than the pain itself. Therefore, it is essential to acknowledge the specific hindrance and deal with it before learning can take place.

This chapter has focused on the patient's psychological reaction to disability, his or her responsibility for health care, and the influence pain and medications can have on the learning process. This focus was chosen because these issues are often overlooked in the teaching session and are neglected in the literature on education for the arthritis patient, and because these factors need to be considered preliminary to initiating patient instruction. The structure of the actual teaching process has been mentioned only briefly but is equally important for a successful educational/instructional program.

GUIDELINES FOR PATIENT INSTRUCTION

The following guidelines identify the key factors that provide structure for a successful learning-teaching experience with patients who have arthritis.

A. Preliminary considerations
   1. Does the patient *need* education about arthritis or medical care? Does the patient have incorrect information or misconceptions about these issues? Before any other factor is considered, *the patient's educational needs must be evaluated.*
   2. Is the patient ready or interested in participating in an educational session?
   3. Is the patient's medical condition controlled sufficiently to allow *effective instruction?* If the patient is feeling ill or is in severe pain, instruction should be delayed if possible.
   4. Is the patient's psychological response to the disability conducive to learning more about the disease and treatment? Or is the patient so depressed or angry about the arthritis that he or she is not ready to start taking positive actions to help the arthritis?
   5. Does the patient understand his or her responsibility for health care and his or her role in medical treatment of the condition?
   6. Will the patient's medication interfere with learning (See Chapter 12.)
   7. What are the patient's goals and interests in learning about the disease and medical and health care?
   8. Determine the patient's track record with regard to arthritis education.
      a. Has the patient ever participated in an arthritis education program before? Was it helpful? What helped and what did not? Was the patient able to incorporate the suggestions made? Can the patient identify factors that facilitated or hindered compliance with instructions? (This may be the most valuable information you will receive for structuring the teaching format.)
      b. Has the patient actively sought information about arthritis or read any books on the topic? If the patient is an avid reader and has not sought any information on arthritis, why not? What does reading or learning about the disease mean to the patient?
B. The learning-teaching session
   1. Explain your educational concerns to the patient: the material you think would be helpful for the patient to learn and why it is important. (Your views may alter the patient's personal goals.)
   2. Establish *both* the learning and teaching goals with the patient. Sometimes it is helpful to make a verbal contract with the patient to establish clear expectations and responsibilities. For example, the therapist might say, "I will teach you methods for reducing the stress and pain in your fingers, if you will practice the techniques for two days." The contract may be of any format desired. This can be a very effective method for making roles and responsibilities explicit rather than implicit and therefore subject to confusion.
   3. After the goals are established, the duration and number of educational sessions need to be planned with the patient.
   4. The teaching objectives for each session should be realistic for the learning capabilities of the patient.
   5. The teaching session should be conducted in a location free from distractions.
   6. Family members should be included when appropriate.
   7. Whenever possible, use teaching examples and materials that are relevant to the patient's personal and home situation, to maximize carry-over of the information. For example, if the therapist is teaching a patient with early joint involvement, examples

or slides showing patients with severe deformities may be more distractive than illustrative to the patient.

8. If specific techniques are being taught, provide opportunity, space, and equipment for the patient to practice.

9. Before teaching any techniques, find out how the patient performs the activity. Often the patient's own method is correct or acceptable. Positive reinforcement of the patient's own method validates his or her intelligence and ingenuity. It also encourages correct process and eliminates the need to teach that particular step.

10. Whenever possible use printed handouts to reinforce the material being taught. If a commercial booklet on the topic does not express the full philosophy of your facility, adapt it. Cross out sections that are not relevant to the patient, circle or star the most important section, or add a supplementary page or a favorite diagram. Make the booklet into a dynamic teaching aid. Also, explaining the changes to the patient reinforces the content.

11. All major or key instructions should be provided in writing. This is particularly important if you are teaching a lot of new material in a short period of time.

12. Throughout the teaching process, it is critical to evaluate if the patient has learned the material correctly. This is usually done by having the patient demonstrate the technique or explain the process to the therapist. Positive reinforcement is a valuable tool for helping the patient learn new skills. The therapist should provide support and use positive reinforcement at every opportunity.

    If the patient has not learned the material correctly, it is a signal that the teaching process needs to be modified and repeated. During this process it is important to keep in mind an old adage: "If the student didn't learn, then the teacher didn't teach."

One last word about patient education. In many hospitals and outpatient clinics, therapists spend a great deal of time teaching patients about arthritis and medical or rehabilitative treatment. Often the teaching is done informally, during an interview or while making splints. The therapist provides this information because he or she has determined (by some method) that the patient lacks information and the therapist believes that the patient would be helped by knowing the information. Paradoxically, the same therapist who believes in the value of patient education and in his or her ability to provide it generally does not mention either the assessment or the process in the patient's chart. Consequently, therapists often do a considerable amount of patient education, but no one else on the medical team is aware of the therapist's skills or interest in these areas. Therapists can promote team communication and appreciation for the value of patient education simply by documenting the patient's knowledge about arthritis or his or her information needs in the initial evaluation. This does not have to be an elaborate process. A couple of succinct sentences can suffice; e.g., Patient believes his arthritis (OA) is due to too much calcium and has avoided dairy products for this reason. He is not aware of the side effects of his medication. (There is a strong possibility that a few comments like this in the medical chart will increase the staff's awareness of patient education.) If it is apparent that the patient needs information then patient education, even if it is informal, should be included in the treatment goals and plan. Documentation of the education and learning can also be included in the progress or discharge notes. In many instances, such as the example above, the therapist's educational assessment may reveal that the patient lacks information in an area other than the therapist's area of expertise. In these cases, it is certainly appropriate to document that education will be coordinated with a nurse, dietician, or other health professional.

REFERENCES

1. Wolff, B. B.: *Current psychological concepts in R.A.* Bull. Rheum. Dis. 22:656, 1971.
2. Spergel, P. et al.: *The RA personality—A psychodiagnostic myth.* Psychosomatics 19(2):79, 1978.
3. Boynton, B. L., Leavitt, L. A., Schnur, R. R., Schnur, H. L., and Russell, M. A.: *Personality evaluation in rehabilitation of rheumatoid spondylitis.* Arch. Phys. Med. Rehab. 34:489, 1953.
4. Cleveland, S. E., and Fisher, S.: *Behavior and unconscious fantasies of patients with rheumatoid arthritis.* Psychosom. Med. 16:327, 1954.
5. Cobb, S.: *Contained hostility in rheumatoid arthritis.* Arthritis Rheum. 2:419, 1959.
6. Cobb, S., Bauer, W., and Whiting, I.: *Environmental factors in rheumatoid arthritis.* J.A.M.A. 113:668, 1939.
7. Cobb, S., Miller, M., and Wieland, M.: *On the relationship between divorce and rheumatoid arthritis.* Arthritis Rheum. 2:414, 1959.
8. Fisher, S. and Cleveland, S. E.: *Comparison of psychological characteristics and physiological reactivity in ulcer and rheumatoid arthritis groups.* Psychosom. Med. 22:283, 1960.
9. Hellgren, L.: *Rheumatoid arthritis in both marital partners.* Acta Rheum. Scand. 15:135, 1969.
10. Hellgren, L.: *Marital status in rheumatoid arthritis.* Acta Rheum. Scand. 15:271, 1969.
11. King, S. H.: *Psychosocial factors associated with rheumatoid arthritis.* J. Chronic Dis. 2:287, 1955.
12. King, S. H., and Cobb, S.: *Psychosocial factors in the epidemiology of rheumatoid arthritis.* J. Chronic Dis. 7:466, 1958.
13. King, S. H., and Cobb, S.: *Psychosocial studies of rheumatoid arthritis: Parental factors compared in cases and controls.* Arthritis Rheum. 2:322, 1959.
14. Kirchman, M. M.: *The personality of the arthritic patient.* Am. J. Occup. Ther. 19(3):160, 1965.
15. Lewis-Faning, E.: *Report on an enquiry into the aetiological factors associated with rheumatoid arthritis.* Ann. Rheum. Dis. (Suppl.)9, 1950.
16. Lugwig, A. O.: *Rheumatoid arthritis: Psychiatric aspects.* Medical Insight. Insight Publishing, Dec., 1970.
17. Moos, R. H., and Solomon, G. F.: *Personality correlates of the rapidity of progression of rheumatoid arthritis.* Ann. Rheum. Dis. 23:2, 1964.
18. Mueller, A. D., and Lefkovits, A. M.: *Personality structure and dynamics of patients with rheumatoid arthritis.* J. Clin. Psychol. 12:143, 1956.
19. Mueller, A. D., Lefkovits, A. M., Bryant, J. E., and Marshall, M. L.: *Some psychosocial factors in patients with rheumatoid arthritis.* Arthritis Rheum. 4:275, 1961.
20. Nalven, F. B., and O'Brien, J. F.: *Personality patterns of rheumatoid arthritis patients.* Arthritis Rheum. 7:18, 1964.
21. Polley, H. F., Swenson, W. M., and Steinhilber, R. M.: *Personality characteristics of patients with rheumatoid arthritis.* Psychosomatics 11:45, 1970.
22. Rimon, R.: *A psychosomatic approach to rheumatoid arthritis.* Acta Rheum. Scand. (Suppl.)13, 1969.
23. Robinson, H., Kirk, R. F., and Frye, R. L.: *A psychological study of rheumatoid arthritis and selected controls.* J. Chronic Dis. 23:791, 1971.
24. Robinson, H., et al.: *Psychological study of patients with rheumatoid arthritis and other painful diseases.* J. Psychosom. Res. 16:53, 1972.
25. Ward, D.: *Rheumatoid arthritis and personality: A controlled study.* Br. Med. J. 2:297, 1971.
26. Wolff, B. B., and Farr, R. S.: *Personality characteristics in rheumatoid arthritis.* Arthritis Rheum. 7:354, 1964.
27. Kinnealey, M.: *The relationship between self concept and hand deformity in RA* (thesis abstr.). Am. J. Occup. Ther. 24:294, 1970.

28. Bourestom, N. C., and Howard, M. T.: *Personality characteristics of three disability groups*. Arch. Phys. Med. Rehab. 46:626, 1965.
29. Crown, S., and Crown, J. M.: *Personality in early rheumatoid disease*. J. Psychosom. Res. 17:189, 1973.
30. Meyerowitz, S., Jacox, R. F., and Hess, D. W.: *Monozygotic twins discordant for rheumatoid arthritis: A genetic, clinical and psychological study of 8 sets*. Arthritis Rheum. 11:1, 1968.
31. Solomon, G. F.: *Psychophysiological aspects of rheumatoid arthritis and auto-immune disease*. In Hill, O. W. (ed.): *Modern Trends in Psychosomatic Medicine*, Vol. 2. Appleton-Century-Crofts, New York, 1970, pp. 189-216.
32. Solomon, G. F., and Moos, R. H.: *Emotions, immunity and disease: A speculative, theoretical integration*. Arch. Gen. Psychiatry 11:657, 1964.
33. Shan, L. L.: *The world of the patient in severe pain of long duration*. J. Chronic Dis. 17:119, 1964.
34. Simon, J.: *Emotional aspects of physical disability*. Am. J. Occup. Ther. 25(8):408, 1971.
35. Shontz, F. C.: *Physical disability and personality*. In: Neff, W. S. (ed.): *Rehabilitation Psychology*. American Psychological Association Publication, 1970.
36. Shontz, F. C.: *Physical disability and personality: Theory and recent research*. Psychological Aspects of Disability 17:51, 1970.
37. Kubler-Ross, E.: *On Death and Dying*. Macmillan, New York, 1969.
38. Psychological Aspects of Disability and Rehabilitation. The Menninger Foundation Seminar, Topeka, Kansas. Division of Vocational Rehabilitation, February, 1962.
39. Friedmann, L. V.: *The Psychological Rehabilitation of the Amputee*. Charles C Thomas, Springfield, Ill., 1978.
40. Zaphiropoulus, G., and Barry, H. C.: *Depression in rheumatoid disease*. Ann. Rheum. Dis. 33(2):132, 1974.
41. Wright, B.: *Physical Disability: A Psychological Approach*. Harper and Bros., New York, 1960.

ADDITIONAL SOURCES

Psychological Aspects of Rheumatoid Arthritis

Cobb, S., Schull, W. J., Harburg, E., Kasl, S. V., et al.: *The intrafamilial transmission of rheumatoid arthritis*, I-VIII. J. Chronic Dis. 22:193, 1969.

Edwards, M. H., and Calabro, J. J.: *Patient's attitudes and knowledge concerning arthritis*. Arthritis Rheum. 7:425, 1964.

Ehrlich, G. E.: *Arthritis management: Treating rheumatoid arthritis with behavioral and clinical strategy*. Practical Psychology for Physicians, Harcourt, Brace, Jovanovich, July, 1975.

Geist, H.: *The Psychological Aspects of RA*. Charles C Thomas, Springfield, Ill., 1966.

Hoffman, A. L.: *Psychological factors associated with R.A.: Review of the literature*. Nurs. Res. 23(3):218, May-June, 1974.

Katz, S., Vignos, P. J., Moskowitz, R. W., Thompson, H. M., and Svec, K. H.: *Comprehensive outpatient care in rheumatoid arthritis*. J.A.M.A. 206:1249, 1968.

Medsger, A. R., and Rohenson, H.: *A comparative study of divorce in rheumatoid arthritis and other rheumatic diseases*. J. Chronic Dis. 25:269, 1972.

Meyerowitz, S.: *Psychosocial factors in the etiology of somatic disease*. Ann. Intern. Med. 72:753, 1970.

Meyerowitz, S.: *The continuing investigation of psychosocial variables in rheumatoid arthritis*. In Hill, A. G. S. (ed.): *Modern Trends in Rheumatology*, 2 edition. Butterworth, London, 1971.

Moldofsky, H., and Chester, W. J.: *Pain and mood patterns in patients with rheumatoid arthritis: A prospective study*. Psychosom. Med. 32:309, 1970.

Moldofsky, H., and Rothman, A. I.: *Personality, disease parameters, and medication in rheumatoid arthritis*. Arthritis Rheum. 13:338, 1970.

Moos, R. H.: *Personality factors associated with rheumatoid arthritis: A review.* J. Chronic Dis. 17:41, 1964.

Moos, R. H., and Solomon, G. F.: *Minnesota Multiphasic Personality Inventory response patterns in patients with rheumatoid arthritis.* J. Psychosom. Res. 8:17, 1964.

Moos, R. H., et al.: *Psychological orientations in the treatment of R.A.* Am. J. Occup. Ther. 19(3):153, 1965.

Moos, R. H., and Solomon, G. F.: *Personality correlates of the rapidity of progression of rheumatoid arthritis.* Ann. Rheum. Dis. 23:145, 1964.

Moos, R. H., and Solomon, G. F: *Psychologic comparisons between women with rheumatoid arthritis and their nonarthritic sisters. I. Personality test and interview rating data.* Psychosom. Med. 27:135, 1965.

Moos, R. H., and Solomon, G. F.: *Psychologic comparisons between women with rheumatoid arthritis and their nonarthritic sisters. II. Content analysis of interviews.* Psychosom. Med. 27:150, 1965.

Padilla, G. V.: *Conditions under which an arthritic patient is held responsible and receives negative sanctions for her illness.* Dissertation, University of California, Los Angeles, 1971.

Prick, J. J. G, and Van de Loo, K. J. M.: *The Psychosomatic Approach to Primary Chronic Rheumatoid Arthritis.* F. A. Davis, Philadelphia, 1964.

Rekola, J. K.: *Rheumatoid arthritis and the family. (Psychiatric study comparing families with R.A., schizophrenia and neurosis.)* Scand. J. Rheum. (Suppl. 3)2, 1973,117 pages.

Rimon, R.: *Depression in R.A.* Ann. Clin. Res. 6(3):171, June 1974.

Robb, J. H., and Rose, B. S.: *Rheumatoid arthritis and maternal deprivation: A case study in the use of a social survey.* Br. J. Med. Psychol. 38:147, 1965.

Scotch, N.A., and Geiger, H. J.: *The epidemiology of rheumatoid arthritis: A review with special attention to social factors.* J. Chronic Dis. 15:1037, 1962.

Solomon, G. F., and Moos, R. H.: *The relationship of personality to the presence of rheumatoid factors in symptomatic relatives of patients with rheumatoid arthritis.* Psychosom. Med. 27:351, 1955.

Southworth, J. A.: *Muscular tension as a response to psychological stress in rheumatoid arthritis and peptic ulcer.* Genet. Psychol. Monogr. 57:337, 1958.

Vargo, J. W.: *Some psychological effects of physical disability.* Am. J. Occup. Ther. 32(1):31, 1978.

Vignos, P. J., Thompson, H. M., Fink, S. L., Moskowitz, R. W., Svec, K. H., and Katz, S.: *The effect of psychosocial factors on rehabilitation in chronic rheumatoid arthritis.* Paper read at the 5th Annual Meeting of the Allied Health Professions Section of The Arthritis Foundation, Detroit, June 20, 1970.

Wolff, B. B.: *Rheumatoid arthritis — Assessment.* In Nichols, J. R., and Bradley, W. H., (eds.): *Proceedings of a Symposium on the Motivation of the Physically Disabled.* National Fund for Research into Crippling Diseases, London, 1968, pp. 16-20.

Wolff, B. B.: *Experimental pain parameters and pain perception as predictive indices for rehabilitation of the disabled chronic arthritic patient.* Final Report, SRS Grant # RD-1733-P, 1970.

Psychological Aspects of Systemic Lupus Erythematosus

Cares, R. M., and Weinberg, F.: *The influence of cortisone on psychosis associated with lupus erythematosus.* Psychiatr. Q. 32:94, 1958.

Clark, E. C., and Bailey, A. A.: *Neurological and psychiatric signs associated with systemic lupus erythematosus.* J.A.M.A. 160:455, 1956.

Guze, S. B.: *The occurrence of psychiatric illness in systemic lupus erythematosus.* Am. J. Psychiatry 123:1562, 1967.

Heine, B. E.: *Psychiatric aspects of SLE.* Acta Psychiatr. Scand. 45:307, 1969

Johnson, R. T., and Richardson, E. P.: *The neurological manifestations of systemic lupus erythematosus.* J. Lab. Clin. Med. 74:369, 1969.

Kreindler, S., and Cancro, R.: *An ego psychological approach to psychiatric manifestations in systemic lupus erythematosus.* Dis. Nerv. Sys. Feb. 1970, p. 102.

McClary, A. R., Meyer, E., and Weitzman, D. J.: *Observations on role of mechanism of depression in some patients with disseminated lupus erythematosus.* Psychosom. Med. 17:311, 1955.

Stern, M., and Robbins, E. S.: *Psychoses in systemic lupus erythematosus.* Arch. Gen. Psychiatry 3:205, 1960.

Patient Compliance

Berkowitz, N. H., et al.: *Patient follow-through in outpatient department.* Nurs. Res. 12:16, 1963.

Carpenter, J., and Davis, L.: *Medical recommendations—Followed or ignored? Factors influencing compliance in arthritis.* Arch. Phys. Med. 57(5):241, 1976.

Coomes, E. N.: *Physician's assessment of functional overlay.* Ann. Rheum. Dis. 29:562, 1970.

Davis, M. S.: *Physiologic, psychological, and demographic factors in patient compliance with doctors' orders.* Med. Care 6:115, 1968.

Davis, M. S.: *Variations in patients' compliance with doctors' advice: Empirical analysis of patterns of communication.* Am. J. Public Health 58:274, 1968.

Davis, M. S., and Eichhorn, R. L.: *Compliance with medical regimens: Panel study.* J. Health Hum. Behav. 4:240, 1963.

Diamond, M. D., et al.: *The unmotivated patient.* Arch. Phys. Med. 49:281, 1968.

Feinberg, J., and Brant, K. D.: *Use of resting splints by patients with rheumatoid arthritis.* Am. J. Occup. Ther. 35(3):173, 1981.

Francis, V., Korsch, B. M., and Morris, M. J.: *Gaps in doctor-patient communications: Patients' response to medical advice.* N. Engl. J. Med. 280:535, 1969.

Gersten, H. R., Gray, R. M., and Ward, J. R.: *Patient noncompliance within the context of seeking medical care for arthritis.* J. Chronic Dis. 26:689, 1973.

Gordis, L., Markowitz, M., and Lilienfeld, A.: *Why patients don't follow medical advice: A study of children on long-term antistreptococcal prophylaxis.* J. Pediatr. 75:957, 1969.

Korsch, B. M., Gozzi, E. K., and Francis, V.: *Gaps in doctor-patient communication. I. Doctor-patient interaction and patient satisfaction.* Pediatrics 42:855, 1968.

Lowe, M. L.: *Effectiveness of teaching as measured by compliance with medical recommendations.* Nurs. Res. 19:59, 1970.

Marston, M.-V.: *Compliance with medical regimens: A review of the literature.* Nurs. Res.19:312, 1970.

Mayo, N. E.: *Patient compliance: Pratical implications for physical therapists. A review of the literature.* Phys. Ther. 58(9):1083, 1978.

Moon, M. H., et al.: *Compliancy in splint wearing behavior of patients with rheumatoid arthritis.* N.Z. Med. J. 83(564):360, 1976.

Oakes, T. W., et al.: *Family expectations and arthritis patient compliance to a hand resting splint regimen.* J. Chronic Dis. 22:757, 1970.

Patient Education

An Interdisciplinary Educational Program for Patients with Rheumatic Diseases: A Guide for Professional Staff. Columbia Hospital, Rheumatic Disease Program, 2025 East Newport, Milwaukee, WI 53211.

Arthritis Information Clearinghouse. Provides listings of available print and nonprint educational materials through bibliographies, fact sheets, and newsletters. Arthritis Information Clearinghouse, P.O. Box 34427, Bethesda, MD 20034.

Arthritis Teaching Slide Collection for the Arthritis Health Professional. Contains 198 slides covering comprehensive management of arthritis. Includes a 216-page instructional guide. This is an excellent patient education resource. Available from the Arthritis Foundation, 3400 Peachtree Road, N.E., Atlanta, GA 30326.

Educational Materials Exhibit. Arthritis Health Professions Association Annual Meeting. Each year this exhibit includes all current professional and patient education materials. The catalog for this exhibit is an excellent resource. It is available from the Arthritis Foundation.

Freedman, C. R.: *Teaching Patients.* Courseware, Inc., Department HT-4, 10075 Carroll Canyon Road, San Diego, CA 92131.

Kaye, R. L., and Hammond, A. H.: *Understanding rheumatoid arthritis—Evaluation of a patient education program.* J.A.M.A. 50:57, 1976.

Lawrence, S. V.: *Hospital develops educational program for arthritis patients.* Forum on Medicine July, 1978, p. 34.

Locke, E. A.: *Motivational effects of knowledge of results: Knowledge of goal setting.* J. Appl. Psychol. 31:325, 1967.

Norberg, B., and King, L: *Third-party payment for patient education.* Am. J. Nurs. 46:1269, 1976.

Patient Education in Arthritis — "How to" Packet. Arthritis Foundation, 3400 Peachtree Road, N.E., Atlanta, GA 30326.

Rand, P. H.: *Evaluation of patient education programs.* Phys. Ther. 58(7): 851, 1978.

Wallace, R., Heiss, M. L., and Bautch, J. C.: *Staff Manual for Teaching Patients about Rheumatoid Arthritis.* American Hospital Association, 840 North Lake Shore Drive, Chicago, ILL. 60611. (This also contains the "How to" packet listed above and an excellent bibliography.)

Wright, V.: *What the patient means. A study from rheumatology.* Physiotherapy 64(5):146, 1978.

Vignos, P., Parket, W., and Thompson, H.: *Evaluation of a clinic education program for patients with rheumatoid arthritis.* J. Rheum. 3(2):155, 1976.

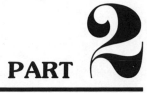

PART

MAJOR RHEUMATIC DISEASES

3

RHEUMATOID ARTHRITIS

Rheumatoid arthritis (RA) is a chronic inflammatory disease of the synovium with a course characterized by exacerbations and remissions. It is a systemic disease and in some clients may involve the lungs, blood vessels, heart, or eyes.

Etiologic Factors

While no etiologic agent has been identified, much has been learned about the inflammatory process involved in RA. The disease seems to be perpetuated by a continued unknown immune reaction in synovial tissue that leads to inflammation, hypertrophy of the synovium, weakening of the capsule, tendons, and ligaments, and eventual destruction of cartilage and bone. Recently, the recognition of histocompatibility antigen HLA-DW4 in a high percentage of patients indicates that genetic factors may also influence the disease.[1]

Age and Sex Affected

Three out of four cases of RA occur in women. It can occur at any age, but the greatest incidence is in the age group of 35 to 45 years.

Diagnosis

The first indication of RA usually is a polyarthritis affecting the small joints of the hands and feet in a symmetric fashion. Large joints and the cervical spine can also be involved, but the thoracic and lumbar spine are usually spared. The diagnosis may be confirmed by the presence of subcutaneous rheumatoid nodules, by radiologic demonstration of cartilage destruction or bony erosions, and by the presence of an antibody in the serum called rheumatoid factor.[2]

The American Rheumatism Association (ARA) has classified the various forms of disease as *classical, definite, probable,* or *possible,* depending on the number of characteristic features present. (See Appendix 1 for classification and criteria.)

Course and Prognosis

The onset may be insidious with slowly progressive symptoms or it may be abrupt with acute joint pain and systemic symptoms requiring hospitalization.

The course of the disease is different for each person. It may range from mild, limited, monoarticular episodes to chronic patterns of complete or incomplete remissions and exacerbations. (See Appendix 2 for classification for progression of RA.)[2]

Joint involvement is usually bilateral (symmetric). That is, the level of joint involvement may be symmetric but the residual deformities can be asymmetric; e.g., a person can have boutonniere deformities on the left hand and swan neck deformities on the right. Peripheral joints are involved more often than proximal ones.

The client's functional ability can vary considerably between exacerbations and remissions. He or she may be independent during remissions and maximally assisted during flare-ups.

SYMPTOMATOLOGY AND IMPLICATIONS FOR OCCUPATIONAL THERAPY

The symptoms of RA fall into three categories:

1. Articular and periarticular symptoms, including those of inflammatory joint disease and associated soft tissue involvement.
2. Systemic manifestations such as fever, malaise, fatigue, anorexia, and generalized stiffness (morning stiffness).
3. Symptoms associated with involvement of organs, including lung, vascular, and cardiac complications.[3]

Articular and Periarticular Involvement

The joint deformities that develop with this disease can also occur in other chronic inflammatory arthritic diseases. For example, a person with systemic lupus or psoriatic arthritis who develops a chronic inflammatory arthritis of the MCP joints can develop the same deformities typically seen in RA.

Since the common hand deformities are not unique to RA they are discussed and referenced in detail in Chapter 21. The following is a discussion solely of the common physical and functional consequences of chronic inflammatory disease of the extremity joints and cervical spine. (Basic treatment for joint involvement is described in Chapter 1.)

The section on surgical rehabilitation (Chapters 13 to 19) also contains a referenced review of the specific pathodynamics for each joint.

The joints are discussed in the order or frequency of occurrence and pattern of involvement in RA, i.e., hands, wrists, feet, ankles, knees, hips, elbows, and shoulders.

HANDS AND WRISTS

Classically the *distal interphalangeal (DIP) joints* are not involved to the same degree as the other hand joints. They may develop a mild synovitis but they are usually spared the severe erosive form. They may lose range of motion (ROM) or develop contractures in conjunction with boutonniere deformities, swan neck deformities, or insufficient excursion of the profundus tendons. They may also become unstable due to weakening of the collateral ligaments. Stretching of the distal attachment of the extensor communis tendon can result in a mallet deformity.

In the *proximal interphalangeal (PIP) joints* the characteristic fusiform-shaped swelling demonstrates that the effusion is confined to the joint capsule. PIP joint synovitis can result in shortening of the collateral or accessory collateral ligaments, producing a flexion contracture; stretching of dorsal capsule and central slip, resulting in volar displacement of the lateral bands and a boutonniere deformity; stretching of the volar capsule, resulting in hyperextension and dorsal migration of the lateral bands, producing a swan neck deformity; and bone erosions and collateral ligament instability, resulting in deviation deformities.

In the *metacarpophalangeal (MCP) joints,* synovitis weakens and distends the joint capsule and ligaments. It is theorized that, in addition, the stretch of the capsule leads to a protective reflex spasm of the interosseus and lumbrical muscles. Intrinsic muscle tightness can lead to a flexion contracture (intrinsic plus) deformity of the MCP joint as well as contribute to a swan neck finger deformity. (See swan neck deformity in Chapter 21.)

Damage to the fibrous flexor sheath (pulley mechanism) that supports the flexor tendons allows the tendons to migrate volar and ulnarward to the joint. This alters the mechanical advantage of the flexor tendons, allowing them to pull the proximal phalanx into ulnar and volar subluxation, during power pinch and grasp activities. These factors, combined with stretching of the radial collateral ligaments, the normal ulnar slope of the metacarpal heads, the power advantage of the ulnar interossei over the radial interossei, and dislocation of the long extensors into the ulnar valleys, make MCP ulnar drift a common sequela in RA. (See Figure 37 in Chapter 21.)

Thumb involvement is similar to finger involvement in that the MCP and carpometacarpal (CMC) joints are the most common sites of inflammation with interphalangeal (IP) joint instability and deformity secondary to collapse of the proximal joints.

The most common thumb deformity (Nalebuff Type I) begins with MCP involvement and results in flexion of the MCP and hyperextension of the IP joints. Other types of deformities can occur in the thumb; they are described in detail in Chapter 21.

Chronic synovitis of the *wrist joint* weakens the supporting ligaments. Loss of ligamentous support combined with the normal volar slope of the distal radius results in volar slippage of the carpal bones on the radius. This volar subluxation may be further enhanced by volar displacement of the extensor carpi ulnaris tendon. Once displaced this tendon loses its effectiveness as an extensor and creates an additional flexor and deviation force on the carpus.

When there is loss of lateral ligamentous support the carpal bones typically sublux in an ulnar direction as well. This ulnar subluxation of the carpal bones typically results in radial deviation of the hand on the forearm. (See Chapter 21 for detailed discussion of finger and wrist deformities.) Ulnar deviation of the hand on the forearm can also occur but is far less common.

Synovitis of the *extensor tendon sheaths* (tenosynovitis) weakens the extensor tendons by direct infiltration and indirectly through pressure, compromising the neurovascular supply of the tendons. Constant movement over the roughened carpal bones can lead to rupture of the finger extensor tendons. Unlike joint synovitis, tenosynovitis may be painless and without warmth during the active phase.

Tenosynovitis of the flexor tendons can occur at three levels: the wrist, palm, and volar aspect of the fingers and thumb. In the wrist (carpal tunnel) it can result in entrapment of the median nerve, impairing sensation to the thumb, index, middle, and ring fingers, as well as the ability to abduct the thumb. Wrist tenosynovitis can also impede flexor tendon excursion, creating either a flexion or extension lag, typically affecting all four digits. If left untreated, this can result in permanent contractures of the digital joints. Flexor wrist tenosynovitis can also directly invade the tendons, making them vulnerable to rupture. Digital tenosynovitis is common and can result in: impaired tendon excursion that initially limits DIP flexion, but if severe, can limit motion in all of the joints; thickening or stenosing of the flexor sheath; proliferative tenosynovium that can impair tendon function; and granulomatous plaques that can build up on the tendon. These plaques as well as tendon nodules can catch on the fibrous bands of the sheath (annular ligaments), creating a "trigger finger." (See Hand Pathodynamics and Assessment, Chapter 21.)

The various combinations of hand deformities are practically boundless. Each hand is unique and the effect of the deformity on hand function depends on the person's daily activities. However, the following disabilities appear to contribute the greatest to functional loss:

1. Wrist pain can severely limit hand strength for functional activities.
2. Decreased PIP and MCP flexion or extension restrict grasp and fine manipulation.
3. Thumb involvement, especially an adductor contracture, and IP instability which limits pinch prehension.

Therapy

Occupational therapy for hand involvement consists of five areas:
1. Evaluation of hand pathology and function.
2. Splinting to reduce pain, reduce inflammation, maintain joint integrity, and improve function.
3. Instruction in joint protection techniques, adaptive methods, and use of assistive equipment to maintain joint integrity, reduce pain, and improve function.
4. Patient instruction in the use of hot and cold compresses to control inflammation, enhance mobility, and facilitate exercise.
5. Instruction in activities or exercises to maintain or improve hand function, joint mobility, and muscular strength.

Specific therapy procedures can be found in the following chapters: Hand Pathodynamics and Assessment, Chapter 21; Splinting for Arthritis of the Hand, Chapter 25; Joint Protection and Energy Conservation Instruction, Chapter 26; Exercise Treatment, Chapter 29; and Positioning and Lying Prone, Chapter 30.

FEET AND ANKLES

Initial RA involvement typically includes the metatarsophalangeal (MTP) joints. MTP joint involvement is painful and is frequently described by the patient as "feels like walking on marbles." It interferes with the push-off phase of ambulation, thereby shifting the effect of weight bearing on other joints.

Synovitis in the MTP joints weakens the joint capsules and supporting ligaments; this makes them extremely vulnerable to the stress of weight bearing. The result of MTP synovitis is flattening of the anterior arch (splayed forefoot), volar subluxation of the metatarsal heads with plantar callosities, spasm of the intrinsic and extrinsic muscles, and secondary cock-up or hammer toe deformities.

Synovium lines the ankle (tibiotalofibular joint) and subtalar joints, the sheaths of the tendons that cross the ankle, and the Achilles bursa. Although it is possible for all of these structures to become inflamed, many (possibly the majority) patients with RA only have involvement for the MTP and subtalar (hindfoot) joints and never develop true ankle joint disease. Subtalar involvement increases the natural tendency of the talus to glide forward, downward, and medially. Subsequent pressure on the calcaneus and spring ligament results in hindfoot pronation (valgus) and flattening of the longitudinal arch. This diminishes inversion and eversion mobility necessary for adjustment to uneven ground. Ambulation with the ankle in this position necessitates medial pressure against the large toe and contributes to a hallux valgus deformity of the first MTP joint and alters weight-bearing forces on the knee.

The true ankle joint is involved less frequently than the subtalar but, when it is involved, it severely limits ankle flexion and extension.

Therapy

Foot and ankle pain diminishes the desire to walk and necessitates walking slowly; thus the time spent performing daily activities is lengthened. This must be kept in mind when planning therapy for patients.

Occupational therapy programs for foot involvement vary considerably. They may consist of (1) evaluation to determine the degree of foot involvement and how the pain affects the person's daily activities; (2) patient education regarding appropriate exercise and rest for the foot and ankle during synovitis, proper positioning in bed, and appropriate shoe support; and (3) fitting of Plastazote shoe liners. In some clinics, particularly in Canada, the therapist's role extends to constructing and fitting shoe adaptations. (See Chapter 26, Joint Protection and Energy Conservation Instruction, for a discussion of foot orthotics and recommended shoe requirements.)

There are numerous canvas and elastic ankle supports available but they usually are ineffective when structural deformities are present. At present, the best external support sturdy enough for structural deformities are polypropylene molded orthoses for the foot or foot-ankle combined and metal arch supports. The plastic orthotics worn inside the shoe are valuable for restricting inversion and eversion, thus reducing stress to the subtalar joints. They can also have a metatarsal lift built in to relieve pressure on the metatarsal heads, and a wedge to correct or accommodate valgus deformity.

The occupational therapist needs to be aware of the skills of other team members such as the physical therapist, podiatrist, and orthotist and of community shoe resources so he or she can make appropriate recommendations for referral.

Specific therapy procedures can be found in the following chapters: Joint Protection and Energy Conservation Instruction, Chapter 26, and Positioning and Lying Prone, Chapter 30.

KNEES

The knee joint contains the largest amount of synovium in an individual joint. Consequently synovitis can produce marked hypertrophy and effusions that distend and stretch the joint capsule and the supporting cruciate and collateral ligaments. Pain and stretch of the joint capsule results in reflex spasm of the hamstring muscles. Patients frequently respond by keeping their knees flexed (usually with pillows under the knee or sleeping side-lying) to relieve the joint tension.

Knee flexion contractures, secondary hamstring tightness, and postural adaptation are severe functional problems that disrupt the stability of the joint for weight bearing and ambulation. (See Chapter 18, Knee Surgery, for a discussion of knee pathodynamics and use of ambulation aids.)

Therapy

The goal of occupational therapy for knee involvement is to educate the client in joint protection and assistive equipment. The latter includes raised chairs and resting splints, which are used to minimize stress and pain and, thereby, reduce inflammation and increase functional ability.

Specific therapy procedures can be found in the following chapters: Joint Protection and Energy Conservation Instruction, Chapter 26; Assistive Equipment, Chapter 27; and Positioning and Lying Prone, Chapter 30.

HIPS

Inflamed synovium confined in a tight fibrous capsule produces pain and muscle spasm of the flexor and adductor muscles of the hip. The most comfortable position for someone with hip synovitis is hip flexion and external rotation. Fibrous contractures in flexion and external rotation are common, if restriction of motion is prolonged. Severe disease can produce extensive destruction of both the acetabulum and femoral head, a condition that can result in the acetabulum being pushed into the pelvic cavity by the femur (protrusio acetabulae). Pain as a result of hip involvement is felt anteriorly in the groin; occasionally the pain is referred to the medial side of the knee.

Pain is the cause of functional limitation, and it impedes all weight-bearing activities. Protective muscular spasm promotes hip flexion contractures in the early stages. This necessitates knee flexion and lumbar lordosis in order to permit a vertical position and, thus, produces additional stress to these areas.

When involvement becomes more intense, limitation of hip flexion and abduction may interfere with sitting comfortably in chairs, walking up steps, positioning during sexual intercourse, and with self-care capabilities, such as those involved with reaching the feet.

Therapy

Occupational therapy for hip involvement is primarily of an educational nature. For example, the client is instructed in protection techniques and use of assistive devices, lying prone to maintain hip extension, and proper positioning at night. Exercises to improve hip abductor and extensor strength and joint mobility are usually prescribed in physical therapy.

Elevated chairs and toilet seats can significantly reduce stress to the hip joint and back as well as increase the patient's comfort when there is severe involvement, such as extension contractures. (See the section on Hips in Chapter 10 for additional information on severe limitations and Chapter 17, Hip Surgery, for a discussion on hip pathodynamics.)

Assistive aids for dressing and hygiene of the lower extremity may also be indicated.

Specific therapy procedures can be found in the following chapters: Joint Protection and Energy Conservation Instruction, Chapter 26; Assistive Equipment, Chapter 27; and Positioning and Lying Prone, Chapter 30.

ELBOWS

The synovial lining is common to both the elbow (humeroradioulnar) joint and the proximal radioulnar joint. Painful synovitis prompts the patient to keep the arm in flexion and pronation with consequent contractures as the main functional limitation.

Flexion contractures up to 30 degrees usually do not interfere with functional ability; however, when the loss of extension is greater, function is affected. A lack of 30 to 60 degrees extension interferes with ability for reach such as that needed for pulling on socks, and a loss of 45 to 90 degrees extension restricts push-off leverage for chair transfers and interferes with mobility required in dressing. Loss of greater than 90 degrees extension is rare but, when it occurs, it seriously restricts reach and ability for dressing, perineal care, and transfer and it necessitates trunk flexion for performance of desk work or feeding.

Extension contractures (diminished elbow flexion) are less frequent; they can severely limit ability for feeding, grooming, and facial hygiene. For example, a person who can only flex his or her elbow to 90 degrees generally will not be able to eat even with regular utensils (unless he or she has a long flexible neck).

When loss of forearm rotation is inevitable, the optimal position for ankylosis depends upon shoulder and wrist function; however, 20 degrees of pronation allows relatively easy substitution of shoulder rotation for forearm motion.

Another problem seen in clients with classic or definite RA is the presence of subcutaneous rheumatoid nodules over the dorsum of the olecranon or shaft of the ulna. (These nodules can also occur over other bony prominences, e.g., ischial tuberosity, occipital bone, and so forth.) They are usually painless but can become painful when irritated by pressure.

Therapy

The obvious treatment of choice is prevention. After permanent contractures develop, the only nonsurgical means to improve function is instruction in adaptive methods and use of assistive equipment.

Night splinting of the elbow to provide local rest and proper positioning or to apply sustained passive pressure to reduce developing contractures is not commonly done but is a valid approach for some clients. A condition in which nodules are aggravated by pressure can be helped through alleviation of the irritating source or redistribution of the pressure with a doughnut pad or an elbow protector pad encased in a knit sleeve that slips onto the elbow. Several brands are available from medical supply distributors. (See Chapter 30, Positioning and Lying Prone.)

Specific therapy procedures can be found in the following chapters: Assistive Equipment, Chapter 27; Positioning and Lying Prone, Chapter 30; and methods of documenting nodule status, in Chapter 21, Hand Pathodynamics and Assessment.

SHOULDERS

The shoulder is a complex structure that depends upon the coordinated movement of four joints (glenohumeral, acromioclavicular, sternoclavicular, and thoracoscapular) and the smooth gliding of tendons, principally the biceps and supraspinatus tendons, which cross over the glenohumeral joints.

Synovitis affects the glenohumeral joint, thereby causing cartilage loss, damage to the capsule, 'and severe limitation of motion and function. However, tendinitis, bursitis, and capsular fibrosis are far more frequent sources of shoulder pain, even in clients with RA.

When there is true RA involvement of the shoulder, it is frequently severe and limits functional ability for hair care and dressing. Several factors contribute to this situation. Prime among these are the facts that shoulder joint involvement usually occurs late in the disease process and that clients, who are concerned with limitations caused by early hand, knee, and foot involvement, frequently neglect shoulder exercises and/or problems. They are not aware of shoulder limitations until significant mobility restrictions occur. Since only about 90 degrees of shoulder flexion and abduction and 30 degrees of external rotation are necessary for most functional activities, a person can lose up to 50 per cent of shoulder mobility before it interferes with his or her daily activities.

Therapy

Three factors limit functional use of the shoulder: pain, decreased muscle strength and endurance, and decreased range of motion (ROM). Any program to improve function must address these issues. Pain and poor endurance usually interfere with function long before decreased ROM is a problem.

Functional activities are often an effective adjunct to improvement of shoulder strength and endurance, since they can be designed to tax muscle power within a pain-free range.

Remedial exercises usually do not help when there is actual bony destruction. Compensatory measures such as use of assistive equipment and instruction in adaptive methods are the only nonsurgical means for improving function. Assistive equipment, such as dressing sticks, reachers and extended combs, brushes, and tableware, is helpful. When prescribing this equipment, however, it is important to assess the entire upper extremity since many extended handle devices can cause damaging stress to the hands.

Specific therapy procedures can be found in the following chapters: Joint Protection and Energy Conservation Instruction, Chapter 26; Assistive Equipment, Chapter 27; Functional Activities, Chapter 28; and Exercise Treatment, Chapter 29.

CERVICAL SPINE

The incidence of radiographic cervical spine involvement is extremely high, if not universal, in advanced cases of RA.

Chronic synovitis attacks the capsules, ligamentous supports, and joint surfaces of the apophyseal and lateral interbody joints (joints of Luschka). The first to fourth cervical vertebral joints are the most common sites of inflammation, but the entire cervical spine can be involved. (See Chapter 16, Spinal Surgery, for a discussion on the pathodynamics of cervical subluxation.)

Initially there is pain and muscle spasm that limits mobility. Progressive involvement leads to subluxation of the joints, particularly the atlantoaxial joint (first to second cervical). Subluxation of the low cervical spine is more likely to produce symptoms of cord-root compression than subluxation of the first to fourth cervical vertebrae because the ratio of the spinal cord to the foramen is less in the upper portion. That is, the cord takes up about half the spinal canal in the first to fourth cervical area but nearly fills the foramen along the fourth to eighth cervical vertebrae.

Although high subluxation can be asymptomatic except for pain, nerve compression can result in radiation of pain to the occipital area, the shoulder, or the upper extremity. Severe cases can lead to quadraparesis or frank paralysis. Compression of the vertebral artery may cause visual disturbances (diplopia, blurring) and lightheadedness. (See Chapter 16 for treatment of cervical subluxation.)

Therapy

Patients with evidence of cervical subluxation, whether it is symptomatic or asymptomatic, should wear a neck collar during high-risk situations such as driving. Neck collars are also helpful in relieving neck muscle spasm that is secondary to pain. Neck protection techniques as outlined in Chapter 26 help reduce the dynamic forces that contribute to subluxation.

Soft neck collars are valuable for providing a postural reminder to maintain desired alignment. Custom Plastazote collars provide greater restriction of flexion but do not completely immobilize the neck. The Somi brace is a widely used commercial four-post brace and is the most restrictive type of brace. Maximal (nearly complete) immobilization is achieved only with a halo apparatus, with a plaster vest, or by pelvic fixation.[4,5]

Cervical pillows can also be effective in reducing muscle spasm and stiffness. (See Chapter 30, Positioning and Lying Prone.)

Systemic Manifestations

The symptoms of fatigue, malaise, subjective weakness, anorexia, and decreased motivation accompany all systemic illnesses to some degree. In addition to these, generalized stiffness is part of RA. The severity of these symptoms usually correlates with the severity of the joint involvement. Severity also tends to increase with energy expenditure. Fatigue and other manifestations often become apparent after about 4 to 6 hours of activity.

The symptoms of systemic disease are identical to those of psychological depression. Distinguishing the two can be a difficult task. A helpful feature is that systemic fatigue is usually related to the person's energy expenditure, whereas fatigue associated with depression is more constant.

Therapy

For fatigue resulting from systemic involvement, instruction in work simplification and energy conservation can improve the patient's endurance for functional activities. Assess the individual's rest patterns and reinforce the need for 10 to 12 hours rest per day to allow the body's restorative processes to help combat disease. Another compounding factor is that pain and stiffness at night often cause the patient to lose sleep and thus further enhance fatigue.

When the disease is under control or in a chronic-active phase, patient participation in a routine community program of body conditioning–exercise can be effective for improving endurance, muscle tone, and posture. However, patients often need guidelines for determining which exercises to do and how to monitor the effects of exercise on their arthritis.

When fatigue associated with depression interferes with the person's daily activities, refer the client to a person (physician, psychologist, or social worker) or agency (community counseling service) which can arrange for ongoing counseling to help him or her work through the depression.

Specific therapy procedures can be found in the following sections: Psychology, Education, and Patient Care, Chapter 2; Joint Protection and Energy Conservation Instruction, Chapter 26; and Evaluation of Activities of Daily Living, Chapter 24.

Associated Organ Involvement

A small percentage of people with RA develop various degrees of pulmonary and cardiac involvement.[3] There are no specific occupational therapy measures for these conditions except to be aware that they can exist. If cardiac or pulmonary involvement may influence the therapy program, it should be verified with the physician before starting a treatment program. This usually does not create a problem since clients sick enough to have significant cardiac or lung involvement normally would not be on a stressful therapy regimen.

There can also be a rare but severe vasculitis associated with RA. (See Arteritis and Vasculitis, Chapter 7, for more information.)

DRUG THERAPY

Anti-inflammatory medications are the mainstay of drug treatment for RA. Aspirin is the drug of choice. Aspirin and aspirin-type medications work as analgesics when given in small doses; they are effective as anti-inflammatory agents when given in large doses. The dosage is adjusted to maintain a blood salicylate level just below toxicity which is evidenced by tinnitus (ringing or sound in the ears). Any of the other nonsteroidal anti-inflammatory drugs (NSAIDs) may be used in place of a salicylate. These drugs have been shown to be as effective as acetylsalicylic acid (ASA) in controlling the inflammation of RA.

When synovitis is nonresponsive to aspirin and other nonsteroidal anti-inflammatory medications, the second line of attack (or defense, depending on one's perspective) is to use remission-inducing drugs (RIDs). These medications are stronger and have the potential for serious side effects, but they also have the potential for controlling the disease and effecting an apparent remission. Medications in this category include gold salts, antimalarial drugs (Plaquenil), and penicillamine. Gold therapy is the most widely used and is generally tried first; Plaquenil is the second choice; and penicillamine is reserved for last, because of the nature of its side effects.

Gold salts given by injection can be an effective form of therapy for some patients, particularly in the acute or subacute stages of their disease. Injections are given weekly for 20 weeks and if there is a good response, they are continued at 2- to 4-week intervals.

Antimalarial medication is in tablet form and does not require weekly clinic visits as does gold therapy; however, it can cause permanent visual loss and patients must be responsible for obtaining appropriate ophthalmologic evaluations every six months.

Steroids such as prednisone are effective anti-inflammatory agents, but their undesirable side effects usually preclude their use in RA, except when all other modalities of therapy have failed.

Experimental drugs such as cyclophosphamide (Cytoxan), azathioprine (Imuran), and chlorambucil are used occasionally and can benefit selected patients. However, these drugs may have an immunosuppressive action as well as an anti-inflammatory effect. Their undesirable side effects frequently preclude their use.

The procedure of removing large quantities of plasma, or plasmapheresis, has been claimed to be effective in reducing inflammation in RA. This treatment must be considered purely experimental until well-controlled studies have been performed.

REFERENCES

1. Harris, E. D.: *Pathogenesis of rheumatoid arthritis.* In Kelley, W. M., et al. (eds.): *Textbook of Rheumatology.* W. B. Saunders, Philadelphia, 1981.
2. Harris, E. D.: *Rheumatoid arthritis: The clinical spectrum.* In Kelley, W. M., et al. (eds.): *Textbook of Rheumatology.* W. B. Saunders, Philadelphia, 1981.
3. Decker, J. L., and Plotz, P. H.: *Extra-articular rheumatoid disease.* In McCarty, D. J. (ed.): *Arthritis and Allied Conditions.* Lea and Febiger, Philadelphia, 1979.
4. Johnson, R. M., et al.: *Cervical orthoses: A study comparing their effectiveness in restricting cervical motion in normal subjects.* J. Bone Joint Surg. 59A:3, 1977.
5. Hart, D. L., Johnson, R. M., Simmons, E. F., and Owen, J.: *Review of cervical orthoses.* Phys. Ther. 58(7), July, 1978.

ADDITIONAL SOURCES

Bulmash, J. M.: *Rheumatoid arthritis and pregnancy.* Obstet. Gynecol. Annu. 8:223, 1979.
Calabro, J. I.: *Rheumatoid arthritis.* Clinical Symposia, CIBA, Vol. 23, No. 1, 1971.
Ehrlich, G. E. (ed.): *Total Management of the Arthritic Patient.* J. B. Lippincott, Philadelphia, 1973.
Polly, H. F., and Hunder, G. G.: *Rheumatologic Interviewing and Physical Examination of the Joints.* W. B. Saunders, Philadelphia, 1978.

SYSTEMIC LUPUS ERYTHEMATOSUS

Systemic lupus erythematosus (SLE) is a systemic inflammatory disease characterized by small vessel vasculitis with a diverse clinical picture. Manifestations of the disease depend on the organ systems involved and may include any or all of the following: fever, an erythematous rash, polyarthritis, pneumonitis, polyserositis (especially pleurisy and pericarditis), myositis, anemia, thrombocytopenia, and renal, neurologic, psychological, and cardiac abnormalities. (SLE is different from discoid lupus. See the Glossary.)

Etiologic Factors

Many of the clinical manifestations can be explained by the deposition of antigen-antibody complexes in the walls of small blood vessels. There is also a hereditary predisposition. Although a viral agent may be linked etiologically, none has been identified to date.[1]

Age and Sex Affected

Four out of five patients are women, primarily in young adult and adolescent age range, but the disease can occur at any age. There is a higher incidence in black women when compared with the incidence in white women.

Diagnosis

Diagnosis is made clinically by the presence of multi-organ system involvement and with a facial rash and glomerulonephritis, which are the most frequent of the diagnostic features. Confirmatory tests include the presence of antinuclear antibodies in the serum, a positive LE prep (see Glossary for definition), or characteristic histologic changes in a kidney or skin biopsy.[1]

Course and Prognosis

This is highly variable and depends on which organs are involved. Long-term survival is uncommon in those patients with evidences of renal, neurologic, or myocardial damage. However, the long-term outlook may be good if the disease is limited to the joints or skin.[2]

SYMPTOMATOLOGY AND IMPLICATIONS
FOR OCCUPATIONAL THERAPY

Patients with an associated arthritis, myositis, neuropathy, or functional psychosis are frequently referred for rehabilitation. Unfortunately, patients with only general systemic manifestations are often not referred because physicians are not aware of occupational therapy measures for these symptoms. Patients limited by fatigue can often benefit from instruction in energy conservation methods and stress management techniques as well as general body conditioning. Biofeedback has proven to be a valuable adjunct in the management of Raynaud's phenomenon.[3,4,5,6]

A word of caution is needed regarding patient instruction with patients taking high-dose corticosteroids. This medication can produce a wide range of side effects, including euphoria and a false sense of well being. This does not occur in all patients, but when it is present, even in mild form, patient instruction is extremely difficult. When a patient is euphoric, he or she cannot perceive the seriousness of the condition or the need for instruction. Many of these patients are in the process of having their medications stabilized. If possible, patient education should be delayed until the medication is reduced. Also, all patient education for patients on high-dose steroids should be reinforced with written instructions.

Polyarthritis

Polyarthritis occurs in 90 percent of SLE patients. The arthritis associated with SLE has the same distribution as rheumatoid arthritis; that is, it is symmetric and affects the small peripheral joints more frequently than the larger joints. Unlike rheumatoid arthritis, the arthritis associated with SLE typically does not erode the cartilage but primarily affects the capsule and supporting structures.[7] Deformities are not as common as in RA, but they do occur and can include all of the typical rheumatoid-type deformities, e.g., ulnar drift, swan neck, or boutonneire. The deformities in SLE are primarily due to capsular and ligamentous involvement, rather than erosive cartilage and bone changes. Therefore, joint instability and subluxation are common sequelae, and contractures and ankylosis are unusual.

Therapy

Treatment for the acute, subacute, and chronic stages is the same as outlined for inflammatory joint disease in Chapter 1. Also, see Rheumatoid Arthritis, Chapter 3, for information on the functional and physical consequences of arthritis in the peripheral joints.

Systemic Manifestations

Symptoms include fever, malaise, fatigue, weight loss, anorexia, and weakness. Fatigue can become very disruptive to the patient's life-style and family and social relationships. Patients may feel too tired to play with their children, maintain a job, have sexual relations, or participate in social events. As with all systemic diseases, these systemic manifestations need to be distinguished, if possible, from the symptoms of depression. See the section on systemic manifestations in Rheumatoid Arthritis, Chapter 3, and the section on depression in Psychological Considerations in Patient Education and Treatment, Chapter 2.

The level of fatigue is also affected by sleeping and rest patterns. Some patients taking high doses of corticosteroids may have a great deal of difficulty sleeping at night, resulting in greater fatigue during the day.[1]

Therapy

It is critical that patients with SLE get sufficient rest. Some patients perform best when they have 10 hours sleep per night; others may need 8 to 9 hours with a nap during the day.

Exercise should be in moderation and not to the point of exhaustion. Yoga and general body toning and stretching exercises can improve endurance and help a patient stay in shape without excessive stress. All exercise programs should be built up gradually, and reduced if they appear to cause an increase in systemic manifestations.

Since this is a systemic disease, it is important to consider the patient's daily hospital or home routine when planning a treatment program. Instruction in energy conservation and work simplification can be of benefit in improving the patient's functional endurance. Specific therapy procedures can be found in Joint Protection and Energy Conservation Instruction, Chapter 26.

Muscle Involvement

The most common involvement is an inflammatory myositis. It presents similar to polymyositis with initial proximal muscle weakness but is usually milder than idiopathic polymyositis. Patients can also develop a noninflammatory myopathy secondary to steroid or chloroquine therapy.[1]

Therapy

Because myositis or myopathy is a relatively common development, a therapist should be alert to the signs of proximal muscle weakness in all patients with lupus or patients on steroid or chloroquine therapy. Typical signs include difficulty in rising from a chair without assistance (not resulting from joint involvement); tiredness or difficulty in stabilizing the neck; waddling gait; drooping of and/or tiredness in the shoulders; difficulty stepping up onto a step or curb; and dysphagia. If these signs are observed in a patient, a group muscle test should be done to determine any actual proximal weakness and the findings should be reported to the physician. Occupational therapy for a myositis is the same as for polymyositis (see Chapter 6, Polymyositis and Dermatomyositis).

Skin Involvement

An erythematous rash, which is often symmetric, occurs over the face, neck, extremities, hands, and elbows. It may form a characteristic butterfly shape when it is over the nose and cheeks. The rash may be episodic or chronic and with or without scarring. In some cases it appears to be a healthy looking blush. Frequently, exposure to sunlight or ultraviolet light can cause the rash or systemic manifestations to flare up. [1,2]

Therapy

If the patient is sun-sensitive, the patient should be advised to report sensitivity to his or her physician, avoid sun exposure when possible, wear protective clothing, and use a sun block lotion containing para-aminobenzoic acid (PABA) over exposed areas. (It is helpful to give the patient some brand names so that he or she does not buy a suntan lotion by mistake. A pharmacist can advise which commercial sun blocks have the greatest amount of PABA. A PABA sun protection factor of 15 or more is recommended.

Neuropsychological Involvement

Psychological reactions may include anxiety, depression, hyperirritability, confusion, hallucinations, and paranoia. Psychotic episodes during exacerbations may be secondary to lupus cerebritis, steroid treatment (drug-induced), or psychological need (functional). Other neurologic findings may include headaches, organic brain syndrome, seizures, and peripheral neuropathy, although the latter is uncommon. Peripheral motor and sensory loss is usually responsive to corticosteroid therapy. [8,9,10]

Therapy

It is important to relay observed neurologic or personality changes to the referring physician.
　　Crafts employed as a therapeutic modality can be effective during psychotic periods to enhance the patient's reality testing and as evaluation tools to assess the patient's psychological status, problem solving ability, or judgment.

Other Manifestations

Other manifestations of SLE may include:

1. Pleurisy and pneumonitis. (Occurs in 50 per cent of patients.)
2. Raynaud's phenomenon. Raynaud's associated with SLE differs from that seen with systemic sclerosis in that it often resolves if the SLE goes into prolonged remission. (Instruct patient in appropriate precautions; see Chapter 5.)
3. Pericarditis or myocarditis. (It is important to determine the patient's cardiac status and observe work tolerance carefully.)
4. Nephritis accounts for 50 per cent of all fatalities.
5. Ulcerations of mouth, pharynx, or vagina. (These ulcers are usually painful; mouth ulcers may make talking uncomfortable for the patient.)
6. Alopecia. (Usually there is eventual regrowth. If the alopecia is severe, purchase of a wig is warranted.)
7. Transverse cord myelopathy is rare but has been reported in 28 cases. It can result in quadriplegia or paraplegia. [11]

Associated Conditions

These include Sjögren's syndrome and avascular necrosis (osteonecrosis), usually of the femoral head.

PREGNANCY AND SLE

SLE primarily affects women of the childbearing years. The concerns about pregnancy—how it will affect the mother, the child, and the lupus—are common ones. Pregnancy may cause an exacerbation of the lupus, most frequently in the last trimester and in the early postpartum period. The effect of an exacerbation varies from patient to patient depending on how extensive the lupus is and which organs are involved. For example, a patient with kidney involvement could be placed at high risk for renal failure. Women with SLE also have a higher incidence of miscarriages, premature births, and stillbirths than women in the general population. Despite these risks patients with mild disease can have a safe and successful pregnancy. For women who are planning to have children it is recommended that conception be planned when the disease is mild or in remission. For many women the disease can be kept under control with corticosteroids during the pregnancy. So far, there is no evidence that steroid therapy affects the fetus.

Another major concern is whether SLE can be genetically transmitted. The answer to this question is uncertain. It appears that people who develop SLE have a genetic predisposition to it. Occasionally SLE will run in families, or various rheumatic diseases will run in a family. It is also possible for people to have a genetic predisposition to a disease but never develop the disease, as demonstrated in studies of identical twins. To date, no specific genetic defect has been detected.[12,13]

The first few months after having a baby are difficult both physically and emotionally for healthy parents. The risk of a lupus flare at this time makes adjustment even more difficult. Patients may need counseling to plan realistically for the child care and psychological support needed during the postpartum period.

DRUG THERAPY

Medications used in SLE depend on the organ systems involved with the disease.

Skin disease may be controlled with local steroid creams or with antimalarial drugs such as hydroxychloroquine sulfate (Plaquenil Sulfate) or quinacrine (Atabrine).

The inflammatory manifestations such as arthritis and pleurisy often can be controlled with anti-inflammatory drugs such as aspirin in high doses. This may be combined with an antimalarial drug or with prednisone if manifestations are not controlled.

For life-threatening conditions, such as with central nervous system, cardiac, or hematologic involvement, steroids such as prednisone are used in high dosages.

In certain types of renal disease, steroids may be combined with an immunosuppressive drug such as azathioprine (Imuran) or cyclophosphamide (Cytoxan).

Some physicians administer steroids in alternate-day doses; for example, 20 mg. every other day or alternating a high and low dose. This is done to encourage the patient's adrenal glands to produce natural steroids on alternate days. Patients on this type of program often vary in their functional ability, depending on the day and dose. An ADL evaluation needs to take this dual functional pattern into account.

See Chapter 12 for precautions and side effects of specific drugs.

REFERENCES

1. Rothfield, N.: *Clinical features of systemic lupus erythematosus.* In Kelley, W. M., et al. (eds.): *Textbook of Rheumatology.* W. B. Saunders, Philadelphia, 1981.
2. Fries, J. F., and Hollman, H. R.: *Systemic Lupus Erythematosus: A Clinical Analysis.* W. B. Saunders, Philadelphia, 1975.
3. Taub, E., and Strobel, C. F.: *Biofeedback in the treatment of vasoconstrictive syndromes.* Biofeedback Self Regul. 3(4):363, 1978.
4. Sunderman, R. H., and Delk, J. L.: *Treatment of Raynaud's disease with temperature biofeedback.* South. Med. J. 71(3):340, 1978.
5. Sedlacek, K.: *Biofeedback for Raynaud's disease.* Psychosom. Med. 20(8):535, 1979.
6. Green, E., and Green, A.: *General and specific applications of thermal biofeedback.* In Basmajian, J. V. (ed.): *Biofeedback — Principles and Practice for Clinicians.* William & Wilkins, Baltimore, 1979.
7. Labowitz, R., and Shumacher, H. R.: *Articular manifestation of systemic lupus erythematosus.* Ann. Rheum. Dis. 33:204, 1974.
8. Gibson, T., and Myers, A. R.: *Nervous system involvement in systemic lupus erythematosus.* Ann. Rheum. Dis. 35:398, 1976.
9. Small, P., et al.: *CNS involvement in SLE.* Arthritis Rheum. 20:869, 1977.
10. Baker, M.: *Psychopathology in systemic lupus erythematosus. Part I. Psychiatric observations.* Semin. Arthritis Rheum. 3(2):95, 1973.
11. Thakarar, P., and Greenspun, B.: *Transverse myelopathy in systemic lupus erythematosus.* Arch. Phys. Med. Rehab. 60:323, 1979.
12. Medsger, T. A., and Chetlin, S. M.: *Lupus and Pregnancy.* Pennsylvania Lupus Foundation, 1978.
13. White, J. F.: *Teaching patients to manage systemic lupus erythematosus.* Nursing '78 8:27, 1978.

ADDITIONAL SOURCES

Dubois, E. L. *Lupus Erythematosus: A Review of the Current Status of Discoid and Systemic Lupus Erythematosus and their Variants,* ed. 2. University of Southern California Press, Los Angeles, 1974.

Patient Education

Dubois, E. L.: *Information for Patients with Lupus Erythematosus.* National Lupus Foundation, 16255 Ventura Blvd., Suite 605, Encino, CA 91316 ($1.00).
Epstein, W. V., and Clewley, G.: *Living with SLE.* Millberry Union Bookstore, 500 Parnassus Ave., San Francisco, CA 94143 ($2.00).
Lupus and You: A Guide for Patients. St. Louis Park, Minn. 55416 ($1.00).

5

SYSTEMIC SCLEROSIS (SCLERODERMA)

Systemic sclerosis (SS), or scleroderma, is a generalized disorder of the small blood vessels and connective tissues, characterized by fibrotic, ischemic, and degenerative changes in the skin and internal organs. Its systemic nature is evidenced by frequent involvement of the alimentary tract, synovium, lungs, heart, and kidneys. SS frequently is associated with calcinosis, Raynaud's phenomenon, sclerodactyly, and telangiectasis (the CRST syndrome).

Etiologic Factors

The cause of the excess deposition of fibrosis tissue is unknown and there is no known hereditary component.[1]

Age and Sex Affected

SS usually occurs during the third to fifth decades and three out of four patients are women. Onset is rare in children and uncommon in the elderly.[2]

Diagnosis

Diagnosis is made by the presence of characteristic tightening of the skin. In the early stages this may involve only the fingers but often it progresses proximally to a more generalized involvement. The presence of Raynaud's phenomenon and abnormalities of esophageal mobility are other diagnostic features.[2]

Course and Prognosis

Onset is gradual and the course is highly variable. The disease is not always fatal, and many clients have a normal life expectancy. Death is usually secondary to visceral involvement.

In some patients the symptoms are confined to the hands for years (sclerodactyly). In others, the skin sclerosis may progress to total body involvement within the first year. Involvement is usually symmetric and occurs in the hands first.

SYMPTOMATOLOGY AND IMPLICATIONS FOR OCCUPATIONAL THERAPY

Characteristic Skin and Joint Involvement

GENERAL

Early changes show edema which gradually is replaced by fibrosis. This gives the skin a tight, hard, smooth appearance. The changes are often symmetric and progress proximally to include the arms, neck, face, trunk, and lower extremities.[1]

Patients usually are referred to therapy when they begin to lose range of motion (ROM), particularly in the hands. Limitation of ROM is secondary to a combination of decreased skin mobility, edema, fibrosis, arthritis, and thickening of the subcutaneous tissues, muscles, tendons, synovium, and joint capsules. The patient usually perceives any of these changes as stiffness. For evaluation purposes, this must be distinguished from any morning stiffness, because the morning stiffness tends to wear off.

Hyperpigmentation or hypopigmentation may occur in spots or blotches. Leathery creaking is often audible where tendons pass over joints secondary to fibrinous deposits on the surfaces of the tendon sheaths and overlying fascia.[2]

Therapy

Because of the nature of the disease, the primary goal in treament is to *maintain maximal ROM* since it is very difficult to increase ROM. In some cases it is possible to increase joint range, but treatment in this area is highly experimental. The possibility of increasing ROM is more favorable when the disease is in the early stages and edema is a major source of range loss. The ideal situation is to have the patient referred to therapy before he or she loses ROM. This allows the therapist to determine the patient's normal measurements and use them as the baseline or objective for treatment.

Many physicians do not refer patients to therapy because they believe it is impossible to prevent joint contractures due to systemic sclerosis. There is partial truth to this concept. Sometimes the sclerosis is so severe that contractures develop despite diligent daily exercises. However, far more frequently contractures develop as a result of disuse, inappropriate ROM or lack of ROM exercise, and improper positioning. *Contractures that develop from these processes are preventable.*

Any method for increasing ROM is applicable. The most effective means for diminishing established contractures is gentle passive, slow stretch applied through exercise or splints. (Precaution: if range limitation is due to active synovitis, excessive or forceful stretching may increase inflammation and fibrosis. Additional information can be found in Exercise Treatment, Chapter 27, and Positioning and Lying Prone, Chapter 30.)

Mild heat applications such as warm water soaks, wrapping the part, use of a heating pad, and the use of massage, can increase circulation and thus help reduce edema and stiffness and increase mobility prior to exercise. A cylindrical facial vibrator is excellent for reducing stiffness, particularly for patients with painful fingers who find massage difficult.

ROM and function can be improved for clients with established range limitations when part of the contracture is recent and when function is limited by multiple joint involvement. To clarify the first point, when a patient presents with a 40-degree flexion contracture of the MCP joint, it is usually not known how long-standing the entire contracture is. The patient might have lost the last 10 degrees in the previous week. The time factor is significant. In the second point, being able to gain 5 degrees of range in a single joint is not significant but, if function is limited by multiple joints, a 5- to 10-degree increase over several joints can be significant. For example, for the patient unable to perform palmar pinch and lacking one inch between finger and thumb pads, a few degrees gained at each finger and thumb joint can make a significant difference. The more joints involved in limiting function the greater the chances of improving functional ability; for example, if a patient is unable to reach his toes for foot dressing, a gain of 10 degrees each in the knees, hips, back, and elbows can make the difference between dependence and independence in this task.

HANDS

The characteristic hand deformities that occur in systemic sclerosis are:

1. Loss of flexion of the MCP joints and loss of extension of the PIP joints. This is probably due to early fibrosis of the delicate dorsal expansion in a shortened position.
2. Loss of thumb abduction, opposition, and flexion.
3. Loss of wrist motion in all planes.

Motion is usually lost in all joints in all planes. In order to preserve hand function, the primary objectives of hand therapy are to maintain MCP joint flexion and thumb abduction and to prevent wrist flexion contractures.

Patients with SS generally do not develop ulnar drift or swan neck deformities unless they have a chronic inflammatory arthritis of the MCP joints prior to sclerotic changes.

Typical skin and vascular changes include painful small ulcerations over the fingertips and Raynaud's phenomenon.[3]

The painful ulcerations over the fingertips are caused by ischemia and tight skin. These can severely limit hand function, especially for fine tasks such as writing, buttoning, sewing, and using zippers, and they impair strong grasp. The ulcers may heal after sufficient atrophy has occurred and the blood flow becomes adequate for the remaining tissue.[2] Calcium deposits may occur in or under the skin, creating a painful pressure area with skin breakdown over the deposit.[2] Later in the disease, bony resorption of the distal phalanges can result in shortening of the fingers.

Handwriting is often a difficult task for patients with painful ulcers. Rubber slip-on pencil holders are often helpful in reducing the pressure required. They are available from stationery stores.

Raynaud's phenomenon is an episodic vasospasm of the digital arteries causing cyanosis or blanching during the spasm and erythema of the skin following the spasm. It is most often precipitated by cold but may be induced by emotional stress. It occurs in 90 percent of all patients with systemic sclerosis.[2]

Therapy

The objective of therapy is not to prevent all contractures, because some limitations are inevitable, but to prevent unnecessary contractures due to inadequate daily ROM, poor positioning, and disuse. It is important that the patient is also aware of these realistic objectives so that they do not have false expectations or false guilt if they develop limitations. (Patients often assume guilt for hand limitations, when in fact they may have developed despite the patient's efforts.)

RANGE OF MOTION. The type of ROM program used with other patients is not sufficient for scleroderma patients. For example, if a patient has a maximum of 80 degrees of MCP flexion, that patient needs to achieve 80 degrees every day to maintain mobility. Typically, two things happen to patients when they do passive exercises: (1) they may achieve 75 degrees one day, 72 degrees the next, and so forth, not realizing that they are not achieving the same amount, or (2) they may waste a lot of energy or time trying to achieve more than 80 degrees, not realizing that they are at their maximum. Since patients with scleroderma have so many exercises to do, the therapist must encourage them to work on the exercises that will bring the most results.

Patients seem to maintain mobility more effectively when they have a precise ROM program with objective goals to aim for and to measure their progress by.

The challenge to the therapist is to help the patient develop a system of applying sustained gentle passive stretch to all affected joints. This is often difficult for patients with sensitive painful fingertip ulcers who are unable to apply pressure with their fingers. Arthritis can also be a limiting factor. Swollen painful joints should be ranged gently, and anti-inflammatory medications should be taken prior to exercising. The ROM program and instruction can be simplified if the patient has already developed an effective method for exercising certain joints; or the therapist can tell the patient the objective of the exercise program and let him or her determine the exercise. If a patient develops his or her own exercise, he or she is more likely to remember it and follow through. It also means less learning and less teaching.

Evaluation. Goniometric measurements should be taken of all joints in all planes of motion, and a tracing of the hand should be made to document digit abduction and thumb web space. Ideally, measurements should be taken before and following a heat and exercise program. Measurements taken before will tell you how much mobility the patient easily maintains; and measurements taken after determines exercise objectives. If a patient has not been exercising, this type of an initial evaluation (especially if it follows the physician's evaluation) may make the patient's hands somewhat sore and stiff the next day. It is helpful to forewarn the patient.

Exercise Programs for Specific Joints and Muscles.

1. MCP joints: MCP flexion is the most important motion to maintain. If a patient is capable of doing only one exercise, this is the recommended one. Some patients can effectively maintain motion by passive manual pressure applied to the dorsum of the proximal phalanges using the heel of the other hand. Others may need the help of a dynamic flexion assistance device, a wrist strap with leather finger cuffs that slip over the proximal phalanges. The tension on the rubber bands should allow gentle pressure for at least a half hour. If the patient can tolerate only 10 minutes, the bands are too tight. For most patients this type of device is most comfortable if the wrist cuff is placed around a simple wrist cock-up splint. One cuff and splint can often be used alternately on each hand. A device like this allows a patient to apply sustained pressure while watching TV or doing other activities. Not all patients can tolerate this type of device. All splints have to be carefully monitored for their effect on edema, decreased

circulation, and skin vulnerability. One method for allowing patients to determine if they are achieving maximal flexion is to have patients use a template, with the desired degree angle cut out of it. These can easily be made out of cardboard or wood. For example, take a 3-inch circle of cardboard and cut a 90-degree wedge out of it. If the patient can fit the wedge over the flexed joint, he or she knows that the goal has been achieved. The amount cut out of the template should correspond with the patient's ROM goals. Many patients need only one or two templates.

2. Finger-thumb abduction: Patients can monitor their abduction and thumb web space by having a copy of their hand tracing at home. They should do active and passive abduction and adduction of each MCP joint, until they achieve their span goal each day. If the fingers are tight, passive stretch can be achieved by wedging a tissue or piece of cloth between each finger for five minutes each or longer. If a patient is starting to loose thumb web space, the only effective method for maintaining it is to use a thumb CMC stabilization splint with a C-bar. The one described on page 345 has worked well with several patients. Wearing it at night is usually sufficient. Patients in an acute episode should also wear it during prolonged bed rest and inactivity.

3. Finger hyperextension: In the early stages finger hyperextension is an important motion to maintain, since it is often the first to be lost. With hands together in a prayer position patients can measure their hyperextension span against a ruler or a marking on an index card.

4. Finger intrinsic muscles: Exercising the interossei and lumbricals is valuable for mobilizing dorsal expansion; for example, resistance applied to PIP extension with the MCP joints flexed; spreading a rubber band apart with the middle phalanges and thumb; active PIP joint flexion with the MCP joints extended; resistance to abduction; or trapping an index card between the fingers to provide resistance to the adductors. It appears that fibrosis of the dorsal expansion creates the characteristic scleroderma hand deformity of MCP extension and PIP flexion.

General Guidelines. When possible, exercises should be done daily to maintain motion in all joints and in all planes. This includes flexion and extension of all the finger and thumb joints; finger and thumb abduction and adduction; thumb circumduction; wrist flexion, extension, deviation, and circumduction; and forearm supination and pronation. It is not feasible to list every possible ROM method that can be used with scleroderma patients. Each program needs to be developed with creativity and sensitivity to the patient's ability to carry out a program. Some patients can only manage three or four exercises despite the twenty or more that could be recommended. It is better that they perform 3 or 4 exercises effectively than none at all.

Other Considerations. When patients have fixed deformities that limit function, the only recourse is to adapt equipment to accommodate the deformity. Typically this includes built-up handles and cuffs. An example of this is a universal cuff (adjustable plastic slip-on handcuff that holds utensils).

There is also increased vulnerability of the skin to infection and irritation. Avoid any abrasive activities, materials, or substances that irritate the skin. Patients should be careful about traumatizing the skin over the dorsum of the finger joints. In some patients the use of thin cotton laboratory gloves helps to protect sensitive skin during housework or routine activities.

If the patient has skin ulcers, it is important to assess hand function in particular for fine tasks such as writing and buttoning.

TREATMENT OF RAYNAUD'S PHENOMENON. Vasospasm of the digital arteries can result in blanching, erythema, or cyanosis of the fingers and hand. The arteries may spasm in various patterns, causing either a uniform color change or the presence of all three shades at one time. The spasm may last from a few seconds to 20 minutes or longer. It can be painless or there may be an associated aching, numbness, burning, or sharp pain.

Arterial spasm in clients with this form of vasomotor instability can occur spontaneously or be triggered by (1) exposure to cold, (2) sudden emotional change, such as excitement, nervousness, or fright, and (3) trauma.

Patients should observe the following precautions:

1. Avoid tobacco (nicotine) and other vasoconstrictors such as amphetamines and ergotamine.[1]
2. Avoid cold:
   a. Wear mittens in cold weather and gloves in the market when touching items from refrigerated sections.
   b. Use oven mitts or potholders when handling frozen foods or ice.
3. Avoid positions that cause venous stasis in the fingers, e.g., allowing the hand to hang motionless to the side for long periods or to hang over the edge of the bed at night.
4. Wear warm clothing on the trunk to help maintain peripheral vasodilatation.[2]
5. Eat modest meals. Eating a large meal reduces peripheral circulation.[2]

Most clients are aware of events that bring on an attack, especially if the event is associated with pain. However, the client may not relate emotional changes or the use of tobacco or various medications to an attack. Nicotine is a major vasoconstrictor. Patients having difficulty giving up smoking may find it helpful to join a community organization devoted to assisting smokers to quit.

These precautions also are important for the therapist to observe in the clinic, especially during Activities of Daily Living (ADL) training in the kitchen or during hand treatment when there is a tendency to work with one hand and let the other hang at the side.

Biofeedback is also a valuable intervention for helping patients to manage Raynaud's phenomenon.[5,6,7,8] Thermal biofeedback provides the most effective method for teaching patients how to raise their peripheral temperature.[9] After biofeedback training, people are able to raise their temperature at will when they experience vasospasm. The relaxation training required for this process is also valuable for the management of stress and developing a greater sense of control over the disease. Several resources are available for the therapist interested in learning biofeedback training.[10,11,12]

FACE

Facial mobility may be lost early in the disease. The skin becomes taut and the lips may atrophy and recede. The face takes on a characteristic mask-like appearance.[2] Facial involvement is one of the most devastating aspects of the disease. It robs the patient of personality and individuality in an unparalleled manner. Facial changes can also create a communication problem in that one cannot always rely on facial expressions as a cue to the patient's emotions or understanding of instruction.

One of the major consequences of facial involvement is the limitation of temporomandibular joint excursion secondary to sclerosis of the skin, subcutaneous tissues, and musculature. Limited excursion restricts oral hygiene, dental care, and ability to chew solid foods and reduces verbal articulation.

Therapy

If lack of facial expression is causing a communication problem, discuss it with the patient. He or she usually is aware of facial changes, but the loss of nonverbal communication may be unsuspected. It is also helpful to have the patient bring in a photograph taken before the onset of systemic sclerosis. A photograph may facilitate discussion about the psychological effects of the facial changes and help the therapist to appreciate the individuality of the patient, as well as changes the patient has experienced.

Where there is decreased jaw mobility, teach the patient how to measure the mouth aperture (distance between upper and lower teeth) in front of a mirror with a ruler at least once a day in order to monitor the excursion. This method provides visual feedback so stretching exercises can be increased if ROM is being lost. It is important to assess the patient's oral hygiene habits and to educate the patient in the importance of maintaining dental health. If the patient does not know appropriate hygiene measures, e.g., how to brush thoroughly or use dental floss, instruct him or her or refer the patient to a dental hygienist for a thorough cleaning and instruction.

If the patient has marked limitation, determine what assistive equipment would facilitate better hygiene, e.g., electric toothbrushes, water jet pics, and dental floss applicators (devices that loop the floss around the tooth).

MAINTAINING FACIAL MOBILITY THROUGH EXERCISE. When planning therapy for facial involvement it is important to keep in mind that fibrosis and atrophy take place in all the soft facial structures including the skin, subcutaneous fat, and muscles in SS. The use of exercises to maintain facial mobility is experimental in that clinic studies to prove efficiency have not been performed. In fact, their efficacy may never be proven because of the variability of the disease. However, considering the consequences of tight facial structures, i.e. limited mouth aperture and altered appearance, along with the lack of any other form of treatment, a logical treatment approach can be followed.

Each of the exercises described here is designed to move a specific muscle or group of muscles in order to mobilize the fluid in the tissue and stretch the facial structures. It is literally a ROM program for the facial muscles, skin, and subcutaneous tissue.

Patients who use this program daily report one or more of the following outcomes: (1) an increase in the number of different exercises performed over time; (2) an increase in the ability to perform the exercises; and (3) a subjective sense of increased flexibility and suppleness following the exercises.

Treatment Approach. A client should not be instructed in these exercises unless there is definite evidence of sclerosis (skin changes or hardness) in the facial, neck, shoulder, or chest areas. If there is sclerosis in the chest or shoulder area the disease is likely to spread to the neck and facial area; however, if there is sclerosis only in the hands or arms there is no way of predicting the disease course. In some clients the disease may affect only the hands; but these patients should be monitored for disease progression.

All the facial and neck muscles should be exercised no matter what the stage of involvement. Obviously many of the muscles will not move in the moderate or severe stages of sclerosis, let alone respond to exercise; therefore the program needs to be individually tailored for each client. A client with severe involvement may be able to do only a couple of the prescribed exercises. The lip and mouth exercises are the most important since a limited mouth opening interferes with eating and oral hygiene.

Instructions to the Client.

1. Do exercises in front of a mirror.
2. Massage (firm touch) the entire face using small circular motions with the fingertips, a warm washcloth, or a vibrator. Then massage each specific area again just before exercising that part.
3. The number of repetitions necessary to get maximal mobility depends upon the individual. One approach is to do the exercise fast for two or three times as a warm up and then do five repetitions holding each stretch position to the count of five. Sustained stretch is more effective for increasing mobility than rapid motions.

Exercises. (These directions are designed to isolate, contract, and stretch the major facial muscles.)

1. Raise the eyebrows as high as possible. Return to the normal position.
2. Bring the eyebrows down and together as hard as possible as if frowning. Then raise eyebrows as high and wide as possible.
3. Wrinkle the bridge of the nose by raising the upper lip and then frowning (as if smelling something bad).
4. Close the eyes very tight. Then release the squeeze slowly and raise the eyebrows as high as possible before opening the eyes.
5. Flare the nostrils; then narrow the nostrils down, pushing the upper lip out.
6. Make an exaggerated tight wink with each eye separately, using the cheek muscles to help close the eye.
7. Cover the teeth with the lips. Then open the mouth as wide as possible without the teeth showing. Close lips and press hard (as if blotting lip gloss).
8. Open the mouth so that the lips are as wide apart as possible.
9. Open the mouth so that the teeth are as far apart as possible.
10. Push the jaw forward to create an underbite (bottom teeth in front of the upper teeth).
11. Make as wide a grin as possible without showing the teeth.
12. Pucker the chin by pushing the lower lip upward.
13. Stick the tongue out as far as possible.
14. Push lower lip down and outward (as in an exaggerated pout).
15. Keep mouth closed and puff cheeks out with air; hold to the count of five and then release the air and suck cheeks inward.
16. Lean the head back as far as possible and open and close the mouth five times.

THORACIC AREA

Chest expansion may decrease secondary to fibrosis of the skin, subcutaneous tissues, and intercostal muscles. In some patients, pulmonary fibrosis may develop, further decreasing vital capacity.[1]

Therapy

The objective of therapy is to maintain normal chest excursion. Treatment includes instructing the patient in deep breathing exercises. Usually this is done in physical therapy. Evaluation of progress or status can be made by measuring the chest circumference during inspiration and expiration at the nipple line or below the breasts.

Mobility is also enhanced by having the patient perform total body/trunk stretching exercises.

Arthritis

Arthralgia and/or arthritis occurs in 90 percent of the cases at some time. About one third of the patients have articular symptoms first.[2]

Typically the arthritis is a polyarticular, inflammatory, small joint, symmetric arthritis. The arthritis is nonerosive and usually self-limited.

Therapy

Treatment for arthritis in SS is the same as outlined for rheumatoid arthritis *except* that people with SS generally *do not* develop the same hand deformities. For example, they usually do not develop ulnar drift or swan neck deformities.

Muscle Involvement

Involvement of the skeletal muscle is insidious and often difficult to detect in the early stages. Pathologic changes in the muscle include atrophy and necrosis of the fibers, fibrosis of the fiber sheaths with increased production of connective tissue, diminished number of capillaries and perivascular infiltrates of lymphocytes and plasma cells, and EMG abnormalities.

Muscle weakness may be due to muscle pathology, it may be secondary to disuse, or it may be due to the inhibition of muscle strength by joint pain.

Patients with SS can develop proximal muscle weakness similar to polymyositis. Difficulty in stepping up on a curb or raising arms overhead is often the first symptom of proximal muscle weakness. (See Chapter 6.)

Calcinosis

There are two types of subcutaneous calcification. The more common occurs as a localized deposit (calcinosis circumscripta) around joints or near body prominences that may become painful if constantly irritated by pressure.[1] This is especially true over the elbows and ischial tuberosity. Rarely, there may be a diffuse encasing calcification of the skin and subcutaneous tissues that may contribute to severe joint contractures.

Therapy

T foam cushions, convoluted cushions, or slip-on foam elbow protector sleeves may help relieve pressure and discomfort.

Telangiectasis

Chronic dilation of capillaries and small arterial branches produces small reddish spots in the skin, called telangiectasia. The condition usually is benign and is an indication of internal vascular changes.[3]

Therapy

No therapy is available; it is primarily a cosmetic concern.

Visceral Involvement

Viscera are usually involved in all patients with SS. The severity, however, ranges from being entirely asymptomatic to causing death.[1]

Gastrointestinal Involvement

Involvement of the alimentary tract most frequently results in a slowing or absence of the peristaltic waves throughout the tract. The esophagus is usually involved first. The effects of this hypomotility are more pronounced in the recumbent position. Hypomotility results in difficulty swallowing (dysphagia), reflux esophagitis, heartburn, bloating, nausea, vomiting, and regurgitation with the risk of aspiration.[2] More extensive involvement of the bowel may lead to malabsorption with consequent severe weight loss and weakness.[1]

Patients with gastrointestinal symptoms are at high risk of developing nutritional deficiencies directly from the symptoms or from a decreased interest in food or from difficulty in planning or preparing full meals. Patients often start omitting foods that are difficult to eat without making appropriate substitutions for the nutritional loss.[13]

Therapy

The symptoms of hypomotility, reflux, and dysphagia can be reduced or alleviated by sitting very erect while drinking or eating in order to optimally align the esophagus and to allow gravity to assist motility; by eating smaller, more frequent meals, chewing food well, and concentrating on the chewing and swallowing process; and by sleeping with the head of the bed elevated eight inches on blocks to allow gravity to assist motility.[2,13]

All patients who have difficulty eating or who cannot eat certain foods should receive counseling from a nutritionist.

Pulmonary Fibrosis

Involvement of the lungs may lead to diminished oxygen uptake and dyspnea.

Therapy

Occupational therapy primarily involves instructing the patient in energy conservation methods. Physical therapy instruction in diaphragmatic breathing may also be helpful. Training in adaptive self-care methods should be correlated to diaphragmatic breathing principles.

Cardiac Fibrosis

The most common forms of cardiac involvement include pericardial effusion, myocardial necrosis with fibrosis, and involvement of the large and small vessels of the coronary arteries. Myocardial infarctions are rare.[2]

The symptoms of cardiac involvement are similar to those of pulmonary involvement, i.e., shortness of breath at rest and dyspnea on exertion. Orthopnea, cardiomegaly, and dependent edema indicate primary cardiac disease.

Therapy

It is important to determine the status of the heart from the physician who is treating the patient, since the overall treatment program should be relevant to this aspect of the patient's condition. Observe work simplification principles in the clinic.

Renal Involvement

Renal failure is the most common cause of death in systemic sclerosis. Patients with proteinuria, hypertension, azotemia, or hyperreninemia are at high risk for developing renal failure.[2]

Therapy

Patients with renal failure are treated with aggressive antihypertensive therapy and with renal support measures of dialysis. Nephrectomy and kidney transplantation have been used successfully with selected patients.[2]

Associated Conditions

Associated conditions in SS are myositis, which is indistinguishable from polymyositis (see Chapter 6), and Sjögren's syndrome, a disease of the lacrimal and parotid glands.

DRUG THERAPY

No single drug or combination of agents has been proven to be valuable. Current drug therapy is symptomatic. Steroids such as prednisone are usually contraindicated except in those patients with inflammatory complications such as polymyositis.

See Chapter 12 for precautions and side effects of specific drugs.

REFERENCES

1. Rodnan, G. P. (ed.): *Progressive systemic sclerosis.* Clin. Rheum. Dis. 5(1):1, 1979.
2. LeRoy, E. C.: *Scleroderma (systemic sclerosis).* In Kelley, W. M., et al. (eds.): *Textbook of Rheumatology.* W. B. Saunders, Philadelphia, 1981.
3. Entin, M. A., and Wilkinson, R. D.: *Scleroderma hand: A reappraisal.* Orthop. Clin. North Am. 4:1031, 1973. (Only specific resource on hand problems.)
4. Winkleman, R. K., Kierland, R. R., Perry, H. O., et al.: *Management of scleroderma.* Mayo Clin. Proc. 46:128, 1971.
5. Taub, E., and Stroebel, C. F.: *Biofeedback in the treatment of vasoconstrictive syndromes.* Biofeedback Self Regul. 3(4):363, 1978.
6. Taub, E.: *Self-regulation of human tissue temperature.* In Swartz, G. E., and Beatty, J. (eds.): *Biofeedback: Theory and Research.* Academic Press, New York, 1977, pp. 245-300.
7. Sunderman, R. H., and Delk, J. L.: *Treatment of Raynaud's disease with temperature biofeedback.* South. Med. J. 71(3):340, 1978.
8. Surwit, R. S., Pilon, R. N., and Fenton, C. H.: *Behavioral treatment of Raynaud's disease.* J. Behav. Med. 1:323, 1978.
9. Keefe, F. J., Surwit, R. S., and Pilon, R. N.: *Biofeedback, autogenic training and progressive relaxation in the treatment of Raynaud's disease: A comparative study.* J. Appl. Behav. (In press)
10. Green, E., and Green, A.: *General and specific applications of thermal biofeedback.* In Basmajian, J. V. (ed.): *Biofeedback—Principles and Practice for Clinicians.* Williams & Wilkins, Baltimore, 1979.
11. Olton, D. S., and Noonber, A. R.: *Biofeedback: Clinical Applications in Behavioral Medicine.* Prentice Hall, Englewood Cliffs, NJ, 1980. (Contains a chapter on the treatment of Raynaud's disease.)
12. Biofeedback Society of America can provide information about resources and training opportunities in your area. Write: Francis Butler, Executive Secretary, University of Colorado Medical Center, 4200 East 9th Ave., Denver, CO 80220.
13. Silverman, E. H., and Elfant, I. L.: *Dysphagia: An evaluation and treatment program for the adult.* Am. J. Occup. Ther. 33(6):382, 1979.

ADDITIONAL SOURCES

Craig, M.: *Miss Craig's Face Saving Exercises.* Random House, New York, 1970. (Written by a physical therapist but designed for the public, this book is an excellent resource regarding facial musculature. However, it is too detailed to be used by patients with SS for the purposes described in the exercise in this chapter.)

Patient Resources

Scleroderma patient groups are being developed around the country. These groups can be invaluable for helping patients cope with the complex psychological and social ramifications of this disease. For information on local groups write: The United Scleroderma Foundation, P.O. Box 724, Watsonville, CA 95076; or The Arthritis Foundation, 3400 Peachtree Road, N.E., Atlanta, GA 30326.

The United Scleroderma Foundation also publishes a newsletter for patients.

6

POLYMYOSITIS AND DERMATOMYOSITIS

Polymyositis is a diffuse inflammatory disease of striated muscle that leads to muscle destruction and symmetric proximal muscle weakness. When any of a variety of skin rashes accompanies this condition it is known as dermatomyositis. Frequently polymyositis is associated with other rheumatic diseases such as systemic lupus erythematosus, progressive systemic sclerosis, and Sjögren's syndrome.

Etiologic Factors

The cause is unknown. In some cases there is a link with visceral malignancies, particularly in older age groups. [1]

Age and Sex Affected

Polymyositis can occur at any age and is found in females in a ratio of 2 to 1 over males. [1]

Diagnosis

Diagnosis is based on proximal muscle weakness, serologic evidence of muscle destruction (indicated by elevated muscle enzymes), heliotrope (purple) rash of the eyelids (not always present), characteristic muscle biopsy, characteristic electromyogram, and a lack of neurologic findings. [1]

Course and Prognosis

This varies in all aspects. Initial symptoms may be muscular, dermal, or articular. Remissions or exacerbations may occur spontaneously. Prognosis is more favorable when onset occurs at a younger age and for those who have a slowly progressive course. [2]

SYMPTOMATOLOGY AND IMPLICATIONS FOR OCCUPATIONAL THERAPY

Proximal Muscle Weakness

Muscle weakness may vary from mild involvement with no functional loss to severe muscle destruction with quadriparesis.

The pelvic girdle, shoulder girdle, and neck flexor muscles are the most obvious groups involved but the abdominal, back extensor, intercostal, and diaphragm muscles are affected also. Weak pelvic girdle muscles cause a characteristic waddling gait. Muscle involvement may become more distal with severity.

Therapy

When the patient is in an *acute exacerbation,* the following protocol is recommended:

1. *Safety precautions against falling should be taken.* Assistive equipment to insure safe ambulation should be used and instruction in safe transfer methods should be started early in the course of the disease. A wheelchair or rolling walker should be used to protect the hip muscles.
2. Weakened muscle groups should not be used beyond tolerance. Only activities that can be done comfortably without muscle fatigue are recommended. A patient should not perform an activity that cannot be stopped immediately if he or she becomes fatigued, e.g., walking down a long hallway or standing in a shower. Heavy resistive tasks should be *avoided;* these include unassisted walking, difficult unassisted transfer, and wheelchair propulsion with the arms. Muscle stress is believed to enhance tissue destruction and thus elevates enzyme levels.
3. Patient education regarding activity and exercise is important. Many patients believe incorrectly that weak muscles should be used as much as possible.
4. Active-assisted or gentle-passive ROM should be performed daily. Lying prone is also recommended to maintain hip ROM.
5. During bed rest (sitting or lying), neck and back support should keep the spine in straight alignment. A soft neck collar may be necessary to support the neck when the patient is sitting up.
6. *If* involvement progresses distally, night splinting may be indicated for the knees, elbows, or wrists.
7. For patients with severe weakness, mobile arm supports (or deltoid aid) can be used to increase functional independence for feeding, facial hygiene, and writing.

As the patient responds to the medication and gains in strength, functional activities can be progressed as tolerated and an active-assistive exercise program initiated. All exercise should be performed to tolerance and the muscles should not be fatigued. The program should be progressed gently with patient response carefully observed.

The strengthening program can be continued and progressed to a resistive one as long as the patient continues to gain in strength. The patient is essentially in a chronic-active phase if the inflammatory process decreases then plateaus at a low level. At that point the program emphasis changes from strengthening to one of (1) activities of daily living to tolerance, (2) instruction in energy conservation and work simplification to improve functional endurance, (3) instruction in proper positioning at night and at leisure (see Positioning and Lying Prone, Chapter 30), and (4) physical therapy with exercise to maintain ROM and strength.

Dysphagia

In polymyositis difficulty in swallowing is a result of inflammation of the striated muscle of the pharynx and upper esophagus. This inflammation creates a major risk of regurgitation and possible asphyxiation.[1]

Therapy

Because the risk of regurgitation is life-threatening, dysphagia secondary to muscle weakness is considered a medical emergency. Advise the treating physician promptly if the patient reports symptoms of dysphagia. Patients with established dysphagia should be advised to have several small feedings instead of three large meals per day; to sit erect while drinking or eating (with back and head supported if necessary) to optimally align the esophagus and maximize gravity assistance; to chew foods carefully; and to avoid dry, hard foods. The head of the bed should be elevated eight inches at night or during rest to provide gravity assistance to muscles for swallowing.

Muscle Pain

When muscle pain occurs, it is most common about the shoulders, upper back, upper arms, and forearms. It is not usually a predominant symptom. Also, a patient may interpret muscle weakness or tiredness as pain.[2]

Therapy

Heat applications often help relieve soreness. (For the inpatient this usually is carried out by physical therapy. The patient at home may need instruction in use of heating pads.)

Muscle Atrophy

Atrophy is common in later stages of the disease. It is secondary to muscle degeneration and other factors such as disuse.[2]

Therapy

Strengthening treatment depends upon the phase of the disease. (See Exercise Treatment, Chapter 29, for a discussion on the relationship between muscle strength and atrophy.)

Joint Contractures

Joint contractures may be due to joint and muscle pain, muscle fibrosis, calcinosis, weakness, or postural adaptations.

ROM may be limited early in the disease, being secondary to pain or inflammation. Fixed contractures are typical of later stages of the disease or in cases in which medical treatment has been delayed. Children with dermatomyositis differ from adults in that they often develop severe joint contractures rapidly in the early stages of the disease.[3,4,5]

Therapy

ROM and muscle strength should be watched closely. The distal muscle groups can also be involved in severe cases.

During the acute or subacute phase, gentle-passive ROM with slight stretch to the point of pain is recommended twice a day to affected joints. If a patient develops contractures in the acute phase, serial splinting is the most effective method for reducing them and should be instituted as soon as the patient is medically stable and can tolerate the procedure. If done early, serial splinting can reduce contractures in a few days. In the chronic-active phase, active or active-assisted exercises are recommended. In the nonactive phase, a standard ROM program to increase ROM is suitable. Lying prone to tolerance is recommended to prevent hip contractures. (See Exercise Treatment, Chapter 29, and Positioning and Lying Prone, Chapter 30.)

Arthritis

An inflammatory type of polyarthritis may occur with polymyositis. It differs from rheumatoid arthritis in that it is nonerosive, usually not chronic, and subsides without residual deformity. If hand deformities do occur, they usually are due to muscle fibrosis and tendon shortening.[1]

Therapy

Treatment is the same as outlined for inflammatory joint disease (see Chapter 1). Additional information on chronic inflammation of specific joints can be found in Rheumatoid Arthritis, Chapter 3.

Skin Rash

Rashes occur in 40 percent of the patients and may occur in various forms. Typically it occurs initially as a scaly erythema over the extensor surfaces of the knuckles and elbows. It may also occur over parts of the body exposed to the sun. The eyelids may be a characteristic helioptrope hue with edema in the periorbital area.[2]

Therapy

The rash *may* be sensitive to the sun, with exposure to sun or ultraviolet light causing it to flare up. The patient should wear protective clothing and sun block lotion with a PABA factor of 15 or more when outside if he or she has a sun-sensitive rash.

Associated Conditions

Malignant neoplasms are common in patients over 40 years of age; however, they are not associated with the childhood form of the disease or when myositis occurs in association with another rheumatic disease. Other conditions that may occur with polymyositis are Sjögren's syndrome, Raynaud's phenomenon, and pulmonary fibrosis.

DRUG THERAPY

The principle of drug therapy in polymyositis is to give an agent that will stop the inflammatory destruction of muscle fibers. Prednisone or other steroid preparations are considered the drugs of choice for this condition. Steroids are initially given in large doses (60 to 100 mg/day) and tapered when signs of activity have abated. Methotrexate, an antimetabolite, has also been of benefit in those patients not responding to prednisone.[2,4]

See Chapter 12 for precautions and side effects of specific drugs.

REFERENCES

1. Bohan, A. and Pelter, J.: Polymyositis and dermatomyositis. N. Engl. J. Med. Part I, Vol. 292, No. 7, p. 344, Feb. 1975; Part II, Vol. 292, No. 8, p. 403, Feb. 1975. (Contains current medical information; does not include aspects of rehabilitation.)
2. Pearson, C. M.: *Polymyositis and dermatomyositis*. In McCarty, D. J. (ed.): *Arthritis and Allied Conditions*, ed. 9. Lea & Febiger, Philadelphia, 1978.
3. Feallock, B.: *Dermatomyositis: Case study*. Am. J. Occup. Ther. 19(5):279, 1965. (Describes OT treatment for an adolescent with severe involvement.)
4. Jacobs, J. C., Jr.: *Treatment of dermatomyositis*. Arthritis Rheum. 20(2):338, 1977. Proceedings of the Conference on the Rheumatic Diseases of Childhood. (Strong advocacy for steroid therapy.)
5. Sullivan, D. B., Cassidy, J. T., and Petty, R. E.: *Dermatomyositis in the pediatric patient*. Arthritis Rheum. 20(2):327, 1977.

ADDITIONAL SOURCES

Fessel, W. J.: *Muscle disease in rheumatology*. Semin. Arthritis Rheum. 3(2):127, 1973.

ARTERITIS AND VASCULITIS (ANGIITIS)

These conditions involve inflammation, which is usually segmental, of the arteries (arteritis) or both arteries and veins (vasculitis) associated with a severe systemic disease process. They present in two ways: (1) as a primary disorder with or without secondary joint involvement, or (2) concomitant with a rheumatic disease (usually rheumatoid arthritis or systemic lupus erythematosus).[1] It is because of this second factor, relationship with the rheumatic diseases, that arteritis and vasculitis are included in Part 2.

Symptoms of arteritis depend upon the severity, duration, and size and location of affected arteries. Each arteritic syndrome tends to involve arteries of a particular size or location in various combinations, resulting in a more or less characteristic symptom complex.

ARTERITIC SYNDROMES

These conditions are less common than the other diseases in Part 2 and are included primarily for definition. Patients are not likely to be referred to therapy unless there is significant or prolonged arthritis, central nervous system involvement, muscle weakness, neuropathy, or a major peripheral ischemic complication such as gangrene.

Polyarteritis Nodosa

Polyarteritis nodosa (periarteritis nodosa) is an inflammatory disease that destroys the wall of medium-sized arteries. It primarily affects males between the ages of 20 and 50 years. Although the cause is unknown, in some patients there is an association with intravenous use of methamphetamine (speed) and with the hepatitis-associated antigen. Prognosis for life is poor, particularly if multiple organs are involved.[2]

The vasculitis that occurs rarely in rheumatoid arthritis (malignant rheumatoid arthritis) has the same pathologic basis and prognosis as polyarteritis nodosa.

Referrals may be made to occupational therapy for treatment of a mild arthritis, peripheral neuropathy,[3] or central nervous system involvement, or for protective splinting for digital gangrene.

Giant Cell Arteritis

Giant cell arteritis (temporal arteritis) is an inflammation of the temporal and cranial arteries. It affects women in the 50- to 70-year age range in three out of four cases. The major consequences are sudden blindness in one eye or a cerebrovascular accident. Various mental disturbances can occur also.[1]

Polymyalgia rheumatica is a more frequent condition affecting the same age group. It is included here because some patients have concomitant temporal arteritis. Polymyalgia rheumatica is characterized by stiffness and pain of the shoulder muscles but *without weakness* and can severely limit the person's ability for activities for daily living. Prognosis is good because these symptoms usually disappear with low-dose corticosteroid treatment.[1]

Wegener's Granulomatosis

Wegener's granulomatosis is a destructive arteritis of the upper respiratory tract, lungs, and kidneys that, when untreated, progresses to death from renal failure. Associated symptoms may include a rash, arthralgias, muscle involvement, peripheral neuropathy, and nephritis.[1]

Henoch-Schönlein Purpura

Henoch-Schönlein purpura (anaphylactoid purpura) is a vasculitis that affects small vessels of the skin, gastrointestinal tract, synovium, and kidneys. The disease is usually self-limited in one to two months, although about 5 percent of the patients progress to terminal renal failure. A mild, self-limited arthritis usually accompanies this condition.[1]

Hypersensitivity Angiitis

Hypersensitivity angiitis is a general term that refers to inflammation of small vessels that results from drug reactions, serum sickness, or other unidentified inciting factors. The skin and synovium are the most frequently involved sites and can result in a mild self-limited synovitis.[1]

Aortic Arch Arteritis

Aortic arch arteritis (Takayashu's or pulseless disease) is an arteritis of the large muscular arteries that arise from the aortic arch. It is a rare disease of young women. Symptoms reflect insufficient circulation to the areas served by the large vessels and can include central nervous system involvement with intermittent claudication secondary to femoral nerve involvement, arthralgias, gangrene, and occasionally arthritis.[1]

REFERENCES

1. Hunder, G. G., and Conn, D. L.: *Necrotizing vasculitis.* In Kelley, W. M., et al. (eds.): *Textbook of Rheumatology.* W. B. Saunders, Philadelphia, 1981.
2. Duffy, J., et al.: *Polyarteritis and hepatitis B*[1,2]. Medicine 52:19, 1976.
3. Besole, R., Lister, C., and Kleinert, H.: *Polyarteritis: A cause of nerve palsy in the extremity.* J. Hand Surg. 3(4):320, 1978.

8

ANKYLOSING SPONDYLITIS

Ankylosing spondylitis (AS) is a chronic joint and bone disease in which the inflammatory process has a predilection for the sacroiliac, spinal apophyseal, and sternal joints. An osteitis of the symphysis pubis, the vertebral bodies, and the attachment of the paravertebral ligaments and muscles is frequent. A peripheral arthritis with asymmetric distribution may also occur.

Etiologic Factors

There is a definite genetic predisposition to the disease. A genetically determined antigen located on the surface of cells has been found in greater than 90 percent of patients with ankylosing spondylitis. This antigen, termed HLA-B27, is present in only 6 percent of normal individuals.[1]

Age and Sex Affected

In the classic presentation of AS described in this chapter, men are affected in 9 out of 10 cases and the onset is usually in the second or third decade. There is recent evidence indicating the disease may have a milder presentation in women without lower spine involvement.[2]

Diagnosis

Ankylosing spondylitis is suspected in a young adult male who presents with low back pain and limited mobility of the lumbar spine. The diagnosis is confirmed by radiologic examination of the sacroiliac joints and spine.[3]

Course and Prognosis

The onset usually is insidious and the course may be either episodic or steadily progressive. If the disease persists, it ascends from sacroiliac involvement to the lumbar, thoracic, and cervical spine, eventually resulting in bony ankylosis of the involved areas.

The disease process may stop at any stage, at which time the patient usually has a pain-free deformity. Prognosis for the relief of pain and functional capacity is good. About 75 percent of persons with ankylosing spondylitis continue full employment.[1]

SYMPTOMATOLOGY AND IMPLICATIONS FOR OCCUPATIONAL THERAPY

BACK AND NECK

Pain often is a result of both the inflammatory process and paravertebral muscle spasm secondary to inflammation. Usually the pain is episodic and may be more severe at night. Stiffness in the morning and after inactivity commonly accompanies the pain and is usually confined to the involved joints.[2]

Typical deformities include a reversed lordotic curve and kyphosis that is compensated for by neck flexion. The vertebrae eventually become joined by bony bridges, forming the characteristic bamboo spine image on roentgenography.[1]

Involvement of the thoracic spine leads to markedly limited chest expansion and is a common factor in the course of the disease.[4]

Therapy

Proper positioning during activities, leisure, and sleep is crucial in preventing back deformities. Posture habits during activities such as watching television, reading, and desk work need careful evaluation. Assistive equipment may be necessary to insure proper posture. (See Joint Protection and Energy Conservation Instruction, Chapter 26, for neck and back protection.) A reasonably functional life can be anticipated if proper posture is maintained.[4]

The patient needs a firm bed. Hospital beds should be kept flat at night and have only the back raised during the day. Do not use the semi-Fowler position (with the head raised and knee gatch partially raised). Ideally the patient should sleep supine or prone rather than side-lying with legs bent.[4] (See Positioning and Lying Prone, Chapter 30.)

Proper neck positioning at night is a critical factor and can literally prevent neck deformity in patients with cervical AS.[4] Ideally the positioning method should support the cervical muscles (to allow relaxation and reduce muscle spasm) and maintain the normal lordotic curve to the neck without causing cervical flexion (i.e., the occipital skull should be touching or close to the mattress).[5] Sleeping without a pillow flattens the lordotic curve.[5] It may be possible to find a cervical pillow that meets the above requirements, but most are too thick or maintain the neck in flexion. The best solution at this time is to adapt a pillow like the Jackson Cervipillo[5] (Trueze) by removing some of the filler to create the correct thickness. (It may be necessary to return the filler later when the pillow becomes compressed because of use.)

Trunk-stretching exercises for posture in the erect and supine positions with emphasis on extension and hamstring-stretching are part of the physical therapy program as well as deep breathing exercises to maintain chest expansion.

Once patients are over the acute phase, they should be encouraged to participate in an ongoing community sports or exercise group. Swimming, volleyball, basketball, skiing, and tennis are all excellent activities. The only sports not recommended are spring board diving (because of the risk of neck injury) and distance bicycling (because of the static flexion posture required).

In England and Europe, the therapeutic approach to AS is far more vigorous than in the United States. At the Royal National Hospital for Rheumatic Diseases in Bath, patients take an intensive three-week group physiotherapy program. In Austria, there are spas that offer a six-week intensive exercise and sports program for people with AS. These programs have demonstrated the value of active exercise.[6]

Activities of Daily Living

Bed mobility often is limited and can be facilitated by grab bars, cloth ladders, or blanket cradles. Electric blankets help reduce stiffness.

Daily activities such as transferring, dressing, hygiene, toileting, driving, and vocational skills need special consideration. The need for training in adaptive methods for performing these activities varies with each person.

Sitting and standing postures during work activities need evaluation. If a person cannot maintain an erect posture during a specific task, a soft neck collar or back support may be valuable solely as a postural reminder during the activity.

For clients with fused backs, special consideration is needed with regard to safety precautions against falling. This is especially true during bending activities (dressing, gardening, or bathing), when a shift in the center of gravity can cause a loss of balance. These patients in particular are vulnerable to neck fractures.[4]

Safety while driving is another factor that needs consideration, since cervical ankylosis reduces the visual driving field. Elongated clip-on rear-view mirrors are readily available in auto supply stores and allow people to see side blind spots without turning around. Wright and Moll describe an ingenious right angle mirror that attaches to the hood of the car, which allows the driver to see cars approaching from both left and right directions, while facing straight ahead.[4]

Patients with fused backs also find it helpful to have a comfortable chair at home with a swivel base. This allows them to face people easily during conversations and to expand their visual field. Executive office chairs (with casters removed) work well for this purpose and often can be purchased at a reasonable cost at used office furniture stores.

Joint Stiffness

Stiffness is often prominent after rest, sitting, or prolonged static positioning. Usually clients are more comfortable if they can change positions frequently and avoid sustained postures. Exercise, repetitive movement, and heat application (hot showers and heating pads) help relieve stiffness and pain secondary to muscle spasm.

HIPS

About 30 percent of all AS patients develop clinically significant arthritis of the hips. The consequences of hip disease in AS are often identical to the problems seen in both rheumatoid arthritis and degenerative joint disease.[4] Many of these patients develop hip-flexion and/or hip-extension contractures and may develop compensatory knee-flexion contractures. To stand vertically, they compensate for the hip flexion by flexing the knees, and thus cause knee contractures.[1] Adduction contractures can also develop and interfere with perineal care and ability for sexual intercourse for women.[4] (Also see the sections on hip involvement in Chapter 3 and Chapter 10.)

Therapy

In addition to proper positioning at rest, as mentioned previously in this chapter, instruction in lying prone to stretch the hip flexors is important. Begin with lying prone to tolerance and progress to at least 90 minutes per day.

Hip involvement often limits ability for transferring and lower extremity dressing. If extension contractures are present, the patient will have difficulty sitting straight in a normal chair.

Treatment for joint inflammation is the same as inflammatory joint disease in Chapter 1 and for rheumatoid arthritis. Specific therapy procedures can be found in the following chapters: Joint Protection and Energy Conservation Instruction, Chapter 26, and Positioning and Lying Prone, Chapter 30.

SHOULDERS

The development of a bicipital or supraspinatus tendinitis occurs quite frequently. Involvement of the sternoclavicular and acromioclavicular joints or glenohumeral joints is seen in some patients.[4]

Therapy

Treatment for joint disease of the shoulders is the same as for rheumatoid arthritis (see Chapter 3).

Peripheral Arthritis

Not all patients with AS develop arthritis in the peripheral or distal joints. When it occurs, it usually affects large joints, often asymmetrically. Outside of the hips, the knees are the most frequently affected. Small joint peripheral arthritis tends to be transitory and seldom causes residual deformity. Occasionally the wrists or an isolated finger joint develops severe disease.

Therapy

Treatment is the same as for rheumatoid arthritis except that for the hands or wrists instruction in joint protection techniques needs to be carefully individualized because people with AS generally do not develop ulnar drift or swan neck deformities.

Other Manifestations

IRITIS

This occurs in 25 percent of patients with AS. Symptoms may involve acute, painful red eyes with blurring of vision, or it may be insidious and progressive, thus leading to visual impairment before it is recognized. Iritis may also continue to be present long after the AS has become inactive.[4]

Therapy

There are no occupational therapy measures for this symptom; however, the therapist needs to be alert for signs of eye involvement and to have the patient report any symptoms to the physician.

CARDIOVASCULAR INVOLVEMENT

Aortic valve disease becomes a complication in about 3 percent of the patients. This is usually a very late manifestation that becomes symptomatic 20 to 30 years after the onset of the disease. [1]

Therapy

The hospital or home program should be planned according to the status of the client's cardiovascular condition.

Associated Conditions: The Rheumatoid Variants *

At one time AS was believed to be a variant of rheumatoid arthritis. AS is now identified as a separate disease and is a member of a group of diseases called seronegative spondyloarthritides. [4,7,8] Other diseases in this classification include psoriatic arthritis, Reiter's syndrome, enteropathic spondylitis (arthritis associated with regional enteritis or ulcerative colitis), and the arthritides of Whipple's disease and Behçet's syndrome. The four major diseases in this classification, ankylosing spondylitis, psoriatic arthritis, Reiter's syndrome and enteropathic spondylitis share the following characteristics: (1) small joint involvement tends to be asymmetric; (2) there is frequent arthritis of the sacroiliac joints and spine similar to ankylosing spondylitis; (3) iritis may be associated with any of these diseases, (4) HLA-B27 antigen is present in a high percentage of these patients; and (5) the overall prognosis in terms of disability is better than in rheumatoid arthritis.

DRUG THERAPY

Indomethacin (Indocin), phenylbutazone, or any of the new NSAIDs are recommended to relieve the inflammatory manifestations of AS. Aspirin, given in anti-inflammatory doses (8 or more per day) either alone or in combination with another anti-inflammatory drug may also be effective.

See Chapter 12 for precautions and side effects of specific drugs.

---

*Some physicians refer to the rheumatoid variants as seronegative spondyloarthritis. However, this classification also includes the arthritides of Whipple's disease and Behçet's syndrome.

REFERENCES

1. Bluestone, R.: *Ankylosing spondylitis.* In McCarty, D. J. (ed.): *Arthritis and Allied Conditions.* Lea and Febiger, Philadelphia, 1978.
2. Calin, A.: *Ankylosing spondylitis.* In Kelley, W. M., et al. (eds.): *Textbook of Rheumatology.* W. B. Saunders, Philadelphia, 1981.
3. Calabro, J. J., and Mody, R. E.: *Management of ankylosing spondylitis.* Am. J. Occup. Ther. 19:255, 1965.
4. Wright, V., and Moll, J. M. H.: *Seronegative Polyarthritis.* Elsevier North-Holland, Amsterdam, 1976.
5. Jackson, R.: *The Cervical Syndrome,* ed. 4. Charles C Thomas, Springfield, Ill., 1978.
6. O'Driscoll, S. L., Jayson, M. I., and Baddeley, H.: *Neck movements in ankylosing spondylitis and their response to physiotherapy.* Ann. Rheum. Dis. 37(1):64, 1978.
7. Hart, F. D.: *The ankylosing spondylopathies.* Clin. Orthop. 74:7, 1971.
8. Haslock, I., and Wright, V.: *The arthritis associated with intestinal disease.* Bull. Rheum. Dis. 24:750, 1974.

9

PSORIATIC ARTHRITIS

Psoriatic arthritis (PA) is a distinct systemic disease in which psoriasis is associated with inflammatory arthritis and a negative serologic test for rheumatoid factor. The arthritis can range from mild to severely erosive and can affect single or multiple peripheral joints as well as the spine. The disease is characterized by exacerbations and remissions.[1]

Psoriasis is a chronic, occasionally acute, recurring, papulosquamous skin disease of unknown etiology characterized by whitish, scaly patches of varying size.

Etiologic Factors

The specific cause of psoriasis or of psoriatic arthritis is not known. The high incidence of psoriasis within families clearly indicates a genetic component to the pathogenesis of the disease.[3] There appears to be subgroups of patients with psoriasis. HLA-B27 is a useful genetic marker, as it is seen in a group of patients with a high rate of affected family members and an early onset of disease. HLA-B27 is seen in a majority of patients with psoriatic spondylitis.[4]

Age and Sex Affected

Psoriasis occurs in about 1 percent of the population, with a peak incidence in the third decade. About 7 percent of the people with psoriasis develop some form of psoriatic arthritis. The male to female incidence is nearly 1:1.[4]

Diagnosis

In the majority of patients (75 percent), the psoriasis precedes the arthritis; in 10 percent, it has an onset sychronous with the arthritis. The diagnosis is based on the presence of an inflammatory polyarthritis in the presence of psoriasis along with a negative serologic test for rheumatoid factor. Certain clinical features, such as arthritis confined to the distal interphalangeal joints, sausage swelling of fingers or toes, asymmetric distribution of the arthritis in the hands and feet, absence of subcutaneous nodules, characteristic peripheral or axial radiographs, and a history of psoriatic arthritis in first degree family members, are supportive of the diagnosis.[1,3,5,6]

In 15 percent of cases in which the arthritis occurs first, psoriatic arthritis can only be suspected if there is a combination of classic signs, such as severe erosive DIP involvement and seronegative test for rheumatoid factor, or asymmetric sausage swelling, negative rheumatoid factor, and a family history of psoriasis.[5,9]

The incidence of psoriasis in patients with seropositive arthritis is similar to the incidence of psoriasis in the general population, about 1 percent. Therefore, it is possible to have a coincidental occurrence of psoriasis and rheumatoid arthritis.[8]

Initially considered a variant of rheumatoid arthritis, psoriatic arthritis is now recognized as a distinct disease that shares features with other forms of arthritis that occur with disease of the skin, urethra, bowel, or spine. These diseases are called spondyloarthropathies and include Reiter's syndrome, ulcerative colitis, regional enteritis, and ankylosing spondylitis, in addition to psoriatic arthritis. Besides asymmetric inflammatory arthritis, these diseases share the following features: (1) negative test for rheumatoid factor; (2) absence of subcutaneous (rheumatoid) nodules; (3) ocular inflammation; (4) sacroiliitis and/or spondylitis; and (5) evidence of HLA-B27 antigen.[3,5]

Course and Prognosis

Joint inflammation in PA occurs in a wide spectrum of presentations, ranging from mild, insidious monoarticular involvement to a rapidly destructive arthritis mutilans.[3] In general, there is no correlation between the severity of the skin disease and the extent of joint involvement. Exacerbations of joint and skin disease may or may not coincide.[3]

The course and prognosis depend on which type of involvement is present. In general, the outcome for functional independence is better for psoriatic arthritis than for rheumatoid arthritis. The following five clinical patterns of joint involvement have been identified by Wright and Moll.[3]

Group 1. Predominant involvement of the distal interphalangeal joints of the hands. This pattern is described as the classic pattern because it was the first type of arthritis clearly related to psoriasis, even though it represents only 5 to 10 percent of patients with psoriatic arthritis.[5,7] These patients may have asymmetric involvement of other joints. The arthritis can range from minimal to severely erosive with osteolysis of the terminal tuft. DIP joint involvement is almost always associated with psoriatic nail changes.[5]

Group 2. Arthritis mutilans (osteolysis of the bones in the involved joints). Typically, this process occurs in the phalanges (hands and feet), metacarpals, metatarsals, and occasionally, the distal ulna. When it occurs in the digits, the ends of the bones resorb and shorten. The overlying redundant skin creates a telescoping appearance to the fingers (opera glass hand). This condition may happen to one or all of the digits.[9,10] When it occurs in several fingers, it may severely limit functional dexterity. This pattern occurs in a minority of cases, approximately 5 percent of all PA patients.[7] These patients also have a high incidence of spinal involvement and are prone to bony ankylosis in joints not affected with mutilans.[5,7,8]

Group 3. Symmetric peripheral polyarthritis similar to the distribution seen in rheumatoid arthritis. Any synovial joints can be affected, including the temporomandibular joint. As in RA, all degrees of involvement can be seen in this group. Some patients with acute inflammation can rapidly progress to ankylosis.[5,10]

Group 4. Asymmetric, oligoarticular arthritis (affecting a single or few joints) of the fingers or toes.[9] This distribution accounts for 70 percent of all cases of PA.[3,5,7]

Group 5. Ankylosing spondylitis associated with psoriasis. This may occur in a pattern similar to idiopathic ankylosing spondylitis or may be in association with *severe peripheral joint disease.*[5] (See Chapter 8.)

This classification describes five typical patterns; it is possible for patients to have mixed patterns of joint involvement.

SYMPTOMATOLOGY AND IMPLICATIONS FOR OCCUPATIONAL THERAPY

Articular Involvement

HAND INVOLVEMENT

Patients in Groups 3, 4, or 5 often present with diffuse swelling of one or more entire digits, typically referred to as sausage swelling to distinguish it from fusiform swelling, which denotes swelling confined to the joint capsule.

This diffuse swelling is attributed to a combination of IP (or IP and MCP) joint synovitis and flexor tendon sheath effusion.[5,8] The swelling is firm or hard when palpated, and it appears to be throughout the entire digit, not isolated to the volar aspect as flexor tenosynovitis is in rheumatoid arthritis. Radiographs often reveal periosteitis along the shaft of the bone, when there is sausage swelling, but this may be a reflection of generalized tenosynovitis rather than a causal factor.[10]

In addition to the sausage digits, hand involvement in PA differs from that seen in RA in the following features.

1. There may be severe involvement of the DIP joints. Mallet finger deformities are common.[3,5]
2. PIP and MCP joint involvement is random or asymmetric.[5]
3. There is a higher incidence of bony ankylosis, particularly in the digits as well as the wrist (bony ankylosis in RA tends to occur in the wrists).[5,11]
4. It is rare to have extensor tenosynovitis and extensor tendon ruptures in PA.[5,11]
5. Ulnar drift is less common and occurs in patients with chronic MCP synovitis.[6]
6. PIP flexion contractures are common, but swan neck and boutonniere can also occur.[11]
7. Marked synovial hypertrophy is less common.[11]
8. The most common deformities are contractures due to periarticular swelling and generalized capsular fibrosis.

OTHER JOINT INVOLVEMENT

Joint inflammation in all joints except the hands, toes, and spine is similar to that seen with RA. (See Chapter 3 for consequences of chronic synovitis in specific joints.) The toes often have a destructive arthritis of the IP joints similar to that in the fingers and can also have the sausage digital swelling. Rarely, the feet may be involved before the hands.[5]

Spinal involvement may encompass the entire spine, identical to ankylosing spondylitis.[5,7] (See Chapter 8 for symptomatology and treatment.) More commonly, the spinal involvement may be asymmetric and even skip vertebrae as the involvement ascends the lumbar spine.

Therapy

Occupational therapy is the same for PA as it is for RA or AS (if the spine is involved), except in the following areas.

1. Some patients with severe arthritis are prone to developing rapid contractures. These patients need to have their ROM carefully monitored. Proper bed positioning, especially for neck, wrists, knees, and ankles is critical. Hand and ankle splints may be the only effective means of preventing nonfunctional contractures. (See Chapter 25, Splinting, and Chapter 30, Positioning).

Splinting is often difficult in the presence of severe psoriasis. A cotton (not nylon) stockingette with foam splint lining worn over the extremity in addition to foam splint lining often increases comfort. Plastic splints should not be applied directly to skin with psoriatic lesions.

2. The diffuse digital swelling seen in PA is one of the most perplexing hand problems with which to work. From personal experience, none of the conventional means of reducing this edema has been effective in diminishing swelling. Methods tried have included string wrapping, Coban* wrapping, and use of Futuro thermoelastic gloves. Neither heat (parafin) nor ice compresses have reduced digit circumference or increased ROM. On a couple of occasions, heat has increased edema and decreased ROM.

When only one or a few MCP or PIP joints are involved, wrapping the joint into flexion with Coban has proven an effective means of applying gentle sustained pressure and maintaining flexion range.

Some patients are able to accomplish gentle sustained ROM manually. Teaching patients how to measure fingertip to crease provides them with an easy method for determining that they have achieved their goal of maintaining or improving motion.

Skin and Nail Changes

Except for the fact that DIP joint synovitis is always associated with nail changes, other forms of PA are not associated with any particular pattern of skin involvement. Within any of the PA groups, the psoriasis can range from a minuscule flake in an unnoticeable area, such as the scalp or umbilicus, to generalized exfoliative lesions covering the entire body.[1]

The psoriatic lesions consist of sharply demarcated erythematous papules or plaques covered with overlapping shiny or slightly opalescent scales. Itching is usually absent or mild but occasionally can be considerable. The lesions heal without scarring.[2]

Psoriasis characteristically involves the scalp (including postauricular regions), the extensor surface of the elbows and knees, the back and buttocks, the nails, eyebrows, axillas, umbilicus, and anogenital region.[2]

The most common nail lesions seen in psoriasis are multiple pits, as if one stuck the nail with a pin, and onycholysis, which is the discoloration and loosening of the nail beginning at

---

*Coban is a soft stretch tape manufactured by the 3M Corporation. It adheres to itself and is reusable. The one-inch width is convenient for gentle, sustained tension to digit joints. It is available through 3M distributors.

the free border. These lesions, however, are not unique to this disease and can be associated with fungal and bacterial infection, trauma, and other conditions.[2,3,11,12]

Therapy

Effective therapy of localized psoriasis for most patients is the use of topical coal-tar preparations, topical corticosteroid preparations (with or without occlusive dressing), and ultraviolet light or sunlight exposure. Systemic treatment with methotrexate may be considered in patients unresponsive to local therapy. Systemic corticosteroids are contraindicated not only because they are ineffective but because the disease may worsen when the dose is tapered.[4]

Ocular Involvement

Ocular inflammation has been identified with all of the seronegative spondyloarthritides. Iritis is the most significant involvement and is identical to that seen in ankylosing spondylitis.[4,13]

Systemic Manifestations

PA may have an onset associated with nonspecific constitutional symptoms such as malaise and fever.[3]

DRUG THERAPY

As in the therapy of RA, nonsteroidal anti-inflammatory medications are the initial drugs of choice in controlling the symptoms of PA. Aspirin or any of the other nonsteroidal anti-inflammatory medications may be used. These medications will control the inflammatory symptoms in most patients.[4]

Gold salts have been reported to be effective in patients unresponsive to the NSAIDs even though some physicians feel that gold injections may aggravate the skin disease. Penicillamine has not received adequate trial, and the antimalarial drugs are probably contraindicated. Patients treated with methotrexate for skin disease may also show improvement in arthritis as well.[4]

REFERENCES

1. Moll, J. M. H., and Wright, V.: *Psoriatic arthritis*. Semin. Arthritis Rheum. 3:55, 1973.
2. Sauer, G. C.: *Manual of Skin Diseases*, ed. 4. J. B. Lippincott, Philadelphia, 1980. (Excellent dermatologic resource for therapists.)
3. Bennett, R. M.: *Psoriatic arthritis*. In McCarty, D. J. (ed.): *Arthritis and Allied Conditions*, ed. 9. Lea and Febiger, Philadelphia, 1979, pp. 642-655.
4. Wright, V.: *Psoriatic arthritis*. In Kelley, W. M., et al. (eds.): *Textbook of Rheumatology*. W. B. Saunders, Philadelphia, 1981.
5. Wright, V., and Moll, J. M. H.: *Seronegative Polyarthritis*. Elsevier North-Holland Amsterdam, 1976.
6. Kammer, G. M., Soter, N. A., et al.: *Psoriatic arthritis. A clinical, immunological and HLA study of 100 patients*. Semin. Arthritis Rheum. 9(2), 1979.
7. Roberts, M. E. T., Wright, V., Hill, A. G. S., et al.: *Psoriatic arthritis: Followup study*. Ann. Rheum. Dis. 35:206, 1976.

8. Baker, H., Golding, N., and Thompson, M.: *Psoriasis and arthritis.* Ann. Intern. Med. 58:909, 1963.
9. Redisch, W., Messina, E. J., Hughes, G., and McEwen, C.: Capillaroscopic observations in the rheumatic diseases. Ann. Rheum. Dis. 29:244, 1970.
10. Forrester, D. M., Brown, J. C., and Nesson, J. W.: *The Radiology of Joint Disease.* W. B. Saunders, Philadelphia, 1978.
11. Belsky, M. R., Feldon, P. G., Millender, L. H., Nalebuff, E. A., and Phillips, C. A.: *Hand involvement in psoriatic arthritis* (abstr.). J. Hand Surg. 5(3):287, 1980.
12. Zaias, N.: *Psoriasis of the nail: A clinico-pathological study.* Arch. Derm. 99:567, 1969.
13. Lambert, J. R., and Wrist, V.: *Eye inflammation in psoriatic arthritis.* Ann. Rheum. Dis. 35:354, 1976.

ADDITIONAL SOURCES

Fassbender, H. G.: *Pathology of Rheumatic Diseases.* New York, Springer-Verlag, 1975, p. 245. (Includes a section on pathology of sausage swelling in the digits.)
Singsen, B. H.: *Psoriatic arthritis in childhood.* Arthritis Rheum. 20:408, 1977.

10

DEGENERATIVE JOINT DISEASE (OSTEOARTHRITIS) *

Degenerative joint disease (DJD) refers to a noninflammatory, slowly progressive disorder of joints caused by deterioration of articular cartilage with secondary new bone formation.

Etiologic Factors and Age and Sex Affected

The common factor in all types of DJD is the deterioration of cartilage. This may be hyaline cartilage in the synovial-lined joints or fibrocartilage in the spine. DJD can be divided into three broad categories: primary and secondary degenerative joint diseases, and degenerative joint disease of the spine. [1]

PRIMARY DEGENERATIVE JOINT DISEASE

The etiologic factors behind cartilage degeneration in this type is unknown. It occurs in women more frequently than in men and often is first symptomatic at the time of menopause. In many cases there is a definite genetic predisposition. People with involvement of the distal interphalangeal (DIP) joints and the carpometacarpal (CMC) joint of the thumb are the most frequently affected; however, the hips and knees may also be involved. [2]

SECONDARY DEGENERATIVE JOINT DISEASE

If the etiologic factors of cartilage destruction are known, the term secondary DJD is applicable. DJD can occur at any age secondary to (1) trauma, inflammation, or infection of joints; (2) excessive joint stress caused by inflammatory arthritis, obesity, occupational use, sports, structural abnormalities, or dysplasias; or (3) metabolic disturbances such as acromegaly. [2]

There is no typical distribution since the involvement of joints depends on the underlying causative factors. However, weight-bearing joints are the most frequently involved. [2]

---

* Both degenerative joint disease (DJD) and osteoarthritis (OA) can be used to describe this condition. Some clinicians prefer DJD because it does not imply an inflammatory component. Patients often prefer OA because it does not imply degeneration.

DEGENERATIVE JOINT DISEASE OF THE SPINE

This condition is also termed cervical or lumbar spondylosis or discogenic disease of the spine. When the intervertebral discs undergo degeneration and secondary compression, not only are new bone growths (osteophytes) generated from the vertebral bodies but also the compression can alter the alignment of the apophyseal joints as well. This leads to wear-and-tear degeneration of these joints.[3]

The most common sites of involvement are the areas of the spine that receive the most stress from movement, that is, the sixth to eighth cervical, the fourth to fifth lumbar, and the first sacral vertebrae. Some degree of DJD of the spine occurs in everyone over the age of forty.[2]

Diagnosis

Clinically diagnosis is made from the presence of the bony enlargement around the involved joints and by the classic distribution in the primary DJD. Radiologic evidence of cartilage loss and osteophyte formation is confirmatory.[2]

Course and Prognosis

Symptoms do not necessarily correlate with the degree of radiologic involvement of the joints. For example, a person can have severe radiographic changes in the joint and not have any pain or discomfort. Likewise someone can have only minor changes in radiographic readings and be disabled.

In general, prognosis for functional use is excellent for the upper extremity and back, fair for the knees, and poor for the hips.[4]

SYMPTOMATOLOGY AND IMPLICATIONS FOR OCCUPATIONAL THERAPY

All Forms of Degenerative Joint Disease

GENERAL SYMPTOMS

Symptoms are common to all forms of DJD; they may occur in any combination but tend to be concurrent. They include (1) joint pain with secondary muscle spasm; (2) aching during cold weather (considered a response to the change in barometric pressure); (3) stiffness after prolonged rest (usually not as pronounced as in rheumatoid arthritis); (4) crepitation upon motion; (5) limited joint motion and joint deformity due to osteophyte formation (bony enlargement); (6) muscle weakness and atrophy as a result of disuse; and (7) joint effusions, which are usually minimal.[2]

Therapy

Treatment goals are to assess functional ability in order to eliminate aggravating factors, reduce pain, maintain range of motion (ROM), maintain or increase muscle strength, reduce joint stress, and increase functional independence.[3,4,5]

Treatment methods are the same as those outlined for noninflammatory joint disease in Chapter 1 except that improving endurance is not usually a primary treatment goal.

Primary Degenerative Joint Disease

Typically the finger DIP and PIP joints and the thumb CMC joint are involved, but other joints can be affected. Treatment of joints other than the thumb and fingers will be discussed in this chapter under Secondary Degenerative Joint Disease and Degenerative Joint Disease of the Spine.

FINGERS

The DIP joints are the most common ones affected; the PIP joints are affected to a lesser degree. Deforming bony protuberances (osteophytes) on the margins and dorsal surfaces of the DIP joints (Heberden's nodes) are characteristic of primary DJD. It is possible for these nodes to appear on the PIP joints also (Bouchard's nodes). Heberden's or Bouchard's nodes usually are not painful but occasionally are associated with acute pain and swelling. Unilateral osteophyte formation, mucous cyst formation, and cartilage degeneration can result in unilateral collapse of the digital joints and lateral deviation deformities. Mallet-type deformities may occur secondary to bony changes at the DIP joint.[2]

The MCP joints and extensor mechanisms seldom are involved; therefore, it is uncommon to see deformities such as ulnar drift, boutonniere, and swan neck.

Therapy

The main functional limitations are pain and joint contractures with diminished finger flexion. Treatment is often limited to ROM exercises and adaptive equipment such as built-up handles. (See Assistive Equipment, Chapter 27.) Use of cotton stretch gloves at night is helpful in reducing stiffness and pain in some patients.[6] Occasionally a Heberden's node will become inflamed. Slip-on splints that immobilize the joint can often reduce pain with motion and protect the joint from further trauma. Since the MCP joints are seldom if ever involved, joint protection principles for such conditions as ulnar drift, MCP volar subluxation, and swan neck deformities are *not* indicated.

THUMBS

The CMC joint is the most common site of involvement and may be the only symptomatic joint.[7,8] Osteophyte enlargement of this joint often results in partial subluxation and characteristic squaring of the joint. (See Chapter 21, Hand Pathodynamics and Assessment for specific evaluative techniques.)

Therapy

If the CMC joint is the only one involved and pain limits hand function, a slip-on hand splint to immobilize the CMC and MCP joints can reduce pain considerably during functional activities.

(See Splinting for Arthritis of the Hand, Chapter 25.)[8,9] There are also several effective operations for this problem. (See Chapter 13, Hand, Wrist, and Forearm Surgery.)

Secondary Degenerative Joint Disease

The weight-bearing joints (back, knees, hips, and ankles) are the most common sites of involvement, but any joint can be involved secondary to trauma, stress, or infection.[2]

KNEES

Second to the back, the knees are the most common site of secondary DJD. Frequently pain may be present only on weight bearing. Varus deformity and mediolateral instability are common because of focal or asymmetric degeneration of the knee compartments.[7]

Discrepancy of leg lengths can also be an aggravating factor for DJD of the knee. Appropriate referral should be made, if this is suspected, to correct length difference with shoe lifts.[6,7]

Therapy

The incorporation of work simplification methods to minimize ambulation and motion and the use of elevated chairs and joint protection principles to minimize stress and pain are priority treatment objectives.[3,10]

Patient education is a crucial issue. Many people have misconceptions about what to do for their arthritis. The classic example of this is the patient with DJD of the knees who continues, by choice, to live in an upstairs apartment because he believes climbing the stairs three or four times a day will keep his legs strong. In fact, this will wear down the cartilage. There are non-weight-bearing ways such as isometric exercise to keep leg muscles strong.[3]

If obesity is an aggravating factor it is important to reinforce diet planning. If the patient lacks nutritional knowledge, refer him to a dietician or community weight control program when possible.

The use of a cane is a valuable aid for reducing stress to a knee.[11] The cane should be used in the hand *opposite* the involved knee. Patients who have difficulty ambulating should be counseled on how to adapt their home to reduce architectural barriers and reduce safety hazards. (See the section on Home Assessment in Chapter 28, Functional Activities.)

Specific therapy procedures are given in Joint Protection and Energy Conservation Instruction, Chapter 26; Exercise Treatment, Chapter 29; and Positioning and Lying Prone, Chapter 30.

HIPS

The most disabling form of DJD can take place with hip involvement.[4]

Hip *flexion* contractures may develop. These will alter the person's ability to stand straight or require the person to keep his knees bent to compensate for hip angle, thereby promoting knee flexion contractures.[4,7]

Hip *extension* contractures may occur also; actually they are a greater functional limitation than flexion contractures. A person who can flex his hip to only 60 degrees (from neutral) will not be able to sit straight in a regular chair. Hip flexion less than 90 degrees can also cause excessive pressure against the spine when the person attempts to sit in a straight-back chair. (This can be a source of complaints of low back pain in patients with DJD of the hip.) Also, lack of hip flexion can cause the patient to drop into a chair rather than sit down, causing additional stress to the spine and hip.

Discrepancy in leg length can influence hip involvement. Referral for evaluation and possible shoe lift correction is indicated if there is a discrepancy. [5,7]

Hip *adduction* contractures (limited abduction) also are of frequent consequence. For women, adduction contractures can interfere seriously with feminine hygiene and positioning during sexual intercourse. [12,13]

See Chapter 17, Hip Surgery, for a detailed discussion of hip pathodynamics.

Therapy

Incorporation of work simplification and joint protection methods to minimize ambulation, standing, and stress are priority treatment objectives. [10]

Lying prone daily is an important adjunct to maintenance of ROM of the hip. However, if there is also back involvement, see back protection methods in Joint Protection and Energy Conservation Instruction, Chapter 26, before advising the patient to lie prone. [5]

Use of a cane can greatly reduce amount of stress to an affected joint. [3,14]

Hip involvement often limits ability for transfer, lower extremity dressing, and perineal care. (See Assistive Equipment, Chapter 27, for solutions to common problems.) When there is interference with sexual activities, discuss alternative positioning methods that minimize stress.

Lack of hip flexion necessitates specially designed chairs or seats (including toilet seats) that will allow the patient to sit upright with less than a 90 degree flexion. (See Assistive Equipment, Chapter 27, for solutions to common problems.)

If there is a decrease in ambulation status and the patient needs to use a crutch, walker, or wheelchair, it is important that the patient receive training in how to do daily activities with the required ambulation aids. Also, patients with thumb adduction contractures secondary to DJD may require an adapted crutch or cane handle to prevent thumb pain or allow a secure grip.

ANKLES

Involvement of this joint is fairly rare, and the role of occupational therapy is minimal. Polyethylene molded supports (UC-BL support), short leg braces, and ambulation aids may be prescribed. Ambulation should be minimized. Counseling on work simplification methods to reduce ambulation may be indicated.

SHOULDERS

Specific DJD of the shoulder occurs in only about 5 percent of all patients with painful shoulder conditions. The majority of shoulder problems (85 percent) are due to periarticular involvement, e.g., tendinitis, bursitis, rotator cuff tears, and adhesive capsulitis. [15]

Therapy

Occupational therapy for shoulder conditions consists of a combination of joint protection methods designed to eliminate unnecessary shoulder motion or stress and activities planned to maintain strength of shoulder muscles and increase ROM in joints.[5,16]

When a painful shoulder condition severely limits shoulder motion Codman exercises are recommended. In these exercises the patient bends from the waist, allowing gravity to assist shoulder flexion to 90 degrees. It is important that effective ROM be done in the acute stages to avoid shortening of the inferior aspect of the capsule and frozen shoulder syndromes. If a patient has subacromion bursitis, exercises such as wall walking and finger ladder climbing are contraindicated since active flexion or abduction against gravity only causes greater impingement of the subacromion bursa.[15] Also during acute flares of bursitis ice compresses are more effective than heat for reducing swelling and pain.[17]

ELBOWS AND WRISTS

Actual DJD of these joints is rare. Elbow pain frequently is due to inflammation at the point of origin of the extensor muscles (lateral epicondylitis, tennis elbow) or flexor muscles (medial epicondylitis, golfer's elbow) rather than DJD.

Therapy

Evaluate self-care or occupation tasks. These tasks may aggravate joint or muscle pain. Instruct the patient in work simplification or joint protection methods to minimize extraneous stressful motion. Leather or canvas wrist gauntlet splints are effective in preventing twisting motion at the wrist while allowing flexion or extension. Wrist splints can also be effective for relieving pain of epicondylitis by reducing stress on the wrist extensor tendons. (See Splinting for Arthritis of the Hand, Chapter 25.)

BACK

Involvement may be of the apophyseal (facet) joints or the costovertebral articulations and is usually secondary to disc disease. The chief complaint is low back pain.

Secondary nerve root involvement may occur; this can cause impairment of bowel and bladder control and lower extremity motor and sensory impairment.

Initial involvement is usually at the fifth lumbar-first sacral joint (the most mobile joint).

Therapy

To relieve pain, the patient should be instructed in low back and abdominal strengthening exercises, proper posture, body mechanics, and work simplification to minimize back motion and stress. (See Joint Protection and Energy Conservation Instruction, Chapter 26, for back protection methods.)

Lumbar supports can also be very effective for low back pain. They are valuable for increasing the patient's awareness regarding proper body alignment and mechanics, and they support the abdomen, reducing anterior stress to the spine. Several lumbar supports are available on the market. Supports that have an elastic binder and thermoplastic insert that can be custom shaped are often fitted in occupational therapy. (These are manufactured by Warm and Form and Roylan.) Standard lace corsets are recommended for obese patients. These are usually obtained through orthotic services.[21] Patients frequently need instruction in adaptive corset or brace dressing techniques.

DRUG THERAPY

Since DJD is not usually an inflammatory disease, medicines that relieve pain (analgesic drugs) are prescribed. Thus, aspirin, in much lower doses than those used in rheumatoid arthritis, or acetaminophen is usually effective in giving symptomatic relief of pain. Indomethacin is particularly effective in relieving pain related to DJD of the hips, shoulders, or knees. All of the NSAIDs have been shown effective for treating the symptoms of DJD.

See Chapter 12 for precautions and side effects of specific drugs.

Degenerative Joint Disease of the Spine

NECK

Usually the symptoms include pain, stiffness, muscle spasms, and decreased range of motion. Occasionally bony changes, spurs, or disc protrusions may cause neurologic symptoms secondary to compression of motor and sensory nerve root fibers or may interfere with the blood supply to these fibers.[18,19]

Therapy

It is important to assess any stressful factors such as:

1. Posture during reading, writing, driving, watching television, work, and recreation.
2. The use of eyeglasses, e.g., if bifocals necessitate constant head adjustment to read or see.
3. The placement of work and of lighting.
4. Emotional factors which can significantly contribute to muscle spasm.[18]

Instruct patient in neck protection methods. (See Joint Protection and Energy Conservation Instruction, Chapter 26 for list of methods.) If soft or semi-rigid (Plastazote) neck collars are issued, evaluate whether they interfere with the patient's functional ability, e.g., bathing and driving, and evaluate the benefits of assistive equipment to minimize any interference.

Sensory evaluation is indicated if any neurologic signs are present.

The sleep position and type of pillow that a patient uses at night can have a strong influence on neck pain and stiffness. Patients with cervical arthritis should not sleep on their stomachs, since this position requires prolonged positioning at the extreme of range. If a patient complains of greater neck pain at night or upon awakening than during the day it may be due to the type of pillow he or she is using. When a person uses a regular pillow the shoulders and occipital area of the head are supported. This positioning causes a flattening of the normal lordotic curve of the cervical spine and places stress on the cervical joints and ligaments. A pillow that supports the neck in a normal lordotic curve and provides support to the cervical muscles can be very effective in reducing muscle spasm and associated pain and stiffness. [18]

The Jackson Cervipillo was designed for this purpose. [18] A survey of patient response to using the pillow revealed that the majority of patients found the pillow reduced symptoms. Fifty patients were surveyed; thirty-one returned the questionnaires. Of those who responded, 30 stated that the pillow was beneficial and thirteen out of 30 rated their pain as severe with a regular pillow and minimal to absent with the Cervipillo. [20]

Not all patients need a special pillow. Patients may be attaining sufficient support if they have a soft feather pillow that they can shape around the neck. Also the cervipillo is not effective for all patients. Compliance appears to be the highest when the concept of cervical support is explained to the patient and the patient determines to try the pillow on an experimental basis. [20]

REFERENCES

1. Brandt, K. D.: *Pathogenesis of osteoarthritis.* In Kelley, W. M., et al. (eds.): *Textbook of Rheumatology,* Vol. II. W. B. Saunders, Philadelphia, 1981. (Detailed discussion on cartilage degeneration and osteophyte formation.)
2. Bland, J. H., and Stulberg, S. D.: *Osteoarthritis: Pathology and clinical patterns.* In Kelley, W. M., et al. (eds.): *Textbook of Rheumatology,* Vol. II. W. B. Saunders, Philadelphia, 1981.
3. Robinson, W. D.: *Management of degenerative joint disease.* In Kelley, W. M., et al. (eds.): *Textbook of Rheumatology,* Vol. II.W. B. Saunders, Philadelphia, 1981.
4. Stevens, J.: *Osteoarthritis of the hip. A review with special considerations of the problem bilateral malum coxae senilis.* Clin. Orthop. 71:152, 1970.
5. Wickersham, B.: *Physical therapy management of the patient with DJD.* Arthritis Foundation (newsletter), Vol. 13, No. 1, Spring, 1979.
6. Ehrlich, G., and DiPierro, A. M.: *Stretch gloves: Nocturnal use to ameliorate morning stiffness in arthritic hands.* Arch. Phys. Med. Rehab. 52:479, 1971.
7. Polley, H. F., and Hunder, G. G.: *Rheumatologic Interviewing and Physical Examination of the Joints.* W. B. Saunders, Philadelphia, 1978. (Sections on evaluation of the shoulder, hand, and knee.)
8. Dell, P. C., Brushart, M. D., and Smith, R. J.: *Treatment of trapeziometacarpal arthritis: Results of resection arthroplasty.* J. Hand Surg. 3(3):243, 1978. (Includes a description of conservative treatment.)
9. Melvin, J. L.: *Splinting for DJD of the thumb.* (In press)
10. Haviland, N., and Jette, A. M.: *Joint Protection for Osteoarthritis.* Audiovisual program from University of Michigan Media Library, G1302, Towsley Center, University of Michigan Medical Center, Ann Arbor, Mich. 48109. (Program includes booklet.)
11. Tillman, F., and Haviland, N.: *602 Elm Street: Overcoming Barriers to Independence.* Audiovisual program from University of Michigan Media Library, G1302, Towsley Center, University of Michigan Medical Center, Ann Arbor, Mich. 48109. (Program includes booklet.)
12. Currey, H. L. F.: *Osteoarthritis of the hip joint and sexual activity.* Ann. Rheum. Dis. 29:488, 1970.
13. Todd, R. C., Lightowler, C. D., and Harris, J.: *Low fraction arthroplasty of the hip joint and sexual activity.* Acta Orthop. Scand. 44(6):690, 1973.
14. Petty, B., and Harrison, S.: *Compliance with Medical Instruction.* Audiovisual program from University of Michigan Media Library, G1302, Towsley Center, University of Michigan Medical Center, Ann Arbor, Mich. 48109. (Program includes booklet and examples of using a cane and taking medications.)
15. Bland, J. H., Merrit, J. A., and Boushey, D. R.: *The painful shoulder.* Semin. Arthritis Rheum. 7(1):21, 1977.

16. Cailliet, R.: *Shoulder Pain.* F. A. Davis, Philadelphia, 1964.
17. Rocks, J. A.: *Intrinsic shoulder pain syndrome: Rationale for heating and cooling in treatment.* Phys. Ther. 59(2):153, 1979.
18. Jackson, R.: *The Cervical Syndrome,* ed. 4. Charles C Thomas, Springfield, Ill., 1978.
19. Cailliet, R.: *Neck and Arm Pain.* F. A. Davis, Philadelphia, 1964.
20. Melvin, J. L.: *Cervical support pillow to reduce neck pain: Follow up survey of patient response.* Unpublished article, presented at the Physical Disabilities Specialty Section Meeting, San Antonio, 1981.
21. Jacobs, B.: *The arthritic spine.* In Ehrlich, G. (ed.): *Total Management of the Arthritic Patient.* J. B. Lippincott, Philadelphia, 1973.

11

GOUT

Gout is characterized by acute episodes of arthritis associated with the presence of sodium urate crystals in the synovial fluid or deposits of urate crystals (tophi) in or about the joints and other tissues.

Etiologic Factors

Primary gout is the most common form and is the type that may lead to chronic tophaceous gout. It occurs alone and is not secondary to any other major disease. It results from elevation of serum uric acid levels (hyperuricemia) and deposition of urate crystals in the tissues and joints. Hyperuricemia develops because too much uric acid is being produced, too little is being excreted in the urine, or both.[1]

Secondary gout occurs when hyperuricemia is directly due to an underlying disease, e.g., leukemia or chronic renal disease. This form rarely develops tophi because of the decreased life span resulting from the underlying disease.[1]

Age and Sex Affected

Primary gout is found primarily in males (9 to 1); it occurs most commonly in the fifth decade but it can present any time after puberty. It rarely occurs in women until after menopause.[2]

Diagnosis

Diagnosis is confirmed by the presence of monosodium urate crystals in the synovial fluid and hyperuricemia. In patients who present with tophi, the presence of crystals in the tophus establishes the diagnosis.[3]

Course and Prognosis

With appropriate medication: Typically the initial acute attack lasts for a few days; further acute attacks and the development of tophi are prevented.

Without medication: Typically there are recurrent episodes of acute inflammatory monoarticular arthritis that subside spontaneously in about two weeks. If the hyperuricemia persists, tophi may develop. These accumulations of urate crystals can erode into the joints, bones, and periarticular structures, causing functional impairment.[2,3]

SYMPTOMATOLOGY AND IMPLICATIONS FOR OCCUPATIONAL THERAPY

Acute Gouty Arthritis

The acute attack of gout is an excruciatingly painful arthritis, usually affecting a single joint. Lower extremity joints are most commonly affected, particularly the first metatarsophalangeal joint. The onset is rapid with swelling, heat, and erythema in the affected joint.[1]

Historically gout was thought to be caused by the overindulgence of food or alcoholic beverages; however, with the advent of drugs to control the hyperuricemia, severe dietary restrictions are rarely indicated. Patients are advised to eat a regular diet, avoiding only those foods that are particularly high in purines (purines break down into uric acid) such as fish eggs (caviar) and sweetbreads.[3]

Therapy

Occupational therapy is rarely indicated for an acute attack of gout. However, protective or resting splints may be helpful, especially if the site of the attack is the wrist or hand.

Chronic Tophaceous Gout

Five to ten years after the onset of gout, tophi (deposits of urate) may develop. These usually appear as subcutaneous lumps, most commonly in the olecranon bursa and along the cartilage of the ear. When they occur around joints, they may lead to cartilage and bone erosion with residual joint deformity or decreased range of motion secondary to mechanical interference.[2]

The most frequent hand limitations are decreased finger flexion and decreased grip. Other problems related to urate deposition are renal stones and nerve entrapment syndromes; the former are common but the latter, rare.

Tophi can often be reduced or eliminated by proper medication but this usually takes a considerable amount of time—months or even years.[3]

Therapy

The main symptom that would indicate referral to occupational therapy would be decreased hand function secondary to tophi. Physical measures are generally not indicated for deformities directly caused by tophi. Occupational therapy is usually identified in terms of adapted equipment and assistive devices.

DRUG THERAPY

Drugs that reduce inflammation are usually prescribed for acute attacks. Colchicine, indomethacin, and phenylbutazone are the drugs most frequently used for this purpose. After the acute attack is controlled, therapy is directed at lowering the serum uric acid.[2]

Sulfinpyrazone or probenecid lowers serum uric acid by increasing the renal excretion of uric acid. High fluid intake is urged with these drugs to minimize the risk of uric acid renal stone formation. Allopurinol effectively lowers serum uric acid by blocking an enzyme needed for the production of uric acid.[2]

See Chapter 12 for precautions and side effects of specific drugs.

REFERENCES

1. Gutman, A. G. (ed.): *Gout: A Clinical Comprehension*. Burroughs Wellcome Co., Research Triangle Park, North Carolina, 1971.
2. Kelley, W. M.: *Gout and related disorders of purine metabolism*. In Kelley, W. M., et al. (eds.): *Textbook of Rheumatology*. W. B. Saunders, Philadelphia, 1981.
3. Wyngaarden, J. B., and Holmes, E. W.: *Clinical gout and the pathogenesis of hyperuricemia*. In McCarty, D. J. (ed.) *Arthritis and Allied Conditions*, ed. 9. Lea and Febiger, Philadelphia, 1979.

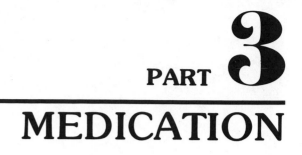

PART **3**

MEDICATION

12

DRUG THERAPY

Drug therapy for arthritis is constantly changing and, in fact, is going through a considerable evolution from a standard sequential selection of five to seven drugs in the 1960s to a current armamentarium of twenty or more effective medications.

Over the last ten years the development of nonsteroidal anti-inflammatory drugs (NSAIDs) has created a new classification of antirheumatic medications and greatly extended the flexibility of medical management.

There have been over 100 variations of these NSAIDs developed internationally. As each drug is developed, it is compared with aspirin and/or placebo. This extensive comparison process, particularly in the last five years, has generated extensive data on drug therapy and resulted in a greater appreciation of individual patient response to medication and dosage regimens, as well as a greater appreciation of the benefits and limitations of aspirin. [1]

Drug therapy, like painting a picture or rearing a child, is a creative process. There are basic rules that are essential to each activity, but no single method is recommended over all other methods. The variables in drug management are always changing. Patients and their needs and concerns change; more information about the use of medications becomes available; and physicians change in response to their patient care experience. It is congruent with this total picture that drug therapy for rheumatic diseases varies widely across the country among medical schools and among rheumatologists. Each physician develops his or her own philosophy and systematic approach to medical management of rheumatic diseases. Therapists and other arthritis health professionals need to understand the medical protocols used by the rheumatologists, internists, and family practitioners at their facility.

Understanding medical management is critical to effective rehabilitative treatment planning, particularly since medications can significantly alter objective measurements, such as grip strength, hand function, range of motion, muscle strength, dressing time, and so forth. The fast-acting anti-inflammatory and analgesic drugs, such as aspirin, indomethacin, phenylbutazone, propionic acids, steroids, and propoxyphene hydrochloride (Darvon) can *influence objective assessments* in as short a period of time as a half hour. Slow-acting medications, such as gold, antimalarial drugs, and penicillamine, which take three to four months to effect change, can influence longitudinal assessments. Therefore, prior to each assessment, it is important to note the type, amount, and time of the last medication dose. This should be checked even with

TABLE 1 Nonsteroidal anti-inflammatory medications

Name: Trade and Generic*	Dosage	Precautions	Additional toxic side effects†
SALICYLATES			
Acetylsalicylic Acid (ASA) aspirin (ASA) Ecotrin (enteric coated ASA) Ascriptin (ASA + antacid) Bufferin (ASA + antacid)	Adult: Start with 8-12 (5 grain) tablets per day.	Take with food or milk. Should not be used by people with a history of gastric ulcer or with bleeding tendencies. (True of all NSAIDs.)	CNS: tinnitus, deafness (reversible). Acute toxic reaction to high salicylate levels can include vomiting, psychosis, hyperventilation, alkalosis, and metabolic acidosis.
Cation Salicylates Arthropan (choline salicylate) Trilisate (choline magnesium trisalicylate) Disalcid (salicylsalicylic acid) Magan (magnesium salicylate)	Children: determined by weight.		
PROPIONIC ACIDS Motrin (ibuprofen) 300 mg (white, round), 400 mg (red, round) and 600 mg (orange, oblong) tablets	900 to 2400 mg daily 3-4 divided doses		
Naprosyn (naproxyn) 250 mg (yellow, round) tablet and 375 mg (orange, oblong) tablet	500 to 750 mg daily 2-3 divided doses		
Nalfon (fenoprofen) 300 mg (yellow) capsule and 600 mg (yellow) tablet	900 to 3200 mg daily 3-4 divided doses	Use with ASA not recommended.	Mouth ulcers (stomatitis); there are occasional reports of tinnitus.
TOLECTIN (tolmetin) 200 mg (white, round) tablet 400 mg (red) capsule	600 to 1800 mg daily 3-4 divided doses		

Drug	Dosage	Notes	Side Effects
CLINORIL (sulindac) 150 mg, 200 mg tablets (Both yellow hexagon tablets)	300 to 400 mg daily 2 divided doses	Use with ASA not recommended.	Main complications are diarrhea and abdominal cramps.
MECLOMEN (meclofenamic acid) 50 mg, (two-tone gold) capsule 100 mg (gold and white) capsule	200 to 400 mg daily 3-4 divided doses		
INDOCIN (indomethacin) 25 mg, 50 mg capsules (Both are blue and white)	50 to 200 mg daily 1-4 divided doses	Should be taken with food or milk.	CNS: headache, dizziness, detached feelings, drowsiness, and hallucinations.
BUTAZOLIDIN ALKA (phenylbutazone) 100 mg (red, round) tablets	100 to 400 mg daily 2-3 divided doses	Should not be used with sulfa drugs and their derivatives, and some anticoagulants.	Occasional GI bleeding. Serious side effects such as aplastic anemia, agranulocytosis, and thrombocytopenia are rare.
TANDEARIL (oxyphenbutazone) 100 mg (tan, round) tablets	100 to 400 mg daily 2-3 divided doses	Should not be used by patient with liver or renal disease.	

*Purpose: All of these medications serve the same purpose or function to some degree. They all have anti-inflammatory, analgesic, antipyretic, and anticoagulant properties.

†Toxic Side Effects: Since all of these medications inhibit prostaglandin production, they share similar side effects. Some of the side effects have a higher incidence with certain medications, but all of the following side effects can occur with each drug. Gastrointestinal: indigestion, heartburn, nausea, abdominal pain, diarrhea, ulcers, constipation. (2) Fluid retention. (3) Anemia. (4) Decreased clotting ability. (5) Lightheadedness, nasal stuffiness. (Patients with asthma can be sensitive to these symptoms.) (6) Allergic skin rash. (7) Possible mild stimulant or depressant effect.

patients who are on a constant medicine regimen, since they may take additional analgesic drugs on bad days. Additional medication can result in significant measurement changes. *Thus, quantitative assessments may reflect only the benefits of medication and not the results of rehabilitative treatment.* The converse situation may also occur. If a patient comes to the clinic complaining of increased discomfort, his or her medication pattern should be investigated. He or she may have delayed or missed the morning medication dosage.

Another issue to consider is that joint exacerbations may be chronic and last for months, or they may be responsive to fast-acting medications in a couple of days. Equipment such as assistive devices or splints and instruction in adaptive methods may not be necessary if the flare is responsive to medications.

Therapists can also play an important role in facilitating patient compliance by reinforcing the rationale for anti-inflammatory medications and adherence to the prescribed regimen. Even when physicians do a thorough job of patient education, patients often have questions after they leave the physician's office. Patients frequently raise these questions in therapy, providing an opportunity for the therapist to correct misunderstandings or reaffirm accurate information. *However, this aspect of patient education can only be done if therapists are familiar with the referring physician's medication protocols.* Excellent articles are available on patient drug education, methods of increasing compliance, and drug usage in the elderly.[2,3,4,5]

Additionally, therapists can facilitate medical care by being alert for serious medication side effects in patients and advising patients to report the symptoms to their physician. For example, if a rehabilitation outpatient is noticeably pale and complaining of tiredness, it is appropriate to recommend that the patient see his or her physician because these symptoms may be related to anemia. The medication side effects to be alert for are outlined in Table 1.

The rationale for drug use for specific diseases is described at the end of each chapter in Part 2, Major Rheumatic Diseases. This chapter discusses the specific drug properties, side effects, and implications for arthritis health professionals.

NONSTEROIDAL ANTI-INFLAMMATORY DRUGS (NSAIDs)

Salicylates (Aspirin and Aspirin-Containing Compounds)

Salicylates are the oldest and most widely used of the antirheumatic drugs and are still the first drugs of choice in the treatment of rheumatoid arthritis and most other inflammatory arthritides. These drugs are popular because they are effective and inexpensive and have a tolerable incidence of side effects.[1] Aspirin (acetylsalicylic acid) is the most commonly used derivative of salicylic acid (Table 2). There are four other derivatives, referred to as cation salicylates, that have become increasingly popular over the past few years.

Salicylates offer an advantage over other antirheumatic drugs in that their level in the blood can be measured by a simple laboratory test. Measurement of salicylate levels is valuable for determining proper blood absorption of the drug. A therapeutic anti-inflammatory level is between 20 to 30 mg per deciliter (dl). Many patients develop side effects that require discontinuation of the drug before a therapeutic blood level is achieved.[1]

Table 2 Common forms of aspirin

Arthropan (liquid aspirin)
Ascriptin (aspirin plus Maalox)
Bufferin
Ecotrin (enteric-coated aspirin to reduce gastrointestinal side effects)
Measurin (long-acting aspirin)

These are prescribed in a dosage equivalent to aspirin. Common aspirin contains 5 grains per tablet, equal to 300 mg or 0.3 gm. Average anti-inflammatory doses are 12 to 24 (5 grain) ASA tablets per day or 3.6 to 7.2 gm per day.

Aspirin

When aspirin is used in large doses (12 to 20 tablets a day), it is effective as an anti-inflammatory agent. Used in low doses (less than 9 tablets per day) it works as an analgesic (pain reliever).[6]

Toxicity from high dosage of aspirin is indicated by tinnitus (persistent ringing or buzzing sound in the ears). The recommended dosage is the amount just lower than that which causes tinnitus. For example, if 16 aspirin a day produces tinnitus, the patient is advised to reduce the dosage one tablet per day until the tinnitus stops. In most people tinnitus corresponds to a serum salicylate level of 20 to 30 mg per deciliter. (Tinnitus is not used as a guideline for monitoring aspirin in children.) In all patients, therapeutic anti-inflammatory levels of salicylates (approximately 25 mg per dl) cause a totally reversible 20 decibel hearing loss at all frequencies. This hearing loss may be unacceptable to individuals with pre-existing hearing impairment. Occasionally deafness occurs when aspirin reaches a toxic level. Normal hearing returns when the aspirin dosage is reduced.

Gastrointestinal symptoms such as nausea and heartburn are the most common side effects of aspirin. Since patients often have to be on aspirin for long periods of time, it is important that they take measures to prevent GI side effects. They should take the aspirin with milk or with meals and never on an empty stomach. For some patients buffered aspirin reduces these symptoms. Enteric-coated aspirin is another useful alternative for some patients, since it is not dissolved until the table reaches the small intestine. More serious complications include gastrointestinal bleeding and allergic reactions such as asthma and hay fever. Aspirin should not be used by patients with documented peptic ulcer or with bleeding tendencies.[7]

Cation Salicylates

These salicylate derivatives have gained increasing popularity because compared with aspirin they may be better tolerated and have fewer side effects; they are often more readily absorbed; and they deliver almost twice as much salicylate per dose than aspirin, making the medication easier to take. Their main disadvantage is that they cost more than aspirin.[1] The drugs in this category are magnesium salicylate (Magan, Mobidin), choline salicylate (Arthropan, a liquid salicylate), choline magnesium trisalicylate (Trilisate), and salicylsalicylic acid (Disalcid).[1]

Most physicians try aspirin first. If the patient has problems with absorption or side effects, the physician may try another salicylate preparation as an alternative. However, many physicians are using cation salicylates as the first drug of choice for RA, unless financial concerns are a predominant factor.

Propionic Acids

Like salicylates, these medications reduce but usually do not completely stop the signs and symptoms of joint inflammation. They are fast-acting medications, in that initially they take effect within two to five days. They are effective only while therapeutic blood levels are maintained.[7,8] While chemically diverse, all the NSAIDs (and salicylates) share the property of inhibiting the production of prostaglandins. This property not only accounts for some of their anti-inflammatory action but also explains why these drugs produce similar side effects such as gastric distress, ulcer formation, fluid retention, bleeding tendencies, and the rare occurrence of asthma and renal failure.[7,9]

The more expensive NSAIDs are selected over salicylates when patients cannot tolerate salicylates or when the individual prefers the convenience of taking two to four tablets per day rather than 12 to 15 aspirin tablets per day.[9]

Many patients who do not respond to aspirin or one of the NSAIDs may respond to another NSAID. There is no way to predict which will be the most efficacious drug for an individual except by trial usage. The third or alternate drug is usually selected from a different chemical class. For example, if one of the propionic acid derivatives does not work, it is not likely that another will, so the next trial drug would be from outside of that group.[9]

Other Drugs

See Table 1 for dosage and side effects of other NSAIDs.

INTRASYNOVIAL STEROID INJECTIONS

Intrasynovial injections of steroids have different purposes, goals, and consequences than daily oral administration or intramuscular injections of steroids.

Steroids injected into a joint, bursa, or tendon sheath provide *localized* suppression of inflammation in a specific area. They are given intermittently, no more than six times a year, to a specific joint.[9] Negative consequences are related to the effect of the drug on surrounding joint and tendon structures.[10] The classic steroid side effects such as cushingoid features, osteoporosis, and so forth do not occur with local intrasynovial injections. Injections can have a slight systemic effect at the time of the injection, but it is not significant enough to produce negative systemic side effects.

Local injections do not cure or stop the inflammation, but they can control it in some patients. Response to local injections is variable. Some patients get relief of pain and swelling for six weeks or longer; for others relief may last only a few days. If the benefit is transient, lasting less than a week, repeated injection is usually not helpful and not advisable.[11] In small joints such as the PIP joint, a single trial is often sufficient to determine effectiveness of this approach. Larger joints, such as the shoulder and hip, may be responsive to a third injection even if the first two have failed.[10,11]

Intrasynovial steroid injections are particularly valuable in the following situations.[10]
1. Severe inflammation of one or a few peripheral joints, especially if the joint inflammation is preventing function or restricting motion to the point that a deformity is likely to occur if the inflammation is not resolved.
2. Severe flexor tenosynovitis of the wrist or digits and extensor tenosynovitis of the wrist.
3. Acute bursitis. (Injections are helpful in this condition but not in chronic adhesive capsulitis.)

Injections are not given in a joint if there is a possibility of infection or fracture near or around the joint, since steroids reduce healing potential. It is also impractical to use injections when multiple joints are inflamed; in these instances systemic medications need to be used.

Complications include:
1. Infections, which are infrequent. They may occur despite rigid sterile technique and are generally due to resistant staphylococcus.
2. Occasionally injections result in a postinjection flare lasting up to 24 hours. This is considered an aseptic process resulting from synovitis induced by corticosteroid crystals. (Ice compresses are recommended until the delayed effect of the corticosteroid reduces the inflammation.)
3. One of the more serious complications is instability in a weight-bearing joint following repeated injections. In the hip this has been seen along with aseptic necrosis of the femoral head.
4. Tendon rupture can occur if the injection is given into the tendon rather than into the tendon sheath, but this is rare. Athletes have been known to rupture tendons following strenuous exercise of tendons or joints that have been repeatedly injected (for instance, weekly).[10,11]

REMISSION-INDUCING DRUGS (RIDs)

When synovitis persists despite the use of NSAIDs and conservative measures, it becomes necessary to use stronger medications. Gold salts, antimalarial drugs, and penicillamine are slow-acting medications that can modify RA and related diseases and in some patients actually induce remission.[12,13,14]

Gold salts are the most widely accepted RID. Most physicians will try gold first. If it is unsuccessful, they will then try an antimalarial drug or penicillamine. Some physicians highly experienced with antimalarials will start with these drugs in selected patients and then try gold as the second option.[13]

Gold Salts (Myochrysine, Solganal)

The value of gold for rheumatoid arthritis was a serendipitous discovery in the 1920s during an experimental trial using gold for tuberculosis. It was found that joint disease improved in tuberculous patients who also suffered from rheumatoid arthritis. (Gold is no longer considered beneficial for tuberculosis.)

Although gold has been used to treat rheumatoid arthritis since about 1930, the reasons for its effectiveness are still unknown. Nevertheless, gold provides beneficial anti-inflammatory results in a majority of patients who can tolerate the drug. There is a definite price to pay for these benefits, since patients must be seen weekly for 20 weeks for blood and urine analyses to detect signs of toxicity. This can pose a problem for patients who are employed or want to return to work, since the clinic visits usually necessitate taking off a half day from work.[13]

Side effects of gold toxicity include skin rashes and mucous membrane ulcerations in the mouth (stomatitis). These may be controlled by stopping or lowering the dosage. More serious complications that may lead to death include bone marrow depression (thrombocytopenia or agranulocytosis) and kidney damage (hence the need for weekly urinalysis). Whenever any of these side effects are noticed, they should be reported promptly to the physician.[13]

Because of the seriousness of the side effects, gold therapy is reserved only for patients with rheumatoid arthritis who are dependable and have a persistent synovitis that is not responsive to other, more conservative management.

Dosage is 50 mg weekly for 20 weeks, then once every three to four weeks. A positive therapeutic response is often not noticeable until 9 to 12 weeks after therapy is started.

Antimalarial Therapy

Hydroxychloroquine (Plaquenil) is the drug of choice among the antimalarials for the treatment of rheumatic diseases because of its effectiveness and low toxicity compared with other antimalarials. This drug appears to be particularly effective in SLE patients with sun sensitivity and skin rashes. It is also used successfully in both adult and juvenile RA and the spondyloarthropathies.[12]

Antimalarial therapy is not used as widely as gold therapy primarily because of its potential for causing permanent visual disturbances or blindness. It can be used safely only in prescribed doses and in conjunction with proper ophthalmologic monitoring. Patients should have an eye examination before starting the drug and approximately every six months thereafter. The drug is discontinued if visual changes occur. The visual symptoms to be alert for are impaired reading ability, poor distance vision, night blindness, blurred vision and halos around lights, and scotomas (spots in the visual field without vision). Since the eyes can become sensitive to the sun, it is recommended that patients wear sunglasses outdoors.[12,15]

Other side effects include a wide range of neurologic conditions, including migraine-like headaches, tinnitus, vestibular problems, dermatologic conditions, and gastrointestinal disorders. Essentially any unusual symptom in these categories could be related to the drug.

A factor that often influences the selection of this drug over gold salts is the method of administration. Hydroxychloroquine is in tablet form and does not require weekly clinic visits as does gold therapy.

Dosage is 200 to 400 mg per day, taken with food. Overdoses can be fatal.[12]

Penicillamine

This medication is generally used as the third RID alternative for the treatment of RA and chronic juvenile polyarthritis. In selected patients with extra-articular manifestations (internal organ involvement), it may be the first drug used because of its effectiveness in controlling these conditions.[14]

The toxicities and side effects that may be produced by penicillamine are many and diverse and have limited its clinical use. These side effects can be severe and include:

1. Hematologic changes, including acute bone marrow depression with neutropenia, thrombocytopenia, and aplastic anemia.
2. Renal changes, including nephropathy and nephrotic syndrome.
3. Dermatologic changes. A wide range of skin rashes can occur and appear similar to the rashes seen with gold therapy.
4. Mucous membrane lesions can occur (both oral and genital) and are dose related.
5. Secondary immune complex diseases can result from penicillamine, including SLE, myasthenia gravis, polymyositis, Goodpasture's syndrome, pemphigus, and Sjögren's syndrome.
6. Hypogeusia (blunting or loss of taste perception) is another common side effect. This may persist for up to three months following onset. It gradually clears, even with the continuation of therapy.
7. Delayed wound healing, which may prolong postoperative recovery and therapy.[14]

Dosage is 250 mg per day, *taken on an empty stomach.* This amount is taken for 12 weeks. If there is no response, it is increased by 250 mg. Maximum is 1 gram per day. It is contraindicated during pregnancy.[14]

STEROIDS

Steroid preparations are the most powerful anti-inflammatory agents known. Their use may be lifesaving in polymyositis and in certain manifestations of systemic lupus erythematosus; however, their rational use on a long-term basis for other inflammatory joint diseases is restricted to patients who would be severely disabled without them.[15]

Cautious use of these drugs is essential, since long-term use produces serious and undesirable side effects. These include cushingoid features, such as moon facies and buffalo humps, secondary to deposition of subcutaneous fat, obesity, purpura, and skin striae; severe osteoporosis that can lead to compression fractures of the spine or other pathologic fractures; avascular necrosis of the femoral or humeral head; cataracts; peptic ulcers and nausea; and a myopathy similar to polymyositis. In addition, steroids can cause hypertension, exacerbate diabetes, lower the body's resistance to infection, and decrease the ability to heal. These drugs can also affect the central nervous system by diminishing the psychological awareness of pain or by enhancing a sense of well being. They can also produce aberrant psychological states, such as euphoria or severe psychosis.[15] Probably the most depressing and significant consequences for the patient are the side effects altering physical appearance.

The occupational or physical therapist and nurse should keep several conditions or consequences in mind:
1. If there is severe osteoporosis, transfers and passive range of motion should be done cautiously.
2. Effects of steroids on the central nervous system can significantly affect the patient's ability to learn and comply with instructions. All instructions need to be written out.
3. For patients on long-term steroid therapy, the signs of myopathy, i.e., drooping shoulders, and difficulty stepping up steps and arising from a chair (not resulting from joint problems), should be noted.

Steroids are used in the lowest dose for the shortest period of time needed to achieve the desired clinical effect. Prednisone in various combinations of 1- to 5-mg tablets currently is the most commonly used oral preparation. As a rough guide, less than 10 mg is considered a low dose, 10 to 30 mg a moderate dose, and 30 to 100 mg a high dose. Other drugs used include cortisone, triamcinolone, dexamethasone, and methylprednisolone.

ANALGESICS

These are drugs that have no anti-inflammatory action of their own but may be used in combination with other medications to help in pain relief. Addictive analgesic drugs should be used with caution in chronic diseases. Analgesics are most rationally used for pain relief in noninflammatory joint disease, such as degenerative joint disease and chronic-inactive rheumatoid arthritis.[6]

Table 3 Common medications used with rheumatic diseases

Generic name	Trade name
Acetaminophen	Datril, Tylenol
Acetylsalicylic acid (ASA)	Aspirin (See Table 2)
Allopurinol	Zyloprim
Azathioprine	Imuran
Chlorambucil	Leukeran
Chloroquine	Aralen
Colchicine	Colchicine
Cortisone	(Several names)*
Cyclophosphamide	Cytoxan
Dexamethasone	Decadron
Fenoprofen calcium	Nalfon
Gold salts	Myochrysine, Solganal
Hydrocortisone	Cortef, Solu-Cortef
Hydroxychloroquine	Plaquenil
Ibuprofen	Motrin
Indomethacin	Indocin
Methotrexate	Methrotrexate
Methylprednisolone	Medrol
Naproxen	Naprosyn
Oxyphenbutazone	Oxalid, Tandearil
Penicillamine	Cuprimine, Depen
Phenylbutazone	Butazolidin
Prednisone	(Several names)*
Probenecid	Benemid
Propoxyphene	Darvon
Quinacrine	Atabrine
Tolmetin sodium	Tolectin
Triamcinolone	Aristocort

*See Physicians' Desk Reference for various names.

Patients with inflammatory arthritis should not be treated with analgesics alone because the inflammatory process will continue to damage surrounding tissues despite pain relief.

Mild analgesics include acetaminophen and low doses of aspirin. More potent and addicting analgesics should be avoided, including propoxyphene (Darvon), codeine, Dilaudid, Percodan, Demerol, and morphine.

See Table 3 for a list of common medications used in the treatment of rheumatic diseases.

DRUGS USED TO TREAT GOUT (COLCHICINE, BENEMID, ALLOPURINOL)

The use of and rationale for these drugs are discussed in Chapter 11, Gout. Side effects vary for each drug. Colchicine may cause nausea, vomiting, and diarrhea. Benemid has almost no side effects except possibly minor skin rashes. Allopurinol on the other hand can result in skin rashes and, rarely, a severe form of hepatitis.

REFERENCES

1. Roth, S. H.: *New Directions in Arthritis Therapy.* PSG Publishing Co., Littleton, Mass., 1980.
2. Simonson, W.: *Medication of the elderly—Effect on response to physical therapy.* Phys. Ther. 58(2):178, 1978.
3. Hussar, D. A.: *Patient noncompliance.* J. Am. Pharm. Assoc. NS15:183, 1975.
4. Ward, M., and Blatman, M.: *Drug therapy in the elderly.* Am. Fam. Pract. February, 1979, pp. 143-152.
5. Hendrix, J. L., and Keith, T. D.: *A comprehensive drug education program for the hospitalized patient with rheumatic disease.* AHP Arthritis Newsletter, 13(4):9-11, Winter, 1980.
6. Wilske, K. R.: *A therapeutic approach to the use of drugs in the treatment of rheumatoid arthritis.* AHP Arthritis Newsletter, 13(4):1-9, Winter 1980.
7. Paulus, H. E., and Furst, D. E.: *Aspirin and nonsteroidal anti-inflammatory drugs.* In: McCarty, D. J. (ed.): *Arthritis and Allied Conditions.* Lea and Febiger, Philadelphia, 1979.
8. Weissmann, G.: *Rheumatoid arthritis: How the new nonsteroidal anti inflammatory drugs work.* Resident and Staff Physician, December, 1976, pp. 48-55.
9. Dick, W. C., and DeCeulaer, K.: *Nonsteroidal antirheumatic drugs.* In *Textbook of Rheumatology.* Kelley, W. M., et al. (eds.): W. B. Saunders, Philadelphia, 1981.
10. Hollander, J. L.: *Arthrocentesis and intrasynovial therapy.* In McCarty, D. J. (ed.): *Arthritis and Allied Conditions.* Lea and Febiger, Philadelphia, 1979, pp. 402-141.
11. Millender, L. H., and Nalebuff, E. A.: *Evaluation and treatment of early rheumatoid hand involvement.* Orthop. Clin. North Am. 6(3):704, July, 1975.
12. Stillman, J. S.: *Antimalarials.* In Kelley, W. M., et al. (eds.): *Textbook of Rheumatology.* W. B. Saunders, Philadelphia, 1980.
13. Zvaifler, N. J.: *Gold and antimalarial therapy.* In McCarty, D. J. (ed.): *Arthritis and Allied Conditions.* Lea and Febiger, Philadelphia, 1979, pp. 355-367.
14. Jaffee, I. A.: *D-Penicillamine.* In Kelley, W. M., et al. (eds.): *Textbook of Rheumatology.* W. B. Saunders, Philadelphia, 1980.
15. Axelrod, L.: *Steroids.* In Kelley, W. M., et al. (eds.): *Textbook of Rheumatology.* W. B. Saunders, Philadelphia, 1980.
16. Wallace, R., Heiss, M. L., and Bautch, J.: *Staff Manual for Teaching Patients About Rheumatoid Arthritis.* American Hospital Association, 840 North Lake Shore Drive, Chicago, IL 60611.

ADDITIONAL SOURCES

A Primer on Medicines. FDA Consumer December 1973-4. Government Printing Office, Superintendent of Documents, Washington D.C. 20402. DHEW Publication No. (FDA) 74-3014.

Physicians' Desk Reference. Medical Economics Co., Litton Industries, Inc., Oradell, NJ 07649 (published annually).

The Truth About Aspirin for Arthritis. A patient pamphlet distributed by the Arthritis Foundation.

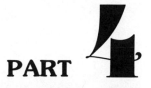

PART 4

SURGICAL REHABILITATION

INTRODUCTION AND OVERVIEW

Reconstructive orthopedic surgery has made revolutionary strides during the last ten years in the treatment of patients with joint diseases. Progress in this field can be attributed to a better understanding of the pathophysiology of the disease, the development of new prosthetic implants, including total joint replacements, and a greater emphasis on postoperative rehabilitation.

Historically, orthopedic surgery has been considered a last resort, to be tried after all else has failed, or reserved for joints that are nonfunctional. This is no longer true. Reconstructive surgery is now considered a part of total care for the person with chronic destructive joint disease. Consultation with an orthopedic surgeon *early*, before severe joint destruction occurs, allows the patient more surgical options and optimal timing of both preventive and corrective surgery.

The decision to perform surgery for arthritis must take into account a series of factors. The criteria common to all major surgery must be considered, including the patient's age, the diagnosis, secondary diagnoses, pain tolerance, postoperative complications, medications, family support, lifestyle, and psychological response to surgery. Ideally, all of these conditions should be favorable to the surgery being considered. In addition to these factors the decision to operate is based on several factors specific to the nature of chronic rheumatic disease.

A key consideration is how the surgery will affect the person's functional ability and, in turn, how the person's functional ability will affect the final surgical outcome. For example, the ability to ambulate and perform knee-strengthening exercises is critical to the success of total knee replacement surgery. If the patient also has painful hip disease that prevents ambulation or participation in therapy, he or she may not achieve satisfactory results from the knee surgery. The patient may possibly develop an extensor lag, instability, or a flexion contracture that could preclude ambulation, even if hip surgery were to be performed at a later date. To avoid these problems it would be preferable to operate on the hip first and the knee second. This can be done during either one or two hospitalizations.

The number of joints involved, the severity of the joint disease, and how the surgery will affect adjacent or contralateral joints all have critical implications for the decision regarding surgery for arthritis.

The extent of associated systemic involvement (particularly cardiac, pulmonary, and vascular systems) may preclude major surgery or the use of general anesthesia. In many facilities upper extremity surgery is performed under a regional block, and lower extremity surgery, including total hip and knee replacement surgery, can be carried out under a spinal anesthesia, without the risks of a general anesthesia. Anesthesia provided in this manner makes surgery possible for patients who have severe cervical spine disease and cannot be safely intubated for general anesthesia. It reduces the surgical risk for patients having multiple surgeries; it eliminates the unpleasantness of recovering from general anesthesia; and it is attractive to many patients who are fearful of being made unconscious.

Several surgeries require the active participation of the patient in postoperative therapy to achieve the desired results. There has been little research evaluating psychological factors in relation to the outcome of orthopedic surgery. A few years ago, a study of patients receiving total knee surgery at Rancho Los Amigos Hospital demonstrated that patients with significant depression attained poorer results than patients without depression.

To encourage or insure appropriate patient motivation for surgery, orthopedic surgeons generally do not try to convince patients to have surgery. They explain the options—risks and gains—and require the patient to make the decision. If a patient waits until the joint is so painful that he or she "can no longer stand it," surgery is often viewed as a positive experience; the patient looks forward to life without debilitating pain. A patient talked into surgery when he or she has only moderate pain may view the pain and stress of surgery with less enthusiasm. Having doubts about the value of surgery does not help to motivate a patient to participate fully in postoperative therapy.

A question that often arises is: How early should surgery be performed? Although the specific timing is different for each surgery, most surgeons are in agreement that surgery should be performed only after all conservative measures have been given a fair trial and the patient is stabilized on a medication regimen. Appropriate conservative treatment for rheumatoid arthritis would include adequate trials of both nonsteroidal anti-inflammatory drugs and remission-inducing drugs, steroid intra-articular injections, splints, ice and heat modalities, joint protection, and possibly biofeedback. Patients who have persistent synovitis and pain for 3 to 6 months, despite conservative measures, are considered possible candidates for joint surgery.

The role of the therapist in surgical treatment varies widely among medical facilities. Occupational therapists play a primary role in (1) *Functional evaluation,* before and after surgery; (2) *Rehabilitation,* before and after surgical procedures for the upper and lower extremities, through splinting, exercise, and selected functional activities; (3) *Patient education,* regarding joint protection, the use of splints, edema reduction, safety measures, and assistive equipment; (4) *ADL training,* instruction and practice in methods for incorporating postoperative precautions and restrictions in activities of daily living.

The protocols for OT and PT surgical assessment vary across the country. In some facilities, the referral to therapy occurs on the day intervention is required; in other facilities, the surgical protocol includes a preoperative OT and PT assessment with intervention scheduled as indicated. Having a routine preoperative assessment enables the therapist to evaluate the patient's preoperative functional ability and to appreciate the severity of the joint involvement and the impact that the surgery will have on the patient's functional ability. The preoperative assessment of ROM of the nonoperative joints provides a rational goal for postoperative ROM and edema reduction. Additionally the preoperative assessment enables the therapist to develop a rapport with the patient and to orient the patient to postoperative exercises and protocols when the patient is not experiencing surgical pain. This greatly enhances the patients ability to learn exercises following surgery.

The following surgical chapters outline the timing for postoperative management. These programs are designed to provide general guidelines and not to provide a ready made treatment protocol. Each treatment program should be modified to answer the patient's individual needs or to suit the personal philosophy of the surgeon. It is essential that the surgeon and therapist have direct communication and that together they establish the specific timing for preoperative and postoperative therapy.

13

HAND, WRIST,
AND FOREARM SURGERY

Hand and wrist surgery for rheumatoid arthritis can be divided into five groups: (1) synovectomy, (2) tenosynovectomy, (3) tendon surgery, (4) arthroplasty, and (5) arthrodesis.[1]*
Forearm surgery is limited to resection and replacement of the distal end of the ulna and the
proximal end of the radius. Resection of the distal ulna is usually done in conjunction with wrist
surgery and is discussed in this section, whereas radial head resection is frequently combined
with elbow synovectomy and is reviewed in Chapter 14, Elbow Surgery.

Since most of the muscles in the upper extremity cross more than one joint, there is considerable synchronization of function throughout the upper extremity. Arthritis in a single joint
affects all other joints to a greater or less degree. For example, decreased mobility in wrist flex-
ion/extension or forearm supination/pronation alters the biomechanics imposed on the elbow
and shoulder during functional activities. Thus, if a patient cannot supinate his or her wrist, he
or she can only position the palm by abducting and externally rotating the shoulder. All surgical
and splinting procedures must take into account the effect the process will have on adjacent
joints.

The wrist, particularly the area over the distal ulna, is often the most frequent site of involvement in RA and juvenile chronic polyarthritis and a common site in PA, SLE, SS, and
post-traumatic arthritis. The wrist provides the foundation for hand function. Pain solely in the
wrist can severely limit grip, pinch, dexterity, and functional use of the fingers. Often one of the
goals of wrist surgery is to improve function of the fingers.

Preoperative assessment of ROM, strength, sensation, and function prove extremely
valuable for establishing realistic goals for ROM and edema reduction following surgery.

The most extensive surgery is often performed on patients with rheumatoid arthritis;
therefore, RA will be used as a prototype for discussing hand surgery. Patients with other
diagnoses may require only one or a few of the surgeries used for RA.

The surgeries in this chapter will be listed according to the type of procedure and the
level of the lesion, distal to proximal, i.e., hand, wrist, forearm. This is done to impart some
sense of order and not to imply that surgery is necessarily performed in this sequence.

---

*References are listed at the end of each group.

SYNOVECTOMY

In the hand, synovectomy is performed on the wrist, MCP joints, and PIP joints.

Originally, the synovectomy procedure was developed on the concept that removal of the diseased tissue would prevent progression of the arthritis. Over the years, clinical experience and studies have shown that it is impossible to remove surgically all of the synovium in a joint and that it grows back.[2] Occasionally, it regenerates in a healthy form; more often, the synovitis reoccurs. Recent studies clearly indicate that there is a higher rate of reoccurrence in patients who have a more destructive arthritis.[2]

All deformities, joint destruction, and pathologic anatomy encountered in RA are the result of the way in which hypertrophied synovial tissue affects its surroundings. The excessive synovium stretches the joint capsule and adjacent structures. Additionally, the diseased synovium causes enzymatic destruction of articular cartilage and has the capacity to locally invade subchondral bone.[1]

Synovial tissue is the site of the inflammatory process. Removal of the synovium eliminates (at least temporarily) the inflammation, reduces intra-articular pressure, and eliminates tension placed on surrounding structures.[2]

Although a synovectomy cannot prevent progression of disease, it can play an important role in relieving symptoms and forestalling joint destruction in selected patients. This operation appears to be the most valuable to patients with low-grade, uncontrolled inflammation who have minimal or absent destruction of cartilage and bone.[2]

INDICATIONS

1. Pain and decreased function secondary to persistent, uncontrolled boggy synovitis of at least 3 months duration that is nonresponsive to corticosteroid injection and shows no evidence of cartilage destruction.
2. To protect joint structures.

OCCURRENCE

All inflammatory arthritides.

SURGICAL AND FUNCTIONAL GOALS

Postsurgical expectations are relief of pain, decreased inflammation and swelling, return of ROM loss due to the swelling, and improved function due to the elimination of pain.

SURGICAL PREREQUISITES

1. Smooth joint motion, absence of crepitus, or x-ray changes of cartilage destruction.
2. Absence of infection.

Wrist Synovectomy

SURGICAL PROCEDURE

1. Approach: Dorsal, slightly curved, or longitudinal incision.
2. Dorsal retinaculum is reflected.
3. Dorsal tenosynovectomy is performed as necessary.
4. Transverse capsular incision is made.
5. Synovium is removed from the radiocarpal and involved intercarpal joints. (Total or complete synovectomy is not possible due to anatomic restraints.)
6. A portion of the retinaculum is relocated deep to the extensor tendons.
7. A drain is used for 24 hours to prevent hematoma.

POSTOPERATIVE MANAGEMENT

Average hospitalization: 3 to 5 days.
1. Initially, the hand is in a voluminous compression bandage and elevated to reduce edema. A plaster splint is used to immobilize the wrist in neutral to allow capsular healing; it should not interfere with MCP joint or thumb motion.
2. Second or third day: Bandage is reduced. Active and passive finger ROM is started. (Patient may have difficulty with active finger extension due to swelling around the tendons.)
3. Approximately twelfth to fourteenth day: Dressing and sutures are removed. Gentle active and passive wrist ROM is started. (ROM is done to tolerance; it is not as critical to push for full ROM in the wrist as it is in the digits.) Warm water soaks facilitate motion. Lotion massage reduces induration, improves skin tone, and helps decrease skin sensitivity. Patient may use a thermoplastic or commercial wrist splint as needed for comfort.

MCP Joint Synovectomy

SURGICAL PROCEDURE

1. Approach: Transverse incision is used for multiple joints and a longitudinal incision is used for single joint.
2. Extensor mechanisms are incised along the ulnar border.
3. The ulnar intrinsic muscles are released if they are tight.
4. Extensor tendons are retracted radialward.
5. Joint capsules are incised longitudinally.
6. Synovium is removed; attention is given to the areas deep to the collateral ligaments.
7. Capsules are closed. This may be combined with a radial collateral ligament repair or shortening.
8. Extensor tendons may be centralized if necessary.
9. A drain is used for 24 hours to prevent a hematoma.

POSTOPERATIVE MANAGEMENT

Average hospitalization: 3 to 5 days.
1. Initially, the hand is in a voluminous compression dressing with a volar plaster splint. The splint should maintain the wrist in approximately 20 to 30 degrees of extension and the MCP joints in approximately 30 degrees of flexion; it should not block PIP joint or thumb motion.
2. Second day: Gentle active and passive ROM is started for the MCP, PIP, and DIP joints. During hospitalization, the patient should have exercises supervised by a therapist 2 or 3 times a day. The splint can be removed during the exercises. When the splint is on, the patient is encouraged to actively move the PIP joints as much as possible to help reduce edema.
3. Fouth day: A dynamic MCP extension splint may be used to support the digits in extension and radial deviation if necessary. Care should be taken not to splint the fourth and fifth MCP joints in full extension, since maintaining full flexion is critical in these joints for tight grasp. The dynamic splint is used during the day, and the plaster splint is used at night. A dynamic splint is the most effective way to maintain alignment and encourage motion. (See Chapter 25 for information on postsurgical splinting.)
4. Twelfth and fourteeth day: Dressing and sutures are removed. Warm water soaks and massage can be added to the program to increase mobility. ROM and strengthening exercises should progress as tolerated. The goal of therapy is full active and passive ROM.

PIP Joint Synovectomy

SURGICAL PROCEDURE

1. Approach: Exposure of the PIP joint is more difficult than exposure of the MCP joint due to the extensor mechanism and snug collateral ligaments. The extensor mechanism can be divided longitudinally or reflected along one margin. Some surgeons routinely divide a collateral ligament and spread the joint laterally to facilitate exposure.[3] (This method would necessitate a delay in beginning active postoperative motion.)
2. Synovectomy is performed.
3. Divided and incised structures are repaired, and the wound is closed.

POSTOPERATIVE MANAGEMENT

Average hospitalization: 3 to 5 days.
1. Initially, the digit is in a voluminous compression dressing with the joint held in slight flexion (approximately 10 to 15 degrees).
2. Second or third day: Dressing is reduced. Active motion is encouraged but is usually limited by pain and swelling. Active and passive exercises are delayed until pain and swelling decrease and the exercises can be tolerated.
3. Fifth day: The main risks of this surgery are stiffness (i.e., loss of active motion because of immobilization and swelling) and lack of full extension because of damage

to or stretching of the extensor mechanism. Flexion is usually regained easier than extension, so the goal of early therapy is to regain extension and then focus on gaining flexion.

For patients with an extensor lag, a dynamic PIP extension splint (such as an LMB Spring Extension Splint[4]) is used during the day, and an aluminum and foam static splint is used at night. Gentle ROM and strengthening exercises are progressed to tolerance. Strengthening of both the extensor communis muscle and the interossei muscles should be done.

4. Twelfth to fourteenth day: Stitches are removed. Splints are used until lag is resolved.

References (Synovectomy)

1. Nalebuff, E. A.: *Present status of rheumatoid hand surgery.* Am. J. Surg. 122:304, 1971.
2. Gschwend, N.: *Synovectomy.* In Kelley, W. M., et al. (eds.): *Textbook of Rheumatology.* W. B. Saunders, Philadelphia, 1981.
3. Lipscomb, P. R.: *Synovectomy of the distal two joints of the thumb and fingers in rheumatoid arthritis.* J. Bone Joint Surg. 49A:1135, 1967.
4. LMB Hand Rehab Products, Inc., P.O. Box 1181, San Luis Obispo, CA 93406.

TENOSYNOVECTOMY

Tenosynovectomy is considered preventive as well as corrective surgery. Several large series have supported the use of tenosynovectomies to prevent tendon rupture and other complications of chronic tenosynovitis.

There are four locations in the hand where the tendons pass through synovial lined sheaths. The purpose of the sheath is to facilitate gliding, particularly where the tendon must slide over several joints. The four locations are the dorsum of the wrist, the volar aspect of the wrist, flexor surface of the fingers, and the volar aspect of the thumb, which contains the sheath for the flexor pollicis longus. The clinical symptoms vary at each site due to the anatomic differences at each level.[5]

The synovium lining the tendon sheaths is similar to the synovium in the joints and subject to the same changes. When synovitis occurs, excess fluid builds up in the sheath. The sheath has a closed double wall construction, and the fluid becomes trapped between the inner and outer walls. If the synovitis becomes chronic, the synovium will become thickened and hypertrophied. The inflammatory process through an enzymatic process weakens the integrity of the tendons, making them more susceptible to rupture. In confined areas, the excess tissue may cause sufficient pressure to compromise the vascular supply to the tendon, resulting in ischemic areas. Additionally, chronic synovitis can result in granulomatous plaques (tendon nodules) forming on the surface of the tendons. These plaques can invade the inner substance of the tendons, causing tendon disruption and increasing the risk of rupture.[5,6,7]

Dorsal Wrist Tenosynovectomy

At the dorsum of the wrist, the finger and wrist extensor tendons pass through six separate compartments. The tendons in each compartment are surrounded by a synovial sheath, which extends approximately one-half inch proximal and distal to the retinaculum. The dorsal retinaculum ligament forms the dorsal surface of the tendon compartments. Vertical septa extend from the retinaculum to the radius and ulna, forming the walls of the tendon compartments.[6] Tenosynovitis can occur in a single compartment or in all six. In the early stages, the swelling usually conforms to the boundaries of each sheath. Tenosynovitis of compartments two through five is generally not painful.[7] (If a person has wrist pain, it is usually due to concomitant radiocarpal or radioulnar joint pain.) However, tenosynovitis of the first compartment (de Quervain's syndrome) or the sixth compartment can be very painful. It is believed that these two compartments are painful because they are adjacent to the dorsal branches of the radial and ulnar nerves. Dorsal tenosynovitis is readily apparent because the skin over the hand is thin and conforms to the swelling. (See Figure 52.)

The main consequence of chronic dorsal tenosynovitis is rupture of the finger and thumb extensors. The tendons most frequently ruptured are the extensor digiti quinti, extensor communis (four and five), and extensor pollicis longus. Rupture results from infiltration of the disease into the tendons and attrition or wearing away of the tendon over bony spurs or rough edges of subluxed joints. Most extensor tendon ruptures occur at the wrist level.[8]

Chronic tenosynovitis of the sixth compartment threatens the integrity of the extensor carpi ulnaris tendon, considered a key tendon for maintaining the stability of the wrist.[9] If the ligaments that maintain the alignment of the tendon become stretched, the tendon can migrate volar to become a strong flexor force contributing to volar subluxation of the carpus.[9]

Dorsal tenosynovectomy with retinacular relocation is considered the treatment of choice for persistent dorsal tenosynovitis. Ideally, it should be performed before tendon rupture occurs.[7]

INDICATIONS

1. Persistent dorsal tenosynovitis despite 3 to 6 months of adequate medical management.
2. Extensor tendon rupture.
3. Rapid proliferation of the tenosynovitis.

OCCURRENCE

Rheumatoid arthritis and chronic juvenile polyarthritis.

SURGICAL AND FUNCTIONAL GOALS

Prevention of further destruction by removing the inflamed tenosynovium and protection of the tendons by relocating the synovial lined retinacular ligament beneath the tendons.[8]

Postsurgical expectations are decrease in swelling, improved comfort, particularly if combined with a wrist synovectomy, improved appearance, and possibly an increase in wrist ROM.

SURGICAL PREREQUISITES

No specific prerequisites.

SURGICAL PROCEDURE

This procedure may be combined with a wrist synovectomy, wrist fusion, extensor tendon repair, or excision of the distal ulna.

1. Approach: Slightly curved longitudinal incision over the dorsum of the wrist.
2. Dorsal retinacular ligament is reflected.
3. Diseased tenosynovium is removed from around the extensor tendons and from beneath the retinacular ligament.
4. Synovium is removed from the wrist joint.
5. Dorsal retinacular ligament is placed beneath the extensor tendons to protect them from further damage.
6. Distal ulna may be resected at the same time (Darrach procedure). Silastic ulnar head prosthesis may or may not be implanted.

POSTOPERATIVE MANAGEMENT

Average hospitalization: 3 to 5 days.

1. Initially, the hand is immobilized in a compression dressing with a volar plaster splint to hold the wrist in extension and the MCP joints in 40-degrees of flexion.
2. Second day: Dressing is reduced. Active and passive MCP extension, PIP, DIP, and thumb ROM is started.
3. Tenth to fourteenth day: Sutures and dressing are removed. Active wrist flexion, extension, pronation, and supination exercises are started. Exercise is modified if additional surgical procedures are carried out simultaneously. If a patient has an MCP extension lag, consider using a dynamic MCP extension splint. (See Chapter 25.) Care should be taken not to splint the ring and little finger in full extension.
4. Third to fourth week: If a wrist synovectomy was also done, a volar wrist splint should be used between exercise periods.

Wrist Volar Tenosynovectomy

At the wrist level, the nine long flexor tendons of the fingers and thumb are enclosed in tendon sheaths as they pass through the narrow carpal tunnel. The tunnel is formed by a concave formation of the carpal bones on three sides and the transverse carpal ligament on the fourth or volar surface.[7] The tunnel is very narrow and affords a passageway for the four tendons of the flexor digitorum profundus and four tendons of the flexor digitorum superficialis enclosed in one sheath and the flexor pollicis longus in a separate sheath and the median nerve. The position of the median nerve between the flexor tendons and the unyielding volar carpal ligament makes it very susceptible to compression or entrapment (carpal tunnel syndrome), if there is any swelling in the carpal tunnel.[10] Hypertrophy of the tenosynovium can cause sufficient pressure to compromise the blood supply to the nerve resulting in ischemia and loss of nerve function.[10] Distal to the transverse carpal ligament, the recurrent motor branch on the median nerve supplies the abductor pollicis brevis and the opponens pollicis, the flexor pollicis brevis (superficial head), and the first and second lumbricals.[7] The sensory branch supplies the volar aspect of the thumb, index, and middle fingers and the radial half of the ring finger. Damage to this nerve can severely reduce hand dexterity and function. The ulnar nerve is superficial to the transverse carpal ligament and, therefore, is not vulnerable to compression from flexor tenosynovitis.

The transverse carpal ligament is covered by the volar carpal ligament and thick palmar fascia at the distal edge. Therefore, tenosynovitis in the palmar sheaths or deep in the tunnel can be extensive without the obvious swelling. Tenosynovitis generally occurs without pain. If there is wrist pain, it is usually due to concomitant radiocarpal synovitis or compression of the median nerve.[7] In addition to nerve entrapment, chronic tenosynovitis can invade the tendons and result in tendon rupture. The flexor pollicis longus and profundus tendons are the most likely to rupture, since they lie next to the carpal bones. However, rupture of the flexor tendons is less common than rupture of the extensor tendons.[7]

A common and often overlooked complication of flexor tenosynovitis is limited tendon excursion or "bound down" tendons. If this occurs, it can limit *active flexion* or *passive extension*. If excursion in a proximal direction is limited, the person will have incomplete active flexion but greater or possibly full passive flexion. Whenever a person has a ROM lag in all four digits, binding of the finger flexors at the wrist level should be evaluated. If excursion of the tendons is limited in a distal direction, the patient will not be able to achieve full active or passive extension of all digit and wrist joints. They will have a tenodesis action in the hand, e.g., the digits will be able to extend fully only when the wrist is flexed. If this problem is not treated promptly, first by conservative measures (i.e., steroid injection and ice compresses) or by surgery, the muscle can become fibrosed in a shortened position and the digits can develop fixed contractures due to the lack of active motion.

Flexor tendon excursion can become limited at the wrist level or at the digit level. When all four digits are limited, the problem can usually be traced to the wrist. If only one or two fingers are limited, they are most likely in the digital sheath.

The most frequent problem that necessitates flexor tenosynovectomy is median nerve entrapment (carpal tunnel syndrome). Initially, patients complain of tingling and numbness at night. They should be treated by conservative measures in the early phase,[10] i.e., splinting or steroid injection and splinting. A patient is a candidate for surgery if a three-month trial of conservative measures has not alleviated the symptoms; if the symptoms are constant day and night; if there is diminished two point discrimination; and if there is weakness of the abductor pollicis brevis muscle (this muscle will show motor impairment first). Once the impingement is severe enough to cause motor or significant sensory loss, conservative measures will not help. Prompt surgery improves the possibility of full return of nerve function.

INDICATIONS

1. Carpal tunnel syndrome, secondary to flexor tenosynovitis, that is nonresponsive to conservative treatment or presents with median nerve motor and sensory loss.
2. Rupture of a long flexor tendon at the wrist level.
3. Decreased excursion of the flexor tendons.
4. Decreased excursion of the flexor pollicis longus tendon secondary to wrist flexor tenosynovitis.

OCCURRENCE

Rheumatoid arthritis and chronic juvenile polyarthritis.

SURGICAL AND FUNCTIONAL GOALS

To relieve pressure on the median nerve. When nerve impairment has not been of long duration, full sensory and motor recovery is expected. The surgery can prevent further destruction or rupture of the tendons by removing the diseased synovium. [7]

SURGICAL PREREQUISITES

Carpal tunnel syndrome needs to be clearly established. Nerve impingement at the cervical spine level needs to be ruled out as a possible cause of sensory and motor loss in the hand.

SURGICAL PROCEDURE (for rheumatoid arthritis)

1. Approach: Curved incision along the thenar crease with a zigzag incision proximal to the wrist (to minimize scarring across transverse wrist crease).
2. Palmar fascia divided longitudinally. (Terminal branches of the palmar cutaneous nerve should not be cut; damage may result in persistent local tenderness.) [12]
3. Median nerve identified proximal to wrist.
4. Transverse carpal ligament divided along the ulnar border, exposing contents of carpal canal.
5. Diseased synovium removed from the superficialis tendons. They are cleaned sufficiently to allow independent action. Adhesions between the profundus tendons may not be extensively removed, since independent action is less important in these tendons.
6. Internal neurolysis of the median nerve may be carried out for severe cases of compression.
7. Any bony spicules are removed from the floor of the canal.
8. Traction is applied to individual tendons to evaluate digital tendon motion. If the tendons are not pulling through, a digital flexor tenosynovectomy may be done.
9. The transverse carpal ligament is *not* repaired, so pressure cannot reoccur in the canal.
10. The wound is closed and a drain is used for 24 hours to prevent a hematoma.

POSTOPERATIVE MANAGEMENT

Average hospitalization: 3 to 5 days. (Patients are usually kept in the hospital until swelling has decreased and the tendons are moving smoothly.)
1. Initially, the hand is in a voluminous compression bandage with a plaster splint. The splint should maintain the wrist in approximately 25 degrees of extension to keep the flexor tendons in the carpal tunnel and thus prevent bowstringing during the healing process.
2. Second or third day: Dressing is reduced. Active and passive finger motion is started three times a day to tolerance. Excessive bleeding occasionally occurs and can delay

exercises, although some gentle motion should be done each day. The profundus and superficialis tendons for each finger should be exercised individually. (This is done by using the same positioning procedures as for individual muscle testing.)

3. Tenth to twelfth day: Dressing and sutures are removed. Begin warm water soaks and massage to increase mobility. Light strengthening exercises can be started, using a soft sponge ball or soft Theraplast. A Futuro or thermoplastic wrist splint is recommended for a few weeks for support and comfort.

Digital Flexor Tenosynovitis

The tendon sheaths for the long finger flexors start at the volar aspect of the MCP joints and extend the length of the finger. The sheath for the flexor pollicis longus extends the entire length of the tendon from the IP joint of the thumb to one inch proximal to the volar carpal ligament.[13]

The sheath and tendons are held in place by fibrous bands. At the point where the tendons cross the digit joints, the bands become thick and are referred to as annular ligaments or pulleys. Their primary function is to prevent bowstringing of the tendons during pinch and grip activities.[13,14]

Granulomatous masses (nodules) may form on the surface of the tendons with or without tenosynovitis. These nodules can be particularly troublesome, since they can catch on annular ligaments during tendon motion and prevent tendon excursion, a condition commonly referred to as trigger finger. Tendon nodules or excessive tenosynovium can get caught in the annular ligaments and cause the digit to painfully lock in flexion or extension. This occurs most frequently at the level of the MCP joint, but it can occur at the PIP level in the fingers and the IP level in the thumb.[7,14]

In the early stages of tenosynovitis, just the sheath effusion alone can limit full excursion of the profundus tendon. Patients may have swollen fingers, without pain or warmth and may not be able to actively flex their DIP joints fully. If the condition becomes chronic, the tenosynovium hypertrophies and crepitus with motion is common. The excess diseased tissue may prevent the tendon from gliding or it can infiltrate the tendon and result in a rupture.[7]

It is not uncommon for people with normal PIP joints to develop PIP joint contractures secondary to the flexor tenosynovitis. These contractures remain after the tenosynovitis resolves.[15]

INDICATIONS

1. Persistent, painful, or dysfunctional trigger finger that does not respond to conservative treatment.
2. Marked tenosynovial hypertrophy, resulting in limited tendon excursion. (This is demonstrated by a discrepancy in active and passive ROM.)

OCCURRENCE

Rheumatoid arthritis and chronic juvenile polyarthritis.

SURGICAL AND FUNCTIONAL GOALS

For trigger finger, the goal is to relieve pain and restore function. For chronic tenosynovitis, the goal is to improve ROM and function and to protect the tendons from further damage and prevent tendon rupture.[7]

SURGICAL PREREQUISITES

Intact tendons.

SURGICAL PROCEDURE

1. Approach: For multiple digits, an incision is made along the distal palmar crease (see Fig. 80) to expose the tendons. It may be possible to remove sufficient synovium from this incision; if not, a zigzag incision is made along the volar aspect of the digit to expose the tendon distally.
2. The tendon sheath is opened, and diseased tenosynovium and adhesions between the tendons are removed. Any nodules (localized granulomas) are also removed.

POSTOPERATIVE MANAGEMENT

Average hospitalization: 3 to 5 days.

1. Initially, the hand is in a voluminous compression dressing with a volar plaster splint. The splint should maintain the wrist in approximately 20 degrees of extension and the MCP joints in about 30 degrees of flexion. The MCP joints should be blocked to encourage tendon function at the PIP joints. If this is not done, patients tend to flex their MCP joints using their intrinsic muscles and then have difficulty using their long flexors in this position.
2. Second day: Dressing is reduced. Active and passive ROM exercises are started for the PIP and DIP joints. Slight resistance to flexion, applied at the finger pad, provides additional proprioceptive feedback and encourages active motion. The profundus and superficialis tendons should have active ROM exercise separately for each. This is performed in the same manner as individual muscle testing.
3. Third day: Splint should be removed at least three times a day for ROM of the wrist and MCP joints. Tendon ROM exercises are progressed to tolerance.
4. Tenth to twelfth day: Dressing and sutures are removed. Warm water soaks and massage are added to the program to encourage motion. The splint is discontinued. An MCP block may be used during the exercise sessions. Strengthening exercises are progressed to tolerance. Exercises are continued until there is no lag in digit motion and grip strength is at an appropriate level for the patient.

References (Tenosynovectomy)

5. Nalebuff, E. A.: *Present status of rheumatoid hand surgery.* Am. J. Surg. 122:304, 1971.
6. Linscheid, R. L., and Dobyns, J. H.: *Rheumatoid arthritis of the wrist.* Orthop. Clin. North Am. 2:3, 1971.

7. Millender, L. H., and Nalebuff, E. A.: *Preventive surgery: Tenosynovectomy and synovectomy.* Orthop. Clin. North Am. 6(3):76, 1975.
8. Kessler, L., and Vainio, K.: *Posterior (dorsal) synovectomy for rheumatoid involvement of the hand and wrist. A followup study of sixty six procedures.* J. Bone Joint Surg. 48:1048, 1966.
9. Flatt, A.: *The Care of the Rheumatoid Hand,* ed. 3. C. V. Mosby, St. Louis, 1974, pp. 102-103.
10. Phalen, G. S.: *Reflections on 21 years experience with carpal-tunnel syndrome.* J. A. M. A. 212:1365, 1970.
11. Clawson, D. K., and Convery, F. R.: *Surgery in rheumatoid arthritis of the wrist.* In Cruess, R., and Mitchell, N. (eds.): *Surgery of Rheumatoid Arthritis.* J. B. Lippincott, Philadelphia, 1971.
12. Nalebuff, E. A., and Smith, J.: *Preservation of terminal branches of the median palmar cutaneous nerve in carpal tunnel surgery.* Orthopedics 2(4):370, 1979.
13. Doyle, J. R.: *Anatomy of the flexor tendon sheath and pulleys of the thumb.* J. Hand Surg. 2(2):149, 1977.
14. Ferlic, D. C., and Clayton, M. L.: *Flexor tenosynovectomy in the rheumatoid finger.* J. Hand Surg. 3(4):364, 1978.
15. Millis, M. B., Millender, L. H., and Nalebuff, E. A.: *Stiffness of the PIP joints in rheumatoid arthritis.* J. Bone Joint Surg. 58A(6):801, 1976.

TENDON SURGERY

Surgical procedures performed on or with tendons are considered restorative or corrective procedures, since they are performed *after* a specific deformity occurs. Synovectomy and tenosynovectomy are considered prophylactic surgical procedures, since they are often done to prevent certain consequences of chronic synovitis.[16]

Restorative tendon surgery for arthritis includes tendon relocation, tendon repair and adjacent suture, tendon transfer, tenotomy, and tendon release.[16]

Extensor Tendon Relocation

Migration or dislocation of the long finger extensor tendons into the ulnar valleys between the MCP heads is a common sequela of chronic synovitis of the MCP joints. When this occurs, the extensor tendons become ulnar deviators of the MCP joint and lose their mechanical leverage for extending the joint.[17] Once the tendons have slipped volar to the axis of the MCP joint, the patient is unable to actively extend the fingers at this level. However, the patient *is* able to maintain the joints in active extension, if the joints are passively aligned. Having the patient maintain passive extension then becomes a specific maneuver or test for ruling out the possibility of ruptured extensor tendons, the primary differential diagnosis.

If this migration process occurs in a patient with moderate MCP ulnar drift, the ulnar placement of the tendons can become a major dynamic force contributing to severe ulnar drift. In most cases the tendon slippage occurs after severe ulnar drift is in existence. In these cases, it is considered a consequence of MCP ulnar drift, not a causal factor.[18] (Prior to 1960 and E. M. Smith's work[18] on the role of the flexor tendons in ulnar drift, ulnar dislocation of the extensor tendons was erroneously thought to be a prime *causal* factor of MCP ulnar drift.)

INDICATIONS

Tendon relocation as a sole surgical procedure is done in a selected group of patients who have well-preserved joint cartilage and in whom the condition can easily be passively corrected.[1]

OCCURRENCE

Rheumatoid arthritis, systemic lupus erythematosus.

SURGICAL PREREQUISITES

Intact tendons and well-preserved joint surfaces and easy passive correctability.

SURGICAL PROCEDURE

This surgery is often combined with MCP synovectomy.
1. Dorsal transverse or longitudinal incision.
2. Shortened transverse fibers on the ulnar side of the extensor mechanism are divided.
3. The ulnar intrinsic insertion is released.
4. Extensor tendons are relocated and held in position by reefing stitches in the elongated radial transverse fibers.
5. In severe cases of MCP ulnar drift, the radial collateral ligaments are shortened.
6. In certain cases, extensor tendons may be sutured to the base of the proximal phalanx.
7. A drain is used only if the surgery is done in conjunction with a synovectomy.

POSTOPERATIVE MANAGEMENT

Average hospitalization: 3 to 5 days.
1. First to third day: Immobilization in a compression dressing with a volar plaster splint to support the MCP joints in maximal or neutral extension and the PIP joints in moderate flexion.
2. Gentle active assistive ROM to all hand and wrist joints.
3. Dynamic MCP extension assist splint is applied to maintain the MCP joint in extension during the day. This splint is recommended for at least 6 weeks. A thermoplastic wrist MCP stabilization splint should be used for 6 to 8 weeks at night to support the MCP joints in a functional position and prevent prolonged full flexion.

Tendon Repair and Transfer

The most frequent causes of tendon rupture are tenosynovitis compromising the integrity of the tendons (attentuation or compression) or attrition over rough edges of carpal bones (Fig. 2).[19]

Rupture of the finger extensors usually occurs at the distal end of the ulna. The extensor pollicis longus tendon commonly ruptures at Lister's tubercle, where the tendon turns towards the thumb. Flexor tendons most frequently rupture over the scaphoid bone. However, they can rupture at the digit or palm level.[19,20] (See Fig. 2.)

The following tendons have the highest incidence of rupture (listed in order of most frequent occurrence): extensor digitorum quinti (EDQ), extensor communis (EC) [fifth and fourth are the most frequent], extensor pollicis longus (EPL), flexor pollicis longus (FPL), flexor

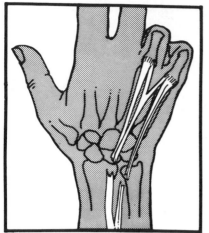

FIGURE 2. The digit extensor tendons typically rupture at the wrist level because of attrition. The extensor digiti quinti and the extensor communis tendons to the little and ring fingers are often the first to rupture.

digitorum profundus (FDP) to the index finger. Rupture of the extensor indicis proprius (EIP) is rare.[20]

In some cases, it is possible to complete an end-to-end repair of the ruptured tendon. But in most cases, the rupture is too long-standing, the gap between the ends cannot be reduced, or the proximal motors adhere or retract with loss of their normal excursion. For these reasons, in rheumatoid arthritis, tendon function is restored by attaching the distal stump to a healthy adjacent tendon or by transferring another musculotendon unit to the distal stump. With either procedure, a tenosynovectomy is also performed to protect the repaired tendon and adjacent tendons from further damage.[20]

Adjacent suture is the method of choice for single extensor tendon ruptures. Tendon transfers provide a better solution when multiple tendons are ruptured.[20]

One of the most commonly used tendon transfers is the use of the extensor indicis proprius. The EIP is ideal since it is expendable, has independent action, and can reach any digit including the thumb. It also can be used for extensor tendon ruptures of the fourth and fifth digits. The EIP tendon is transferred to the distal stump of the EDQ tendon and the EC tendon of the ring finger is sutured to the adjacent intact extensor of the middle finger.[20] It is not uncommon to find patients who have ruptured the EDQ and the third and fourth EC tendons. In these cases, one of three transfers might be considered: an FDS tendon can be used; if the patient has limited wrist motion or is to have a wrist fusion, the extensor carpi radialis longus tendon is a possibility; or if the thumb MCP joint requires fusion, the EPL can be spared.

Ruptures of the flexor tendons pose special problems because of the tendency for tendon adhesions to form within the tendon sheath. If one of the profundus tendons ruptures and the proximal end retracts, it may not be possible to perform an end-to-end repair. In these cases, the treatment of choice may be to excise the FDP tendon and fuse the DIP joint. For a rupture of the sublimus tendon in the digit sheath, the treatment of choice is to excise the remaining FDS tendon and perform a synovectomy of the tendon sheath to protect and insure smooth gliding of the healthy profundus tendon. (In these cases, repair of the FDS may only increase the risk of adhesions, while not improving function.)[20]

Rupture of both the FDP and FDS tendons can occur, usually in the index finger, and results in loss of control of the index PIP and DIP joints. Patients with this problem tend to have severe hand involvement. The most reasonable approach may be to fuse the PIP and DIP joints in a functional position and strengthen the intrinsic muscles for MCP flexion. This provides the patient with a stable post for writing, pinch prehension, and so forth. If fusion is not desired, a two-stage tendon graft or tendon transfer can be performed. But these procedures are complex and generally reserved for trauma cases and rarely indicated in RA.[20]

INDICATIONS

Ruptured or attenuated tendon.

OCCURRENCE

Primarily rheumatoid arthritis.

SURGICAL AND FUNCTIONAL GOALS

The extensor mechanism is restored by reattaching the distal stump to an adjacent intact musculotendon unit or by transforming another musculotendon unit to the distal stump.
Postsurgical expectation is restoration of active joint extension.

SURGICAL PREREQUISITES

1. Normal passive motion of the joints distal to the rupture.
2. Intact adjacent musculotendon units or units that can be transferred.
3. Patient motivation to follow through with an exacting, often slowly progressive, rehabilitation course.

SURGICAL PROCEDURE

There are several surgical options for repair, depending on the status of adjacent tendons or available motor units for transfer. These options include suture to an adjoining tendon, tendon transfer, or tendon graft.[20]
1. For rupture of the extensor communis tendon:
    a. Approach: Dorsal, slightly curved or longitudinal incision.
    b. Dorsal tenosynovectomy (the removal of synovium from around the extensor tendons and relocation of synovial lined retinacular ligament beneath tendons to avoid recurrence).
    c. Suture of the distal stump of the ruptured tendon to an adjacent musculotendon unit or transfer of another tendon to the ruptured distal stump.
    d. Procedure is frequently combined with complete or partial resection (modified Darrach procedure) of the ulnar head and wrist joint synovectomy when rupture was due in part to attrition by the distal ulna.

2. For rupture of the extensor pollicis longus: The extensor indicis proprius is transferred to the extensor pollicis longus and sutured over the dorsum of the thumb MP joint.

POSTOPERATIVE MANAGEMENT

Average hospitalization: 2 to 5 days.
1. First four weeks:
   a. For communis repairs, initial immobilization: short arm splint with wrist in moderate (approximately 25 degrees) extension and MCP joints in slight flexion.
   b. For extensor pollicis repairs, splint wrist in slight ulnar extension and thumb in extension. The thumb in midrange between abduction and extension.
2. About fourth week:
   a. Splint can be removed intermittently to begin therapy.
   b. When surgery involves tendon transfer, muscle re-education is started with repetitive active extension (with or without splint). The amount of muscle re-education required depends upon the tendon transferred. If the flexor digitorum superficialis is transferred to an extensor, re-education can be extensive. (See section on muscle strengthening in Exercise Treatment, Chapter 29, for specific techniques.) Active or passive flexion is avoided. Electrical stimulation may be helpful if there is excessive scarring. Electromyogram (EMG) biofeedback can facilitate the re-education process.
3. About fifth week:
   a. Muscle re-education is continued.
   b. Active flexion can be started.
   c. Use of the resting splint may be continued between exercise sessions and at night.
4. About fifth to sixth weeks:
   a. Splint is discontinued.
   b. Hand can be used in light functional activities.
   c. Muscle re-education may or may not be needed.
   d. Functional activities are gradually increased. Strong resisted flexion and extension should be avoided for an additional two to three weeks. Activities such as transferring with pressure on a dorsum of the hand should always be avoided.
   e. Active and light resistive exercises to strengthen the repaired tendons.

References (Tendon Surgery)

16. Millender, L. H., and Nalebuff, E. A.: *Preventive surgery — Tenosynovectomy and synovectomy.* Symposium on Rheumatoid Arthritis. Orthop. Clin. North Am. 6(2):765, 1975.
17. Flatt, A.: *The Care of the Rheumatoid Hand,* ed. 3. C. V. Mosby, St. Louis, 1974, pp. 72-74.
18. Smith, E. M., Juvinall, R., Bender, L., and Pearson, J.: *Role of the finger flexors in rheumatoid deformities of the MCP joints.* Arthritis Rheum. 7:467, 1964.
19. Boyes, J. H.: *Tendons.* In Boyes, J. H. (ed.): *Bunnell's Surgery of the Hand,* ed. 5. J. B. Lippincott, Philadelphia, 1970, pp. 393-436.
20. Nalebuff, E. A.: *The recognition and treatment of tendon ruptures in the rheumatoid hand.* American Academy of Orthopedic Surgeons: *Symposium on Tendon Surgery in the Hand.* C. V. Mosby, St. Louis, 1975, pp. 255-269.

ADDITIONAL SOURCES

Cohen, J.: *Occupational therapy following hand tendon surgery.* In American Academy of Orthopedic Surgeons: *Symposium on Tendon Surgery in the Hand.* C. V. Mosby, St. Louis, 1975, p. 292.

McCann, V. H., Phillips, C. A., and Quigley, T. R.: *Preoperative and postoperative management: The role of allied health professionals.* Symposium on Rheumatoid Arthritis Orthop. Clin. North Am. 6:881, 1975.

SURGERY FOR BOUTONNIERE DEFORMITY

When it is associated with arthritis, the boutonniere deformity results from synovitis in the PIP joint altering the tendon balance in the finger. The complete deformity has three components: (1) PIP joint flexion, (2) DIP hyperextension, and (3) MCP joint hyperextension.[21]

Synovial hypertrophy stretches the extensor mechanism. The central slip becomes unable to support the PIP joint in full extension. The lateral bands become displaced volarly and result in shortening of the transverse retinacular ligaments. This secondary shortening leads to distal joint hyperextension and limited flexion. When the PIP flexion deformity becomes marked, the patient compensates by hyperextending the MCP joint.[21]

In the early stages, functional loss is related as much to the lack of full DIP joint flexion as to the lack of PIP joint extension. Severe deformity resulting in the inability to extend the PIP joint to grasp objects becomes the major hindrance. The recommended surgical procedures vary, depending on the severity of the deformity.

EARLY BOUTONNIERE. An extensor tenotomy (tendon division) is a simple procedure that can correct the DIP joint hyperextension component of the deformity and aids extension of the PIP joint by altering the balance of forces.[22] The procedure is done under local anesthesia and involves a longitudinal incision over the middle phalanx. The extensor mechanism is divided obliquely or transversely. Postoperative management includes active antideformity exercises, i.e., DIP joint flexion with the PIP joint supported in extension; daytime dynamic splinting of the PIP joint with a reverse knuckle bender splint for 4 to 6 weeks; and night splinting of the PIP joint in extension with an aluminum finger splint. If there is a lag in DIP joint extension immediately postoperatively, it can usually be corrected with splinting in extension.

MODERATE BOUTONNIERE. Once the patient loses 40 to 50 degrees of extension of the PIP joint, functional loss becomes more significant. The deformity may be reducible or fixed in this stage. The objective of surgery is to restore PIP joint extension by tightening the central slip and relocating the lateral bands. This extensor reconstruction is combined with an extensor tenotomy to correct DIP joint limitations.[21]

If there is PIP joint synovitis, a preoperative trial of steroid injection and dynamic splinting is done to shrink the capsular structures and to stretch out soft tissues that restrict extension.[21]

The surgery involves a dorsal longitudinal curved incision over the PIP joint. The central slip is divided distally and separated from the lateral bands proximally. Approximately, one quarter of an inch of the central slip is excised and the remaining portion is reattached to the base of the middle phalanx.[21] Two relaxing incisions are made just volar to the lateral bands. These divide the transverse retinacular ligaments and make it possible to bring the lateral bands dorsally so they can be sutured to the central slip or to each other.[21] A tenotomy is done, which essentially places all of the extensor forces at the PIP joint level.[22] The action of the oblique retinacular ligament is considered responsible for preventing a mallet finger from occurring.[23] Following the reconstruction, it should be possible to passively flex the PIP joints 70 or 80 degrees; the remainder is gained in postoperative therapy.[23] A Kirschner wire is placed across the PIP joint to maintain full extension during the early postoperative phase, which lasts three to four weeks.

Postoperative management includes active DIP joint motion; dynamic daytime splinting with a reverse knuckle bender splint for 3 to 6 weeks following removal of the wire; night splinting with a padded aluminum splint; and after the fourth week, heat and gentle sustained passive flexion are started.

SEVERE BOUTONNIERE. This stage includes deformities with greater than a 60-degree loss of PIP joint extension; these deformities are not passively correctable. Surgery to restore the extensor mechanism cannot be done unless the joint can be passively extended without tension. Surgical options for these patients include serial casting of the digit to regain extension followed by extensor mechanism reconstruction and tenotomy; PIP joint arthroplasty with Silastic implant[24]; and PIP joint fusion in a functional position.

The methods for serial finger casting were developed by Judy Bell, OTR, and can be found in two publications.[25]

PIP joint arthroplasty is particularly appropriate for deformities of the ring and little fingers in which PIP joint flexion is critical for functional activities.[24] Arthroplasty may not be feasible in patients with small or osteoporotic phalanges. When the procedure is done for a boutonniere deformity, it is combined with reconstruction of the extensor mechanism as described above.[24]

The position of fusion varies according to the digit involved. Nalebuff and Millender use approximately 25 degrees of flexion for the index finger and gradually increase the flexion to about 40 degrees for the small finger.

The surgical procedures and postoperative management for arthroplasty and fusion are described in separate sections later in this chapter.

References (Boutonniere Surgery)

21. Nalebuff, E. A., and Millender, L. H.: *Surgical treatment of the boutonniere deformity in rheumatoid arthritis.* Orthop. Clin. North Am. 6:733, 1975.
22. Dolphin, J. A.: *Extensor tenotomy for chronic boutonniere deformity of the finger: Report of two cases.* J. Bone Joint Surg. 47A:161, 1965.
23. Littler, J. W., and Eaton, R. G.: *Redistribution of forces in the correction of the boutonniere deformity.* J. Bone Joint Surg. 49A;1267, 1969.
24. Swanson, A. B.: *Flexible implant arthroplasty for arthritic finger joints.* J. Bone Joint Surg. 54A:435, 1972.
25. Bell, J.: *Plaster cylinder casting for contractures of the interphalangeal joints.* In Hunter, J. M., Schneider, L. H., Mackin, E. J., and Bell, J. A. (eds.): *Rehabilitation of the Hand.* C. V. Mosby, St. Louis, 1978. This information is also available in a booklet from the Hand Rehabilitation Center, Philadelphia, PA.

SURGERY FOR SWAN NECK DEFORMITY

Swan neck deformity represents the end result of muscular imbalance caused by synovitis in the MCP, PIP, or DIP joint. The complete deformity consists of three components: 1) PIP joint hyperextension; 2) DIP joint flexion; and 3) MCP joint flexion.[26]

The extent of functional loss due to a swan neck deformity correlates with the loss of *PIP joint flexion,* not the degree of PIP hyperextension present.[26] Patients with severe (40 degrees or more) PIP joint hyperextension but full flexion will have no functional limitations due to the swan neck deformity. Conversely, a patient with 10 degrees of hyperextension but only 50 degrees of flexion could be limited in functional activities.

Nalebuff has devised a classification system for swan neck deformities based on the degree of PIP joint flexion and PIP joint integrity present.[26] This classification provides an organized approach for delineating the myriad of surgical options available for correcting these deformities. Swan neck deformities are complex because they can appear similar in appearance but can have very different causal factors and functional consequences.

TYPE I: SWAN NECK WITH FULL PIP JOINT FLEXION.[26] Deformities included in this group generally originate at either the DIP joint or the PIP joint. DIP joint involvement produces a partial or complete rupture of the distal attachment of the EDC tendon, resulting in a flexion deformity of the DIP joint secondary to hyperextension imbalance at the PIP joint. If the deformity originates at the PIP joint, it is usually due to synovitis stretching the volar capsule or attenuation of the FDS tendon. These patients usually do not have severe MCP joint disease.[26]

The objective of surgery for these patients is to prevent or correct PIP joint hyperextension or restore DIP joint extension or both. Surgical options include:

1. DIP joint fusion in a functional position, approximately 5 to 10 degrees of flexion.

2. Dermadesis. Removal of a wedge of skin over the volar aspect of the PIP joint to use skin tightness as a means of restricting hyperextension.[26] (This method can be used only in very mild cases.)

3. Flexor tenodesis.[27] A slip of the sublimus tendon is cut proximally and attached to the proximal phalanx with the PIP joint in 20 degrees of flexion. The slip then acts as a checkrein to prevent full extension. The objective is to create a slight flexion contracture. Postoperatively, the patient is splinted in a manner that allows full flexion but limits extension to −20 degrees.

4. Retinacular ligament reconstruction.[28] In this procedure, the ulnar lateral band is cut proximally and left attached distally. The band is then brought volar to Cleland's fibers and to the axis of PIP joint motion and sutured to the fibrous sheath under appropriate tension to restore DIP extension and prevent PIP hyperextension. It is effective for increasing DIP joint extension when the primary problem is in the PIP joint and not the DIP joint.

TYPE II: SWAN NECK WITH PIP FLEXION LIMITED BY INTRINSIC TIGHTNESS.[26] It is theorized that pain and swelling in the MCP joints elicit a reflex spasm of the associated interosseous muscles. With chronicity these muscles can become fibrosed in a shortened position. Decreased excursion of the intrinsic muscles impedes PIP flexion when the MCP joints are in extension. Full PIP flexion becomes possible only when the MCP joints are flexed. The insertion of the interosseous muscles exert force directly on the lateral bands to extend the PIP joints. If there is damage to the PIP joint or natural laxity of the volar plate, intrinsic spasm can become a major dynamic force contributing to PIP hyperextension or swan neck deformity.

In these patients, it is not sufficient to restrict PIP joint hyperextension. It is necessary to correct the intrinsic tightness and the MCP joint disorder that initiates and prolongs the muscular imbalance in the finger. This is accomplished by intrinsic release (digital) in patients without active MCP synovitis and with well-preserved MCP joints, and by MCP joint arthroplasty and intrinsic release in others.

Digital intrinsic release (Little procedure)[29] is carried out through a dorsal ulnar longitudinal incision over the proximal phalanx. The oblique fibers of the intrinsics are resected from the extensor mechanism. A triangle wedge is removed from the dorsal mechanism to lessen the chances of recurrence. This procedure results in improved PIP flexion with the MCP joint extended or radially deviated. This procedure may be combined with a DIP fusion, dermadesis, or flexor tenodesis to further restore balance to the PIP and DIP joints.

An MCP joint arthroplasty (Swanson) with resection of the metacarpal heads lengthens the intrinsic muscles. However, some surgeons, in addition, resect the ulnar intrinsic muscles to reduce the risk of recurrent intrinsic tightness and ulnar drift of the fingers.

TYPE III: SWAN NECK WITH PIP JOINT CONTRACTURE AND INTACT CARTILAGE.[26] Initially, it was thought that PIP joint stiffness was due to severe PIP joint disease and the only recourse for correction was arthroplasty or fusion.[30] It is now apparent that many patients are limited by secondary soft tissue changes and the options for treatment of these contractures have expanded. Swan neck deformity with limited flexion but well-preserved joint surfaces are delineated as Type III. Those with severe PIP joint damage are classified as Type IV.[26]

The first objective of surgery is to restore *passive motion* by using one of several release procedures. If the flexor tendons are intact and moving freely, postoperative strengthening exercises will be sufficient for restoring full active motion. However, if the flexor tendons are adherent it is necessary to perform a second procedure such as a tenosynovectomy or tenolysis before full functional ROM can be achieved.

If the contracture is long standing, there is usually fibrosis in all of the surrounding joint structures.[26] The extensor mechanism collateral ligaments and the skin are key structures that restrict passive flexion and are amenable to surgery.[26] If there are additional deformities at the MCP or DIP joints contributing to the swan neck process, these will have to be corrected with additional surgeries such as arthroplasty, intrinsic release, or fusion. Otherwise, the PIP joint limitation is likely to reoccur.[26]

PIP Joint Manipulation and Skin Release.[26] The patient's PIP joint is *gently* manipulated under anesthesia. In many cases, it is possible to achieve 80 or 90 degrees of flexion. The joint is then fixed with a Kirschner wire for two weeks. This is followed by heat and active and passive exercises to increase both flexion and extension and to improve the strength and excursion of the long flexor tendons. Night splinting that maintains the PIP joint in flexion should be continued until the patient can maintain flexion without them, as determined by one-, two-, or three-day trials without the splints. The splints may be needed for as long as 8 to 12 weeks. Taping the finger to padded aluminum splints or LMB wire-foam Flexion Springs is generally well tolerated by patients. This procedure is often combined with MCP arthroplasty. The temporary fixation of the PIP joint encourages flexion of the MCP joints during the postoperative exercise program.[26]

Excessive tension on the skin over the PIP joint can cause ischemia and secondary necrosis. A skin release is done just distal to the PIP joint to reduce tension on the skin during temporary fixation in flexion of a previously stiff joint.[26] The incision is left open and it gradually closes over a two- to three-week period.

Not all patients are candidates for joint manipulation. Patients with severe osteoporosis are prone to fractures. If patients cannot be *gently* manipulated into flexion, they are considered for a soft tissue release.[26]

Lateral Band Mobilization. In a swan neck deformity the lateral bands migrate dorsal and become contracted, losing their ability to shift lateral and volar with flexion. These contracted bands can prevent passive flexion during manipulation. Freeing the lateral bands from the central slip can often make manipulation possible without releasing the collateral ligaments or lengthening the central slip.[31,32]

If the surgery is done under local anesthesia the success of the release can be determined during surgery. The lateral bands should shift during active flexion and extension. If the release of the bands is not sufficient to allow desired flexion, it may be necessary to release the collateral ligaments and central slip as well.

Following the surgery, the patients are splinted or fixed with a Kirschner wire for two weeks. Then active and passive exercises are started to restore ROM, strength, and dexterity. Night taping the PIP joint in flexion should be continued until patients can maintain flexion without the tape. This may take as long as two to three months.

TYPE IV: SWAN NECK WITH PIP JOINT CONTRACTURE AND DAMAGED CARTILAGE. The surgeries described for other swan neck deformities require an intact PIP joint to be successful. If there is evidence of cartilage destruction, these procedures will not work and a salvage procedure such as arthroplasty or fusion needs to be considered. The criteria and procedures for these surgeries are discussed in separate sections of this chapter.

References (Swan Neck Surgery)

26. Nalebuff, E. A., and Millender, L. H.: *Surgical treatment of the swan neck deformity in rheumatoid arthritis.* Orthop. Clin. North Am. 6:733, 1975.
27. Swanson, A. B.: *Surgery of the hand in cerebral palsy and the swan neck deformity.* J. Bone Joint Surg. 42A:951, 1960.
28. Littler, J. W.: *Restoration of the oblique retinacular ligament for correction of hand contractures.* G.E.M.Nol, Paris, L'Epansion, 1966.
29. Littler, J. W.: Quoted by Harris, C., Jr., and Riordan, D.: *Intrinsic contracture in the hand and its surgical treatment.* J. Bone Joint Surg. 36A:10, 1954.
30. Flatt, A. E.: *The Care of the Rheumatoid Hand.* C. V. Mosby, St. Louis, 1968.
31. Nalebuff, E. A.: *Surgical treatment of finger deformities in the rheumatoid hand.* Surg. Clin. North Am. 49:833, 1969.
32. Leach, R. E., and Baumgard, S. H.: *Correction of swan neck deformity in rheumatoid arthritis.* Surg. Clin. North Am. 48:661, 1968.

ARTHROPLASTY

Once there is cartilage loss, instability, and deformity, joint restoration is no longer possible. It then becomes necessary to choose between two salvage procedures—arthroplasty (joint reconstruction) and arthrodesis (joint fusion). Both surgeries relieve pain, provide stability, correct or reduce deformity, and improve function. The arthroplasty provides the additional benefit of motion. The surgery of choice depends on the joint level, integrity of the bone, and the function of the digits.[33]

The first metal hinge finger prostheses were developed in the late 1950s. They were metal hinges, originally created to provide a solution for swan neck deformities of the PIP joint and later adapted for the MCP joint. The metal prostheses for the MCP joints eventually proved unsatisfactory.[34]

The advent of synthetic materials that could be used in the body opened up the field of implant development and revolutionized joint surgery. Alfred Swanson developed the first flexible Silastic digit implants in 1962.[35] They became available to surgeons in major medical centers around 1969. There are other digit implants available, but the Swanson implants are the most widely used and have the most extensive follow-up. The fact that they have been used in over a quarter of a million patients attests to the worldwide acceptance of this procedure.[35] Since the success of the digit implants, a number of flexible Silastic implants have been developed. Implants for the wrist, thumb, carpal bones, and radioulnar joints have gained the widest acceptance.[35] In 1968, Niebauer created a digit prosthesis similar in design to the Swanson implant but added a Dacron mesh to the stems to encourage scarring or fixation of the stems for greater stability.[36] This is in contrast to the Swanson design, in which the stems are loose in the canal and glide slightly during flexion and extension. The Niebauer prostheses are also effective and widely used.[36]

The term implant is used to describe these devices because they are spacers rather than artificial joints. They function as a hinge and do not perform all of the intricate gliding and rotational motions of a normal joint.[37]

Prior to 1970, the only surgery available to correct severe pain or deformity of the MCP joints was a resection arthroplasty, in which the heads of the metacarpals were removed. A short period of fixation followed surgery to encourage tightening of the soft tissues. For many patients, this was an excellent surgery that resulted in pain-free mobile joints.[38] However, results were often unpredictable and ulnar drift frequently reoccurred.[38] Swanson developed his implant as a "dynamic spacer that acts as an interpositional material for resection arthroplasty to make results more predictable, reproducible and durable."[35]

In addition to providing a spacer for the resected bone, the flexible implant provides support for the capsuloligamentous system that develops around it. The collagen, scar-like tissue that forms around the joint following surgery (encapsulation process) can be shaped or trained during the formation process to enhance motion or stability in certain planes as desired. Shaping the capsule is a key aspect of splinting, particularly in the MCP joints.[35,39,40]

This encapsulation process is a major component of the flexible implant arthroplasty and critical to postoperative management.[40] Prostheses that use cement fixation do not rely on the capsule or ligamentous structures for stability. Therefore, the surgical and postoperative protocols for flexible implants are different from those for metal hinge implants.

Since flexible implants are widely used and require the most postoperative therapy, they will be reviewed in this section.

Wrist Implant Arthroplasty

Over the last five years, several different prostheses have become available for replacement of the radiocarpal joint. They vary considerably in design. Some are metal hinges; others are metal to plastic; and others have a ball and socket component for rotation. Each prosthesis has advantages and disadvantages. The flexible radiocarpal implant is dependent upon capsule and ligamentous integrity for stability.[35] It is popular because it does not require cement (methylmethacrylate) for fixation and can be easily removed if an infection occurs.[33]

The all metal and metal and plastic prostheses offer increased stability (some offer circumduction) but carry the risk of using cement fixation. (It is very difficult to remove the prosthesis and the cement, which may be necessary to treat an infection; and loosening of the stem may require a difficult second operation.) It is still too soon to determine the long-term effect of methylmethacrylate cement in the carpal bones.

In addition to the radiocarpal joint, there are Silastic replacement implants for the scaphoid and lunate bones. These are used primarily to relieve pain secondary to trauma or aseptic necrosis (Kienböck's disease) of these carpal bones and nonunion of the scaphoid.[35]

RADIOCARPAL JOINT (Swanson flexible hinged implant)

The radiocarpal flexible hinged implant is a one piece intramedullary stemmed hinge fabricated from Silastic material. The proximal stem of the implant fits the intramedullary canal of the radius and the distal stem passes through the capitate and fits the intramedullary canal of the third metacarpal.[35,39]

Indications[33,35]

1. Chronic wrist synovitis with subluxation or dislocation unresponsive to conservative treatment.
2. Stiffness or fusion in a nonfunctional position.
3. Stiffness in which movement is required for function.

Occurrence

Rheumatoid arthritis, chronic juvenile polyarthritis, traumatic arthritis, and psoriatic arthritis.

Surgical and Functional Goals

The ideal outcome is a pain-free, stable joint with approximately 30 degrees of flexion and 30 degrees of extension and slight radial and ulnar deviation.[33,35]

Surgical Prerequisites

1. Adequate quality bone stock to hold the implant. (Patients with mutilans of the carpal bones are not good candidates.)
2. Intact wrist extensor tendons.
3. Adequate capsular and soft tissue to secure the prosthesis.

Surgical Procedure[35]

1. Dorsal curved longitudinal incision.
2. Capsule and ligaments are preserved.
3. Contractures are released.
4. Distal end of the radius is resected and the scaphoid, lunate, and part of the trique-trum are removed. (The end of the ulna may also be removed if forearm rotation is limited; Figure 3.)

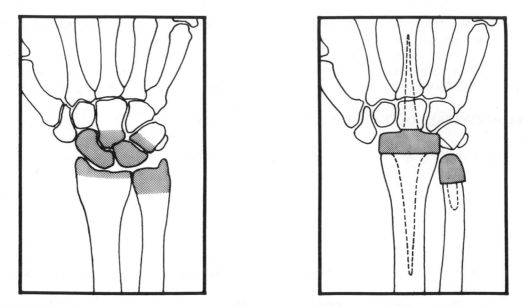

FIGURE 3. Bone resection is required for placement of the Swanson wrist implant and radial head replacement. The dotted line indicates the stem of the implant inside the bones.

5. The capsuloligamentous repair is firmed to allow 45 degrees of flexion and extension and 10 degrees of ulnar and radial deviation.
6. The wrist extensors and retinacular construction are balanced.
7. Ruptured digital extensor tendons are repaired if present.

Postoperative Management

Average hospitalization: 5 days.
1. Second day: Compression dressing is reduced. It is immobilized in a thermoplastic wrist splint. It is necessary to immoblize the wrist for 3 weeks. At the end of hospitalization, it may be desirable to fabricate a thermoplastic splint.
2. Second or third day: Begin daily ROM to digit joints.
3. Three weeks: Begin gentle wrist ROM exercises. A thermoplastic splint or commercial elastic canvas wrist gauntlet are worn as needed to protect wrist during functional activities and to relieve discomfort. It should be gradually discontinued over a period of 6 to 8 weeks. If the patient has excessive lateral motion at 3 weeks, he or she should be fitted with a wrist-hinge splint that allows flexion and extension for use during the daytime for 2 to 4 weeks.

RADIOULNAR JOINT/DISTAL ULNAR RESECTION AND REPLACEMENT (Darrach Procedure)

Chronic synovitis of the radioulnar joint weakens the supporting ligaments and can result in dorsal subluxation of the ulna on the radius. If the subluxation is severe, it can limit supination and pronation. In addition, synovial hypertrophy can limit forearm rotation.

Resection of the ulna eliminates the distal radioulnar joint, thereby eliminating distal radioulnar joint pain and any block to forearm motion. The ulnar head implant is made of Silastic material and is of one-piece construction with an intramedullary stem. (See Figure 3.) The replacement is designed to preserve the anatomic relationship and the physiology of the distal radioulnar joint. Swanson reports that with the use of the replacement less bone needs to be removed and the physiologic length of the ulna is maintained to help prevent ulnar carpal shift and provide greater wrist stability.[35,39]

Indications

1. Pain secondary to destructive arthritis of the distal radioulnar joint.
2. Dorsal subluxation of the ulnar head, threatening the overlying extensor tendons.
3. Limitation of forearm rotation secondary to distal radioulnar joint disease or dorsal subluxation of the ulna.

Occurrence

Rheumatoid arthritis, traumatic arthritis, or chronic inflammatory arthritis of the distal radioulnar joint.

Surgical and Functional Goals

Postsurgical expectations are decreased wrist pain and improved forearm rotation.

Surgical Prerequisites

Stable radiocarpal joint (radioscaphoid-lunate joint), preferably without joint disease, with absence of ulnar displacement of the carpus on the radius.[35]

Surgical Procedure

This procedure may be combined with a dorsal clearance, extension tendon repair, or a wrist fusion.
1. Approach: Slightly curved incision over the dorsum of the wrist or an ulnar midlateral incision.
2. Last $\frac{1}{2}$ to $\frac{3}{4}$ inch of distal ulna is excised.
3. Radioulnar joint synovectomy.
4. Silastic ulnar head prosthesis may be implanted.
5. Periosteum around the last inch of the ulna is closed.
6. Soft tissue closure to prevent dorsal migration of the ulna.

Postoperative Management

Average hospitalization: 3 to 5 days.
1. First two weeks: Immobilization in a compression dressing with a short arm plaster splint or cast that extends to the proximal palmar crease and allows full flexion of the

MCP joints and thumb. (If an ulnar prosthesis is implanted, a sugar tong cast that prevents wrist rotation may be used.)
2. After removal of cast:
   a. Active ROM exercises of the wrist are started with emphasis on supination and pronation.
   b. Gradually increase functional use.
   c. Continue static splinting of the wrist in slight ulnar deviation (10 degrees) to prevent increasing ulnar displacement of the carpus on the radius, which results in radial deviation and wrist deformity. (See Hand Assessment, Chapter 21, for detailed discussion of the dynamics of wrist subluxation and dislocation.)

Implant Arthroplasty of the Metacarpophalangeal Joints (Swanson Silastic Implants)

Prior to the advent of the flexible implant, the most frequent procedure carried out for MCP joint pain and deformity was a resection arthroplasty. This procedure involved resection of the metacarpal head, soft tissue reconstruction, and temporary internal fixation. Resection arthroplasty was often sucessful but the results were at best unpredictable and inconsistent. The flexible implant resolved these shortcomings by providing an internal splint to control the encapsulation process (Fig. 4). The MCP implant arthroplasty is a reliable procedure for relieving pain, correcting deformity, and preserving motion (Fig. 5).

Indications

1. Pain secondary to destructive arthritis of the MCP joints.
2. Ulnar drift not amenable to soft tissue repair alone.
3. Subluxation or dislocation of MCP joints.
4. Stiffness or ankylosis and functional loss of MCP joints.

Occurrence

Primarily in rheumatoid arthritis; occasionally in traumatic arthritis.

Surgical and Functional Goals

Postsurgical expectations are relief of pain, increased joint stability, increased mobility (ideally extension: zero degrees; flexion: from 35 to 70 degrees), improved hand function, and improved cosmetic appearance. Many patients find they are not able to do more or different hand tasks postoperatively but are able to do the same tasks with greater ease and without pain.

Surgical Prerequisites[40]

1. Intact neurovascular supply.
2. Intact flexor and extensor tendons.
3. Patient capable of following precise postoperative splinting and exercise routine.

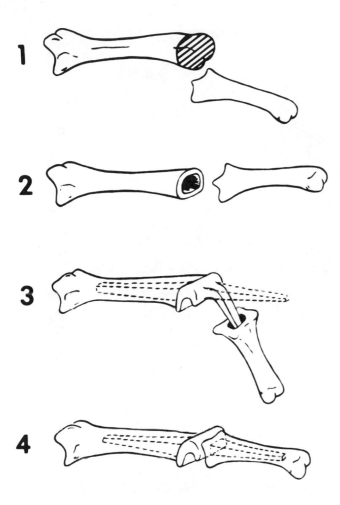

FIGURE 4. Resection of the metacarpal head and insertion of a Silastic Swanson design implant. The stems of the implant are inserted into the intramedullary canals. (Cement is not required.) A comprehensive soft tissue release procedure is necessary to obtain adequate space for the prosthesis. (From Swanson, A. B.: *Silastic finger joint prosthesis.* Dow Corning Bulletin, 1972, with permission.)

4. Absence of infection.
5. Adequate bone density to accept implant.

Surgical Procedure[35]

1. Approach: transverse incision over the dorsum of the MCP joints or dorsal longitudinal incisions between the metacarpal heads.
2. Extensor hood and the joint capsule are incised.
3. Metacarpal heads are excised.
4. Synovectomy of the MCP joints is performed.
5. Contracted soft tissues are released (collateral ligaments, volar capsule, ulnar intrinsic muscles with possible transfer to radial intrinsic muscle).
6. Intramedullary canals of the proximal phalanx and metacarpal bones are broached.
7. Appropriate prosthesis size is selected and installed.
8. Capsular closure is performed.

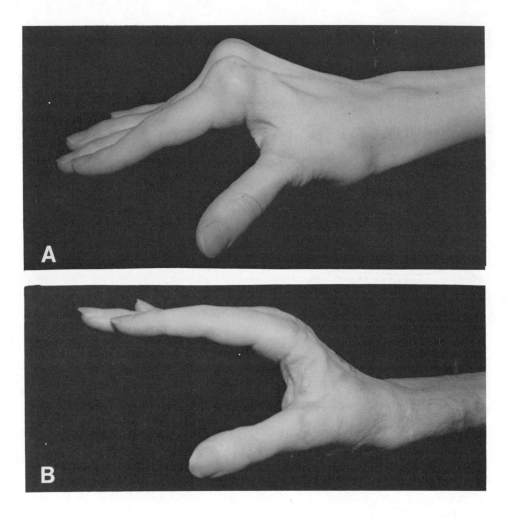

9. Reefing (pleating) of the radial fibers of the extensor hood is done (to maintain alignment of the extensor tendon).

Postoperative Management[35,40,41]

Average hospitalization: 3 to 5 days.
1. First to fifth day: Hand is in a voluminous compression bandage, elevated to reduce edema, with MCP joints extended and interphalangeal joints slightly flexed. Shoulder and elbow should receive daily ROM.
2. Second to fifth day: Compression bandage is replaced with a smaller dressing.
3. Fifth to seventh day:
    a. Postoperative splint is fitted. (See Splinting for Arthritis of the Hand, Chapter 25, for different types of postoperative splints and specific fitting instructions.) Splint should be worn all the time except for ROM of wrist and personal hygiene. Exten-

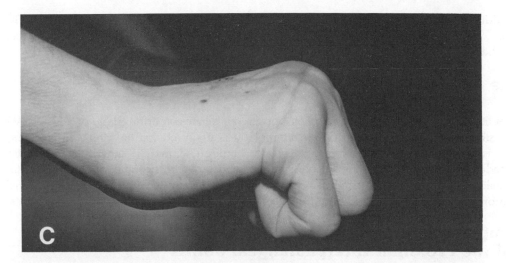

FIGURE 5. MCP arthroplasty and thumb CMC arthroplasty with thumb arthrodesis. (A), Preoperative status: Patient with rheumatoid arthritis has limited MCP extension (− 70°) due to marked MCP subluxation. Her ability for grasp is reduced owing to a Type IV thumb deformity with a CMC joint adduction contracture and lateral instability of the thumb MP joint. (B), Postoperative extension. Her ability for grasp and prehension is significantly improved. MCP extension has gained 40° (now − 30°). (C), Postoperative flexion. Patient has functional, nearly full flexion, although she has lost some flexion compared with her preoperative ROM. This is consistent with the goal of the MCP implant arthroplasty to provide a more functional arc of motion rather than simply to increase excursion or achieve normal ROM. The patient's grasp strength and dexterity skills also improved. Thumb prehension skills are enhanced by the stability provided by the MP arthrodesis.

       sor outriggers should keep the MCP joints in full extension and slight radial deviation and, when necessary, provide a supination assist to the index finger. The wrist is kept in slight (10 degrees) ulnar deviation.

b. To increase MCP joint motion, active sustained flexion and extension exercises of the MCP joints should be performed 4 to 6 times each day for 15 to 20 minutes. These exercises need to be carefully defined and monitored in order that PIP flexion is not substituted for MCP flexion.

c. To avoid recurrent intrinsic contracture, active PIP joint exercises with the MCP joints maintained in full extension should be performed 4 to 6 times each day.

4. Between the tenth and fourteenth day, and then the sixth to eighth week postoperative:

a. Use of flexion assists may be started with about one-half hour flexion alternated with an hour and a half extension and gradually increasing flexion to one hour.

b. The optimal ratio of flexion positioning versus dynamic extension positioning depends upon the range of active motion. Ratio is increased in favor of the range with the greatest deficit.

c. Splinting procedure is continued about 5 to 8 weeks with the extensor assist used at night; the amount of time spent in the splint during the day is gradually reduced, depending on the degree of active motion of the MCP joints with the dynamic splint discontinued at about the tenth week.

(Additional resources: a detailed guide to postoperative treatment is available from Dr. Swanson,[40] and Madden, De Vore, and Arem have published an excellent article describing a comprehensive postoperative rehabilitation program.[42])

PIP JOINT FLEXIBLE IMPLANT ARTHROPLASTY

For stiff swan neck deformities, the choice of surgery is between arthroplasty or a fusion. When possible the mobility provided by an arthroplasty is preferred for the ring and little fingers, where flexion is needed for strong grip. In the index and middle fingers, lateral stability is needed for strong pinch. If the surrounding joint structures are strong enough to insure lateral stability, an arthroplasty is recommended. If the structures are weak or the bones are small, a fusion is often done in the index and middle fingers.[33,43,44]

Implant Arthroplasty of the Proximal Interphalangeal Joints

Indications[43,44]

1. Pain secondary to destructive arthritis of the PIP joints.
2. Instability associated with destructive arthritis of the PIP joints.
3. Stiffness and functional loss of the PIP joints.
4. Stiff swan neck deformity, when adjacent joints and tendons are intact.
5. Boutonniere and lateral deviation deformities.

Occurrence

Rheumatoid arthritis and degenerative joint disease, traumatic arthritis, and psoriatic arthritis.

Surgical and Functional Goals

Pain is diminished by the complete removal of the articular surfaces and diseased synovium. Function is improved by realignment of the joints, increased motion and stability, and decreased pain.[33]

Postsurgical expectations are relief of pain, increased stability or increased mobility (depending upon initial status), improved functional use, and improved cosmetic appearance.[44]

Surgical Prerequisites[44]

1. Intact neurovascular supply.
2. Intact extensor and flexor tendons.
3. Absence of recent infection (6 months minimum).
4. Absence of significant MCP joint flexion deformity. (MCP flexion deformity should be corrected prior to PIP surgery.)

Surgical Procedure

1. Approach: Dorsal or midlateral incision.
2. Extensor tendon mobilized; capsule incised.
3. Excision of the head of the proximal phalanx (synovectomy if indicated).
4. Intramedullary canals reamed and shaped to receive the prosthesis.
5. Selection of appropriate prosthesis and installation.
6. Capsular closure and extensor tendon reconstruction as indicated.

Postoperative Management[35,40,41]

Average hospitalization: 3 to 5 days.
1. First to fifth day: Hand is in a voluminous compression bandage and elevated to reduce edema. ROM of the upper extremity should be done daily.
2. Second to fifth day:
   a. Compression bandage is removed.
   b. Active ROM is started several times per day.
   c. *The exercise program needs to be modified depending on whether or not extensor tendon reconstruction was also performed.* Early motion is contraindicated when tendon surgery is done.
   d. Joint is splinted in extension with a small dorsal aluminum splint, except during exercise periods. If there has been prior swan neck deformity or stiffness, the joint might be splinted into slight flexion. In severe swan neck deformities, the joint can also be taped into flexion at night.
   e. Flexion can be encouraged by stabilizing the MCP joint in extension during active finger flexion, using either a splint or a device like a Bunnell block.
3. Third to fourth week: Splint can be discontinued during the day if the joint is stable; it is usually retained for protective night positioning.
4. About sixth to eighth week: Splint can be discontinued.

THUMB CMC JOINT ARTHROPLASTY

The trapeziometacarpal joint is a common site of primary degenerative joint disease. Cartilage thinning and osteophyte formation can block motion and result in subluxation or dislocation of the CMC joint.[45]

Pain in this joint can be severely debilitating, since 45 percent of hand function is attributed to the thumb.

Patients with episodic pain often are satisfied with using a splint during painful periods. Once the pain becomes unrelenting or is not relieved by a splint, surgery is indicated.

There are several surgeries available for this problem, e.g., resection arthroplasty[47] and hemiartroplasty. The trapezium implant is one of the most widely used. The trapezium implant is similar to other spacers in that it is designed to preserve the anatomic relationships of the basal joints of the thumb after resection arthroplasty. The stem of the implant fits into the intramedullary canal of the first metacarpal. The trapeziometacarpal joint is eliminated and motion then occurs between the implant and the trapezoid and scaphoid bones.[39,45,46,47,48]

Indications[45]

1. Persistent pain of the CMC joint that is nonresponsive to conservative management. (X-ray changes alone without symptoms are not sufficient indication for surgery).
2. Decreased motion that reduces prehension.

Occurrence

Degenerative joint disease, rheumatoid arthritis, and traumatic arthritis.

Surgical Prerequisites

Intact carpal bones (scaphoid).

Surgical and Functional Goals

Pain and crepitation are relieved by elimination of the damaged joint. Prehension and strength limited by pain should return to normal. Full or near full ROM can be expected. Some patients lose mobility due to the postoperative immobilization and require diligent therapy to regain full motion. (See Chapter 22, Evaluation of Range of Motion, for special techniques for measuring CMC joint motion.)

Postoperative Management

Average hospitalization: 3 to 5 days.
1. Immobilization in a thumb spica short arm cast for 6 weeks. The cast should not block digit MCP flexion.
2. About the sixth week: Begin program of hot water soaks, active and passive ROM exercises to increase ROM in all planes. Wrapping the thumb into flexion with Coban tape can provide an effective gentle stretch for increasing flexion. Therapy could be continued until there is a plateau in progress. The length of therapy depends on how much stiffness develops during the 6 weeks immobilization.

References (Arthroplasty)

33. Nalebuff, E. A., and Millender, L. H.: *Reconstructive surgery and rehabilitation of the hand*. In Kelley, W. M., et al. (eds.): *Textbook of Rheumatology*, Vol. II. W. B. Saunders, Philadelphia, 1981.
34. Flatt, A.: *The Care of the Rheumatoid Hand*, ed 3. C. V. Mosby, St. Louis, 1974, pp. 195–221.
35. Swanson, A. B.: *Flexible Implant Resection Arthroplasty in the Hand and Extremities*. C. V. Mosby., St. Louis, 1973.
36. Neibauer, J. J.: *Dacron-silicone prosthesis for the metacarpophalangeal and interphalangeal joints*. In Cramer, L. H., and Chase, R. A. (eds.): *Symposium on the Hand*, Vol. 3. C. V. Mosby, St. Louis, 1971, pp. 96–105.
37. Swanson, A. B.: *Flexible implant arthroplasty for arthritic finger joints: Rationale, technique and results of treatment*. J. Bone Joint Surg. 54A:435, 1972.

38. Robinson, H. S., Kokan, P. V., MacBain, K. P., and Patterson, F. P.: *Functional results of excisional arthroplasty for the rheumatoid hand.* Can. Med. Assoc. J. 108:1495, 1973.
39. Swanson, A. B.: *Reconstructive Surgery in the Arthritic Hand and Foot.* Clinical Symposia, Vol 31, No. 6, 1979. Medical Education Division CIBA Pharmaceutical Co., Summit, New Jersey.
40. *Postoperative Care for Patients with Silastic Finger Joint Implants (Swanson Design): MCP and IP joints.* Compiled by: L. Buchanan, O.T., J. Leonard, O.T.R., A. Swanson, M.D. and G. dG. Swanson, M.D. Available from Orthopedic Reconstructive Surgeons, P.C., Grand Rapids, Michigan, 1979. This is a detailed postoperative guide.
41. Swanson, A. B., Swanson, G. dG., and Leonard, J.: *Postoperative rehabilitation program in flexible implant arthroplasty of the digitis.* In Hunter, J. M., Schneider, L. H., Mackin, E. J., and Bell, J. A. (eds.): *Rehabilitation of the Hand.* C. V. Mosby, St. Louis, 1978.
42. Madden, J. W., Devore, G., and Arem, A. J.: *A rational postoperative management program for metacarpophalangeal joint implant arthroplasty.* J. Hand Surg. 2:358, 1977.
43. Nalebuff, E. A., and Millender, L. H.: *Surgical treatment of the swan neck deformity in rheumatoid arthritis. Surgical treatment of the boutonniere deformity in rheumatoid arhtritis.* Orthop. Clin. North Am. 6:733, 1975.
44. Swanson, A. B.: *Implant resection arthroplasty of the proximal interphalangeal joint.* Orthop. Clin. North Am., 4:1009, 1973.
45. Swanson, A. B., and Swanson, G. dG.: *Disabling osteoarthritis in the hand and its treatment.* In *Symposium on Osteoarthritis,* C. V. Mosby, St. Louis, 1976.
46. Beckenbaugh, R. D., Dobyns, J. H., Linseheid, R. L., and Bryan, R. S.: *Review and analysis of silicone-rubber MCP implants.* J. Bone Joint Surg. 58A:483, 1976.
47. Dell, P. C., Brushart, M. D., and Smith, R. L.: *Treatment of trapeziometacarpal arthritis: Results of resection arthroplasty.* J. Hand Surg. 3(3):243, 1978. (Also includes a discussion on conservative management.)
48. Millender, L. H., Nalebuff, E. A., Amadio, P., and Philips, C. A.: *Interpositional arthroplasty for rheumatoid carpometacarpal joint disease.* J. Hand Surg. 3(6):533, 1978.

ARTHRODESIS

Arthrodesis, or surgical fusion of a joint, is one of the oldest operations for arthritis and, prior to flexible implants, was often the only alternative for severely damaged joints.

So much time and energy are spent trying to maintain mobility in the hand that the idea of an operation that prevents motion permanently often elicits a negative reaction from patients and health professionals alike. But following arthrodesis patients are generally pleased and find that they can do more with a pain-free stable joint than they could with a painful or unstable joint.

Arthrodesis is the treatment of choice in several circumstances and can improve function in severely disabled hands. In cases of mutilans deformity, arthrodesis can prevent the resorption process and maintain the integrity of the bone stock.[49]

In current practice, arthrodesis may be the appropriate procedure to relieve pain, provide stability, and correct nonfunctional deformity in the wrist, PIP, DIP, and thumb joints. In the MCP joints arthrodesis is not recommended because of the need for mobility in these joints and the success of arthroplasty at this level.[50]

WRIST

Arthrodesis of the wrist eliminates flexion and extension but does not affect forearm rotation.[51] The relief of pain and stability of the wrist often result in improved hand function and grip strength. There are basically two clear-cut indications in which arthrodesis is preferred over an arthroplasty: when damage to the carpal bones is so extensive that they cannot accept a prosthesis and when there is loss or rupture of the wrist extensor tendons.[51]

In juvenile chronic polyarthritis, arthrodesis is the most common wrist procedure because the intermedullary canals are often not developed and therefore do not have the capacity to accept the prosthesis. Additionally, these patients often develop intercarpal ankylosis, which makes arthrodesis a logical procedure for a severely damaged radiocarpal joint.[52]

If the patient has sufficient bone stock to receive a prosthesis and adequate motor control, the indications for an arthrodesis versus an arthroplasty are factors external to the joint and based on the surgeon's personal preference. Both advantages and disadvantages of the stability provided by an arthrodesis and the mobility afforded by an arthroplasty need to be carefully considered and evaluated in light of the patient's physical status and functional needs.[50,51] For example:

1. If the wrist is painful and has lost considerable mobility an arthrodesis may be considered over an arthroplasty.
2. When both wrists are involved it may be advisable to do an arthrodesis in one wrist for stability and an arthroplasty in the other for motion—although for some patients it may be preferable to have either procedure bilaterally.
3. For patients who work in vocations with manual labor the stability of a fusion may be desired.
4. If the digital joints are stiff or the proximal upper extremity joints are limited, the motion provided by an arthroplasty may enhance function more than an arthrodesis.
5. For patients who are limited to ambulation with crutches, the stability provided by an arthrodesis is often preferred.

Indications (Definite)

1. Debilitating wrist pain with severe joint destruction.
2. Loss of the wrist extensor muscles.

Occurrence

Rheumatoid arthritis, traumatic arthritis, juvenile chronic polyarthritis, and psoriatic arthritis.

Surgical Prerequisites

No specific prerequisites.

Surgical Procedure

1. Approach: dorsal longitudinal incision.
2. Synovectomy of the extensor tendons.
3. Excision of cartilage from the distal radius and between the carpal bones.
4. If the procedure is unilateral the wrist is usually fused in neutral. When the procedure

is bilateral, one wrist is generally fused in neutral and the other is fused in slight flexion to facilitate self care.

5. A Steinmann pin or Ross rod is inserted between the second and third metacarpals (or within the third metacarpal), across the carpals, and into the intramedullary canal of the radius. Supplementary fixation (staple) and bone graft may be added.
6. The procedure may be combined with an ulnar head resection (with or without an ulnar head prothesis) to improve forearm rotation.

Postoperative Management

Average hospitalization: 3 to 5 days.
1. First to third day: Initial immobilization compression bandage with a volar short arm plaster splint. If a drain is used it is removed on the first day.
2. Third to seventh day:
    a. Compression bandage exchanged for a forearm cast that allows full flexion of the MCP joints, fingers, and thumb.
    b. Active finger motion is encouraged. Techniques for reducing digital edema are applied if needed.
    c. Instruction in ROM exercises for shoulder and elbow.
3. Third week:
    a. Short arm cast is converted to a volar plaster splint.
    b. Active finger motion is continued.
    c. Splint is worn until roentgenography shows evidence of bony consolidation.

PIP JOINTS

Mobility of the PIP joints is important for dexterity and every effort is made to maintain it. The decision to fuse the PIP joint is based on the type and severity of deformity, the digit involved, the condition of the adjacent joints, and the status of the extensor and flexor tendons and structures.[50]

In the boutonniere and swan neck deformities the extent of soft tissue contractures is often the determining factor for an arthrodesis. In the early stages, boutonniere deformities may be reducible and correctable with an arthroplasty. However, if the deformity progresses and becomes fixed in flexion greater than 70 to 80 degrees, shortening of the volar structures may prevent joint restoration and arthrodesis in a functional position may be the only alternative. Similarly, in swan neck deformity, fibrosis of the surrounding soft tissue may be so severe that restoration of balanced motion may not be possible and surgical fusion in a functional position is the most practical solution.[50]

The digit affected can also influence the surgical decision. Flexion of the PIP joint becomes increasingly important in the digits in a radial to ulnar direction. A primary function of the index finger is pinch prehension against the thumb; it also provides a stable post for thumb opposition in lateral pinch. Both of these functions require only slight to moderate flexion in addition to stability. For each of the consecutive fingers slightly increasing flexion is utilized to maximize functional grasp. Flexion of the ulnar fingers plays a more critical role in tight grasp.

For these reasons fusion of the index finger may be less of a handicap than fusion of the little finger.

Another factor that can influence the surgical choice is the degree of mobility present in the MCP joints and secondarily in the DIP joints. The less mobility present in these joints the greater the need for mobility in the PIP joints. The prospect of MCP joint arthroplasty must also be taken into account. When a patient has severe involvement of both the MCP and PIP joints and an MCP implant arthroplasty is indicated (or potential), the length and capacity of the medullary canal is a critical factor and may not be of sufficient length to accommodate prostheses at both levels, necessitating fusion of the PIP joints. Even when it is possible to insert a prosthesis at both levels, most surgeons choose to fuse the destroyed PIP joint when the MCP joint is in need of a replacement.[50]

Indications (definite)

1. Severe fixed boutonniere or swan neck deformities.
2. Ruptured flexor tendons.
3. Severe joint or ligamentous destruction.
4. Beginning mutilans deformity.

Occurrence

Rheumatoid arthritis, juvenile chronic polyarthritis, traumatic arthritis, psoriatic arthritis, and occasionally gout.

Surgical and Functional Goals

Stable motion and relief of pain.

Surgical Prerequisites

No specific prerequisites

Surgical Procedure

1. Approach: Dorsal curved incision; care is taken to preserve the delicate veins over the PIP joint.
2. The extensor mechanism is split and the collateral ligaments are detached.
3. The bone ends are prepared to achieve contact in the desired position.
4. The bones are fixed with K wires, usually two crossed pins.

Postoperative management

Average hospitalization: 2 to 5 days (depending on the number of digits involved and the associated procedures).

1. First to third day: Initial immobilization in a volar splint. If multiple digits are operated on, a full hand resting splint may be used. Dressing is changed.
2. Protective aluminum splints are worn for 4 to 6 weeks. Volar splints provide the greatest protection but limit function, whereas dorsal splints provide sufficient protection and allow the patient to grasp objects.
3. Activity is limited until there is x-ray evidence of bony consolidation, approximately 8 to 10 weeks.
4. The K wires may be left in the bones indefinitely if they do not cause local tenderness.

DIP JOINTS

Arthrodesis is the most frequent surgical procedure performed on the DIP joints. It is used to correct deformity, relieve pain, and provide stability for pinch prehension. It is the procedure of choice in the following conditions.[50]
1. Synovitis can cause bone erosion and laxity of the collateral ligaments resulting in lateral deviation deformity. It can also cause attenuation of the distal attachment of the extensor tendon creating a mallet deformity and possibly a secondary swan neck deformity.
2. A severe boutonniere deformity can result in a hyperextension deformity of this joint.
3. Rupture of the flexor pollicis longus may render the distal phalanx of the thumb useless for prehension if the joint is hypermobile.
4. Osteophyte formation in osteoarthritis is generally painless, but occasionally it can present with inflammation, severe pain, and limited motion.
5. In osteoarthritis, destruction of the cartilage and formation and collapse of mucoidal cysts may occur on one side of the joint and result in unsightly lateral deviation deformities.

Arthrodesis of the DIP joint is carried out through a dorsal incision and primarily includes removal of articular cartilage from the bone ends and removal of osteophytes in a manner that allows the bones to be approximated at the desired angle (neutral or in 5 to 10 degrees of flexion). The position is maintained with wire fixation until the bone ends fuse together. Distal joint fusions are often performed under digital block anesthesia on an outpatient basis.

Arthrodesis has been the only procedure discussed for the DIP joint because it is the most common. It is possible to perform an arthroplasty on this joint and a condylar prosthesis has been developed; however, its use to date has been limited.

THUMB

When thumb deformities progress to a point at which there is marked instability, relentless pain that limits prehension, or MCP/CMC contractures that limit grasp, an arthrodesis is an effective surgical option.

For the IP joint with severe instability or angulation deformity, arthrodesis in a straight or slightly flexed position is the procedure of choice.[50] An IP joint fusion prevents tip to tip pinch, but the gain in stability usually increases the patient's overall functional ability.

For the MCP joint, it is possible to do an arthroplasty. The decision between this procedure and a fusion depends on the status of the adjacent joints. When there is isolated MCP involvement, a fusion in approximately 15 degrees of flexion provides excellent, pain-free stability for function. However, if there is associated IP joint involvement, then an arthroplasty may be preferred to avoid having a fusion in two adjacent joints.[50]

For the CMC joint, there are several successful arthroplasties available that make fusion of the CMC joint a fairly uncommon procedure. A fusion may be considered for this joint in patients with isolated CMC damage as in cases of traumatic arthritis or severe DJD, particularly if the bones are not adequate for an arthroplasty. A fusion may also be considered for patients who have a strenuous vocation in which thumb stability is a key consideration.

In rheumatoid arthritis, isolated CMC joint involvement is rare. An arthroplasty is generally performed to preserve mobility, in the event the patient may need subsequent fusions of the distal joints. The trapezium implant that works well for DJD tends to cause subluxation in patients with RA because of the loss of bone stock in the carpus. For this reason, an alternative type of arthroplasty is performed on the patient with rheumatoid arthritis. This can be a hemiarthroplasty in which either the base of the metacarpal or part of the trapezium is removed and a Silastic spacer is inserted; or a simple resection of the trapezium is performed to improve the alignment of the metacarpal. Any patient limited by thumb instability or deformity should consider surgical options. The functional outcome is usually excellent.

The postoperative management for arthrodesis of the thumb joints is the same as for fusion of the DIP and PIP joints of the fingers described earlier in this section.

References (Arthrodesis)

49. Nalebuff, E. A., and Garrett, J.: *Opera-glass hand in rheumatoid arthritis.* J. Hand Surg. 1(3):210, 1976.
50. Nalebuff, E. A., and Millender, L. H.: *Reconstructive surgery and rehabilitation of the hand.* In Kelley, W. M., et al. (eds.): *Textbook of Rheumatology.* W. B. Saunders, Philadelphia, 1981.
51. Millender, L. H., and Nalebuff, E. A.: *Arthrodesis of the rheumatoid wrist. An evaluation of sixty patients and a description of a different surgical technique.* J. Bone Joint Surg. 55A:1026, 1973.
52. Nalebuff, E. A., Millender, L. H., and Yerid, G.: *The incidence and severity of wrist involvement in juvenile arthritis.* J. Bone Joint Surg. 54A(4):905, 1972.

14

ELBOW SURGERY

In the elbow synovial lining is common to both the elbow (humeroradioulnar) joint and the proximal radioulnar joint. Pain and swelling prompt the patient to keep the arm in a comfortable position of flexion and pronation. The typical consequences are contractures of both joints that limit extension and supination. With severe pain and swelling, motion becomes restricted in all planes. (See Chapter 3, Rheumatoid Arthritis, for a discussion on the relationship of elbow contractures to functional ability.)

In the early phases, elbow synovitis is treated conservatively with systemic medications and local steroid injection.[1] In acute flares, ice compresses and splinting are helpful. When chronic painful synovitis limits function, a person is a candidate for a synovectomy.[1] It can be performed alone but is commonly carried out in conjunction with a radial head resection.[2] Recent studies have shown that elbow synovectomy is successful in relieving pain and improving function in approximately 70 percent of cases for one to three years. Then, radiographic evidence of joint destruction begins to appear. A synovectomy can buy time, but it is not considered a long-term solution.[2,3]

The surgery that shows the greatest promise is total elbow replacement. It is still experimental, but it has been very successful in selected patients. Development of the prosthesis is progressing rapidly towards reducing complications and increasing predictability.

Excisional arthroplasty, once a common surgery for arthritis, is being done only occasionally today and is being supplanted by total joint replacement. It is considered a salvage procedure that relieves pain and allows function (mobility) but reduces stability.

One of the consequences of chronic elbow synovitis and a complication of elbow surgery is entrapment of the ulnar nerve.[4,5] Evaluation of ulnar nerve status is important both before and after surgery. Generally, but not always, one of the first indications of nerve compression is the patient's report of paresthesias along the nerve distribution.[6] Static and moving two-point discrimination on the ulnar innervated fingers should be equal to the median and innervated digits (providing the patient does not have carpal tunnel syndrome). Postoperative swelling may decrease two-point sensitivity, but it should affect all digits equally.[7] (On the finger pads, each person has his or her own norm; generally, it is 3 mm, 4 mm, or 5 mm.) In some patients the ulnar fingers have greater sensitivity than the median fingers. Compression of the ulnar nerve at the elbow can result in weakness of the following muscles: adductor pollicis, flexor pollicis brevis (deep head), all interossei, third and fourth lumbricals, flexor digiti quinti, opponens digiti quinti, abductor digiti quiniti, palmaris brevis, flexor digitorum profundus (ring and little finger), and the flexor carpi ulnaris.[4] If there is weakness, one of the first noticeable signs is weakness in pinch and the inability to adduct the little and ring fingers and/or slight clawing of these digits. The easiest function to monitor is thumb and index pinch adduction of the little finger. (See section on ulnar nerve entrapment in Chapter 21, Hand Pathodynamics and Assessment.)

SYNOVECTOMY AND RADIAL HEAD RESECTION AND REPLACEMENT

This procedure relieves pain and enhances joint motion by diminishing the humeroradial joint and by removing the diseased synovium from the humeroulnar and proximal radioulnar joints.

Supination and pronation can be limited by either the proximal or distal radioulnar joint. Resection of the radial head improves forearm rotation by eliminating restrictions and incongruities between the radial head and its articulation, the ulna.[2] Swanson has developed a Silastic radial head replacement that reduces the amount of instability that often occurs with this surgery; however, the replacement is not universally used.[8]

Some clinicians report that quantitated light touch is the most sensitive assessment for nerve compression. However, two-point discrimination is effective and can be quickly and easily performed at the patient's bedside.[7]

ELBOW SYNOVECTOMY AND RADIAL HEAD RESECTION AND REPLACEMENT

Indications

1. Persistent painful synovitis of the elbow joint.
2. Marked limitations of supination and pronation secondary to proximal radioulnar joint disease.
3. Painful subluxation of the head of the radius.

Occurrence

Rheumatoid arthritis, rheumatoid variants, and traumatic arthritis.

Surgical Prerequisites

1. Absence of severe destructive changes in the humeroulnar joint.
2. Collateral ligament stability.
3. The ability and motivation to follow through with postoperative rehabilitation.

Postoperative Management

Average hospitalization: 5 to 7 days.
1. First to fourth day: Initial immobilization with compression bandage and posterior plaster splint positioning the forearm to neutral rotation and the elbow in 90 degrees of flexion.
2. Fourth or fifth day:
   a. Active sustained ROM exercises can be started in flexion-extension or pronation-supination. Passive exercise should be avoided.
   b. Posterior plaster splint may be used for positioning at night and between exercise periods.
3. Fifth to tenth day:
   a. Cast can be removed during the day.
   b. Active use of the arm is encouraged.
   c. Active sustained ROM exercises can be continued in all planes of motion.
4. After two weeks: Posterior plaster splint can be discarded.

TOTAL ELBOW REPLACEMENT SURGERY

Since the 1920s, there have been numerous attempts to relieve pain and increase mobility and function by replacing either the end of the humerus (hemiarthroplasty) or both the end of the humerus and ulna with metal or synthetic material (total elbow replacement [TER]).[2] The hemiarthroplasties have proven more successful with traumatic elbow problems than with chronic arthritis that affects all joint surfaces, and are currently not being used with patients with RA.[2] The advent of methylmethacrylate fixation cement in the 1960s expanded the options for securing the prostheses and now, the development of TERs dominates the field.

There are a wide variety of designs currently being developed and evaluated in medical centers around the world. Replacements that have been reported in the literature and their design categories include *fully constrained metal hinge replacement:* Dee-McKee and GSB; *full constrained metal-to-plastic hinge replacements:* Stanmore, Link, St. Georg; *flexible elbow replacement:* Mark I, Mark II, Coonrad, Tri-axial; *semi-constrained metal to plastic:* Schlein, GSB (new), Arizona Medical Center radiocapitellum TER, Attenborough, Dee, Mayo; *non-constrained metal to plastic* (with and without intramedullary stems): Kudo, Liverpool, Souter, London, Ishizuki, and Capitello-Condylar TER [Ewald].[2] All of these prostheses are still considered experimental. All have proven effective in *some* patients and all have a higher than desirable rate of complications. Some are so new that sufficient long-term follow-up has not been possible and most are still undergoing design revisions.[2] Therapists interested in a detailed discussion of the above replacements are referred to a recent review by Ewald.[2]

Indications

1. Intractable pain.
2. Destroyed joint.
3. Bilateral elbow limitations of motion that prevent self care.

Occurrence

Rheumatoid arthritis, juvenile chronic polyarthritis, traumatic arthritis.

CAPITELLO-CONDYLAR ELBOW ARTHROPLASTY

The Capitello-Condylar TER was developed at the Robert B. Brigham Hospital in 1974. The current rehabilitative protocol developed for this surgery has been used for over three years and is appropriate for all types of TER replacement surgeries (Fig. 6).[2] However, since these surgeries are experimental, the postoperative management should be closely coordinated among the team members and should reflect the preference of the surgeon.

Surgical Prerequisites

1. Sufficient capsular and ligamentous support to maintain alignment. (Patients with a prior excisional or fasical arthroplasty are not candidates.)
2. Sufficient muscular strength to control the joint.
3. Absence of infection for one year.
4. Adequate bone stock. (Patients with severe osteoporosis or resorption are not candidates.)

Surgical and Functional Goals

The main objective is to have a stable, pain-free elbow with functional ROM. To date, the average postoperative ROM has been 116 degrees arc. A limitation in extension of 20 to 30 degrees is expected. The range of motion should be in the most functional arc.[2] Often the greatest postoperative gains are seen as flexion and pronation rather than extension and supination.[2]

Surgical Procedure[2]

1. Lateral approach between the anconeus and extensor mass.
2. Triceps are partially detached from its ulnar insertion.
3. The extensor mass is elevated from the lateral epicondyle along with the ulnar collateral ligament.
4. The radial head is excised, and synovectomy is performed.
5. The humerus is reamed to accept the fixation stem of the metal component.
6. The ulnar medullary canal is entered and reamed to accept the fixation runners of the polyethylene ulnar replacement.
7. Both components have three major fixation points. These are cemented in place with regard for proper rotation.
8. The soft tissues are reflected back over both epicondylar prominences. The capsule is repaired and the elbow should be able to be flexed to 120 degrees without rupture of the capsule repair.

9. The wound is closed in layers. The triceps are reattached. Both a superficial and deep drain are used for 24 hours.

Postoperative Management

Average hospitalization: 10 to 14 days.
1. Initially, the elbow is in a voluminous compression dressing and splinted in comfortable extension (30 to 40 degrees), and a sling. The elbow is elevated on pillows to decrease edema.
2. Second day: Hand and wrist ROM is started (no forearm rotation). The ulnar nerve is at high risk for being traumatized during surgery or compressed due to swelling or positioning after surgery. Ulnar nerve status should be monitored throughout the postoperative period.
3. Third day: Dressing is changed and reduced.
4. Fifth day: If wound is healing well and there is drainage, active assisted elbow ROM exercises (flexion, extension, forearm rotation) are started. During the exercises, the arm is kept between neutral and internal rotation with the elbow at the side of the body. The exercises are done out of the sling and splint, two times a day. Precaution is needed throughout the postoperative period to protect the triceps repair. The eventual goal of therapy is full ROM with no more than a 30-degree flexion contracture.
5. Seventh to tenth day: The splint is used only at night. The sling is continued during the day. The most stressful force that can be applied to the prosthesis is lateral torque. This occurs when one reaches out, lifts an item, and transports it toward the body with internal rotation of the arm; or when one pushes something away from the body with the hand or forearm using external rotation of the arm. It is lateral torque that is believed to be one of the main causal factors in loosening of the prostheses. To reduce stress to the prosthesis during the vulnerable healing period, patients are instructed not to do any activities that can produce lateral torque for six weeks. Specifically, they are instructed to use the surgical extremity with the upper arm in an adducted position: thus, they cannot reach out to the side to pick up something. Methods for dressing, feeding, bathing, and doing housework that incorporate this precaution are reviewed. Depending on the patient, it may take one to four sessions before the patient can demonstrate observance of appropriate precautions without verbal cues from the therapist. It is important that nursing and physical therapy reinforce precautions with the patient.
6. Twelfth to fourteenth day: Sutures are removed.
7. Fourth week: Splint and sling are discontinued, although some patients prefer to use the sling during the daytime as a reminder to not reach out. Currently, following a total elbow replacement, the patient is restricted from returning to racket sports, golf, baseball, and other competitive sports or heavy labor.

Resection or Fascial Arthroplasty

This surgery involves excision of the ends of the humerus and the ulna. The raw bone ends are either left exposed or covered with fascia lata from the thigh, skin, or synthetic interpositional

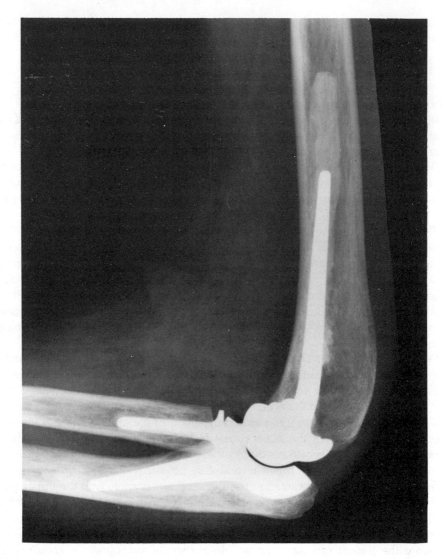

FIGURE 6.   Postoperative x-ray shows placement of a capitello-condylar elbow prosthesis with a radial head replacement. The three intramedullary stems are fixed with acrylic cement. The ulnar component is metal with a polyethylene surface opposing the metal humeral head. On x-ray the polyethylene appears as a gap between the components. The radial head replacement is not used in all total elbow arthroplasties. (Photo courtesy of Dr. Robert Poss and the Journal of Bone and Joint Surgery.)

material.[2] There is also a Silastic implant (Swanson) that is used as a spacer in conjunction with this surgery.[8] The joint is immobilized for a couple of months postoperatively to encourage tightening of the soft tissues.[9]

It is a radical surgery and in the past was done primarily to restore motion and function to ankylosed joints or to relieve intractable pain. The surgery has worked well for many patients, particularly post-traumatic ankylosis.[9] The main problems with the surgery are that it is difficult to predict the outcome and the joint lacks stability sufficient for crutch or cane ambulation or for strenuous work.[9] Thus, it is not an ideal surgery for patients with lower extremity involvement who may need ambulation aids.[9]

Currently, the treatment of choice for an ankylosed joint is a total elbow replacement.[2] The resection arthroplasty has current significance in that this procedure is the alternative the patient is left with if a TER fails, for example due to sepsis, and the prosthesis has to be removed. However, for a patient to have results at least as good as a resection arthroplasty, following failure of a TER, there has to be sufficient length in the bone ends, capsule, and ligaments present.[2] If too many structures have been removed to accommodate the design of the prosthesis, the patient will be left with a completely unstable elbow.

REFERENCES

1. Gschwend, N.: *Synovectomy*. In Kelley, W. M., et al. (eds.): *Textbook of Rheumatology*. W. B. Saunders, Philadelphia, 1981. (Excellent review)
2. Ewald, F. C.: *Reconstructive surgery and rehabilitation of the elbow*. In Kelley, W. M., et al. (eds.): *Textbook of Rheumatology*. W. B. Saunders, Philadelphia, 1981. (Excellent review of TER.)
3. Arthritis Foundation Committee on Evaluation of Synovectomy: *Multicenter evaluation of synovectomy on the treatment of rheumatoid arthritis*. Arthritis Rheum. 20:765, 1977.
4. Nakano, K. K.: *Entrapment neuropathies*. In Kelley, W. M., et al. (eds.): *Textbook of Rheumatology*. W. B. Saunders, Philadelphia, 1981.
5. Broudy, A. S., Leffert, R. D., and Smith, R.: *Technical problems with ulnar nerve transposition at the elbow: Findings and results of reoperation*. J. Hand. Surg. 3(1):85, 1978.
6. Dellon, A. L.: *The moving two-point discrimination test: Clinical evaluation of the quickly adapting fiber-receptor system*. J. Hand Surg. 3(5):474, 1978.
7. Bell, J. A.: *Sensibility evaluation*. In Hunter, J. M., Schneider, L. H., Mackin, E. J., and Bell, J. A.: *Rehabilitation of the Hand*. C. V. Mosby, St. Louis, 1978, pp. 280–283, 289.
8. Swanson, A. B.: *Flexible Implant Resection Arthroplasty in the Hand and Extremities*. C. V. Mosby, St. Louis, 1973.
9. Flatt, A.: *Correction of arthritic deformities of the upper extremity*. In McCarty, D. J. (ed.). *Arthritis and Allied Conditions*. Lea and Febiger, Philadelphia, 1979. (For surgery and rehabilitation of resection arthroplasty.)

15

SHOULDER SURGERY

The shoulder comprises four joints: glenohumeral, sternoclavicular, acromioclavicular, and scapulothoracic. Motion is the result of fourteen muscles acting upon the humerus, scapula, and clavicle.[1,2] Mechanically, the shoulder is extremely complex. None of the joints moves independently. They all move together in a synchronous, rhythmic pattern.[2,3] Because of this complexity and the interdependence of the musculoskeletal structures, the postoperative rehabilitation program is critical to the success of the operative procedure. The role of surgery is also influenced by the functional range of the shoulder and the problems inherent in multiple joint involvement.[4] Approximately 90 degrees of shoulder flexion and abduction and sufficient internal rotation to reach the midline of the body and the opposite axilla are necessary for most functional activities; thus, a person can lose up to 50 percent of shoulder mobility before he or she becomes limited in daily activities. Another factor is that in rheumatoid arthritis, synovitis of the shoulder often comes later in the disease after there is involvement of the hands, feet, and knees.[4] The greatest gains in improving the patient's functional ability often come from surgery of hands and weight-bearing joints. By the time the patient is most concerned about the shoulder, there is severe loss and damage not only to the joint but also to the surrounding musculotendinous support structures.[4]

For patients with rheumatoid arthritis, the functional limitations imposed by a painful and disabled shoulder are dependent upon the involvement of the neck, elbow, and wrist. If these joints have good mobility, the patient will probably be able to do all self-care and daily activities in which reach and lifting can be done in a unilateral manner, e.g., driving. Most patients with shoulder limitations are able to feed themselves, wash their face, shave, and do hair care as long as they have good neck and elbow mobility. If there is severe bilateral shoulder involvement and cervical spine limitations the patient will probably have difficulty in some self-care activities. For patients with multiple joint involvement there is no way of predicting the functional limitations imposed by a painful shoulder without evaluating their actual performance.

Currently, the most common surgeries being performed for problems of the shoulder related to arthritis include synovectomy, bursectomy (with or without an acromioplasty), and total joint replacement.[2,4]

Most cases of bursitis and tendinitis respond to conservative management consisting of anti-inflammatory medication, ice/heat therapy, and steroid injections.[3] Occasionally, some patients develop a severe proliferative synovitis in their subacromial bursa. If the glenohumeral joint is spared, patients can receive excellent results from a bursectomy.[4] In some patients, rheumatoid disease weakens the rotator cuff so that the humeral head continually rides up and impinges upon the acromion, causing pain and further wear on the rotator cuff. Partial removal and shaping of the acromion (acromioplasty) can eliminate this impingment process. In rheumatoid arthritis an acromioplasty is usually done in conjunction with a bursectomy, synovectomy, or total joint replacement.[2,4]

As with total elbow replacement, total shoulder replacement (TSR) is still considered experimental and the prostheses are still undergoing design revisions. TSR surgery is recommended for patients with severe damage to both surfaces of their glenohumeral joints, the most common sequela in rheumatoid arthritis.[4] A humeral head replacement is available for patients who have damage to the humeral surface only, e.g., secondary to trauma or osteonecrosis (aseptic necrosis).[4]

SHOULDER SYNOVECTOMY, BURSECTOMY, AND ACROMIOPLASTY

This procedure is limited to the patient with severe, predominantly bursal shoulder involvement without damage to the surfaces of the glenohumeral joint. The subacromial bursa normally provides a cushion between the head of the humerus and the acromion process. Chronic bursitis may result in swelling and thickening and the production of fibrin bodies within the sac separating the humerus from the acromion, thus preventing elevation of the humerus. The surgery eliminates pain from this source and improves motion and function.[4] Neer recommends a six-month postoperative exercise program to obtain optimal results.[4]

If there is also weakness of the rotator cuff, an acromioplasty is also done.

Indications

1. Thickened subacromion bursa that is nonresponsive to conservative management.

Surgical Prerequisites

1. Preserved glenohumeral joint cartilage.

Surgical Procedure (Neer method)[4]

1. Approach: Across the shoulder from the acromion to the coracoid.
2. The deep fascia is incised and the anterior deltoid is split longitudinally. Part of the deltoid is detached from the acromion.
3. If there is involvement of the acromioclavicular joint, 2 cm of the clavicle may be removed.
4. The clavipectoral fascia is divided.
5. Traction is placed on the arm so the rotator cuff can be inspected and any sharp edges or spurs on the acromion can be detected.
6. If the rotator cuff appears damaged from impingement against the acromion, an

anterior acromioplasty is performed (removal of the anterior edge with beveling of the undersurface).

7. The bursa is excised. (The axillary nerve is at the greatest risk in this surgery.)
8. The subscapularis is detached. The inferior capsule is released and synovectomy of the glenohumeral joint and the sheath of the long head of the biceps is performed.
9. The subscapularis is reattached but may be lengthened by a Z-plasty if it is contracted.
10. The capsule is left open and the deltoid is repaired. The wound is closed and a drain is used for 24 hours.

Postoperative Management[2,4]

Average hospitalization: 10 to 14 days.
1. Initially, the patient is in a voluminous dressing. Patients with preoperative shoulder stiffness are placed in an abduction splint.
2. Second day: Dressing is changed and reduced. ROM exercises to the hand and elbow are started.
3. First week (approximately): When wound healing permits, passive ROM to maintain shoulder rotation and elevation are started two to three times a day. Pendulum exercises with the splint are begun when tolerated.
4. Second week: Gentle isometric exercises are started. Active and resistive exercises are delayed until the reattached muscles have fully healed, approximately three weeks.
5. Third week: The splint can be discontinued if ROM can be maintained.

TOTAL SHOULDER REPLACEMENT

Total joint replacement surgery is indicated when chronic pain and immobility secondary to glenohumeral joint destruction limits functional ability.[4]

The joint prosthesis most frequently used in this country is the Neer prosthesis, originally developed in 1973. The Neer prosthesis consists of a metal humeral head with intramedullary fixation stem. The glenoid component is made of polyethylene and fixed with acrylic cement. New metal-backed glenoid components with polyethylene liners have recently been developed to provide greater humeral contact for severely damaged joints. They function for the humeral head in an acetabulum-like manner (Fig. 7).[4]

In the shoulder, neither bone nor ligaments provide stability. The function of the shoulder after the prosthesis is implanted depends upon the muscles.[4] Postoperative strengthening on the shoulder muscles is critical to the success of the surgery.

In patients with mild to intermediate shoulder RA and with good rotator cuff and surrounding muscles, the following can be expected: pain-free stable motion, full functional use, ROM (flexion and abduction) of about 150 degrees, and nearly full rotation. For patients with severely damaged shoulders, pain relief and functional ROM are the expected results.[4]

Occurrence

Rheumatoid arthritis, juvenile chronic polyarthritis, degenerative joint disease, traumatic arthritis, osteonecrosis, and ankylosing spondylitis.

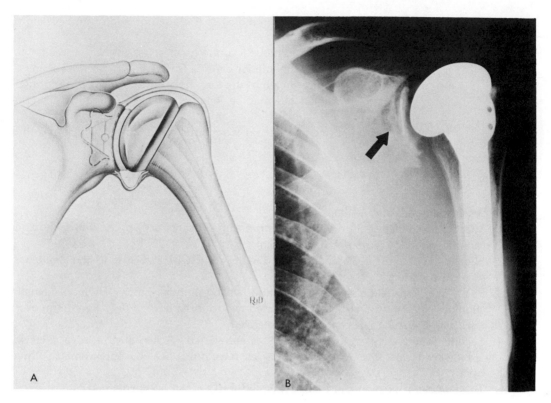

FIGURE 7. The illustration (A) and the x-ray (B) show the standard long head total shoulder resurfacing unit. The polyethylene glenoid component is anchored with acrylic cement (*Arrow*). The metal humeral head has an intramedullary fixation stem, which does not require cement. The humeral stem is available in three diameters and lengths. (From Neer, C. S., II,[4] with permission.)

Surgical Prerequisites[4]

1. Absence of infection.
2. Adequate bone stock to hold the prosthesis.
3. Absence of neurologic impairment to the shoulder muscles. (If there is neurologic impairment, the goals of surgery are reduced to simply pain relief.)

Surgical Procedure

1. Approach: The incision is over the deltopectoral groove, from the clavicle to near the deltoid insertion.
2. The deltoid is retracted, clavipectoral fascia is divided, and the subscapularis tendon is divided.
3. The capsule is released anteriorly and inferiorly. (The biceps is left intact.)
4. The humeral head is rotated into the wound. Diseased synovium is removed from the capsule and bursa. The humeral head is excised at the margin of the articular surface. (On rough edges, osteophytes or granulation tissue is removed from the bicipital groove at this time.)

5. The medullary canal of the humerus is reamed to receive the fixation stem. A trial prosthesis is used to determine proper fit, length, and angle of retroversion (40 degrees).
6. Acromioplasty and acromioclavicular arthroplasty are carried out if needed.
7. The rotator cuff tendons are released from adhesions.
8. The humeral head is inserted; ideally, it fits snugly and cement is not required. In patients with severe RA, the medullary canals are often too soft to hold the stem firmly.
9. The soft tissue repair around the implant is considered of equal importance to the orientation and seating of the prosthesis. The rotator cuff and subscapularis tendons are reattached. (If the subscapularis is tight, it may be lengthened with a Z-plasty.) The wound is closed and two drains are used for 24 hours to prevent hematoma.

Postoperative Management[4,5,6,7]

Average hospitalization: 2 to 3 weeks.
1. Initially, the shoulder is in a compression voluminous bandage. An abduction splint is used if the rotator cuff is repaired. If the splint is of thermoplastic material, it is usually made preoperatively so that it can be fitted by the surgeon in the operating room.
2. The postoperative rehabilitation program is the same as described for synovectomy and acromioplasty except for the following:
   a. If the deltoid is *not* detached from the clavicle, active shoulder exercises can be started in two weeks and progressive resistive exercises can be started about the third week.
   b. If one of the new larger glenoid components is used, the abduction splint is not indicated.

REFERENCES

1. Bateman, J. F.: *The Shoulder and Neck.* W. B. Saunders, Philadelphia, 1972.
2. DePalma, A. F.: *Surgery of the Shoulder,* ed. 2. J. B. Lippincott, Philadelphia, 1973.
3. Bland, J. H., Merrit, J. A., and Boushey, D. R.: *The painful shoulder.* Semin. Arthritis Rheum. 7(1): 1977.
4. Neer, C. S., II: *Reconstructive surgery and rehabilitation of the shoulder.* In Kelley, W. M., et al. (eds.): *Textbook of Rheumatology.* W. B. Saunders, Philadelphia, 1981.
5. Neer, C. S., II: *Arthroplasty of the shoulder: Neer technique.* (Illustrated guide for surgical and postoperative therapy.) Available from: 3M Corporation, Orthopedic Products—Surgical Products Division, 3M Center, St. Paul, Minnesota 55101.
6. Hughes, M. A., and Neer, C. S., II: *Glenohumeral joint replacement and postoperative rehabilitation.* Phys. Ther. 55:850, 1975.
7. Paradis, D. K., and Ferlic, D. C.: *Shoulder arthroplasty in RA.* Phys. Ther. 55:157, 1975.

16

SPINAL SURGERY

CERVICAL SPINE

Subluxation of the cervical spine is common in rheumatoid arthritis, juvenile chronic polyarthritis, and ankylosing spondylitis.[1] In degenerative joint disease the most frequent condition seen is osteophytic formation impinging on the neural structures or limiting apophyseal motion.

Fortunately, in the inflammatory arthritides, the majority of problems related to subluxation can be managed with conservative measures such as medications, pillows, collars, joint protection, exercise, and traction.[2] Surgical fusion is indicated when myelopathy (spinal cord compression) is present and not responsive to conservative measures or if there is persistent debilitating pain.[1,2] When osteophytes create neurologic impairment, surgical removal of the osteophytes or spinal fusion is indicated. When patients with ankylosing spondylitis develop cervical ankylosis in a nonfunctional position, a cervical osteotomy may be performed to correct or reduce the deformity.[1]

ATLANTOAXIAL SUBLUXATION

The unique anatomy of the alantoaxial joint makes it particularly vulnerable to damage and subluxation in the presence of inflammatory joint disease.[1]

There are two synovial joints between the occipital bone and the atlas (C-1). These joints primarily permit nodding of the head. Rotation of the head and atlas takes place upon the axis (C-2) by means of four articulating surfaces—two large joints on each lateral mass and two small joints on the anterior and posterior sides of the odontoid process (dens) between the atlas and the transverse ligament that maintains the alignment of the odontoid process within the atlas. These two small atlanto-odontoid joints are critical because their location allows synovitis to directly erode and weaken the odontoid process and the adjacent transverse ligament that secures the position of the odontoid process.[3] If this ligament becomes stretched or attenuated, subluxation of the atlas on the axis occurs. The atlas differs from other verterbrae, in that it is simply a ring of bone. Within that ring, the spinal cord occupies one-third of the space, the odontoid and transverse ligament occupy one-third of the space, and the remaining one-third

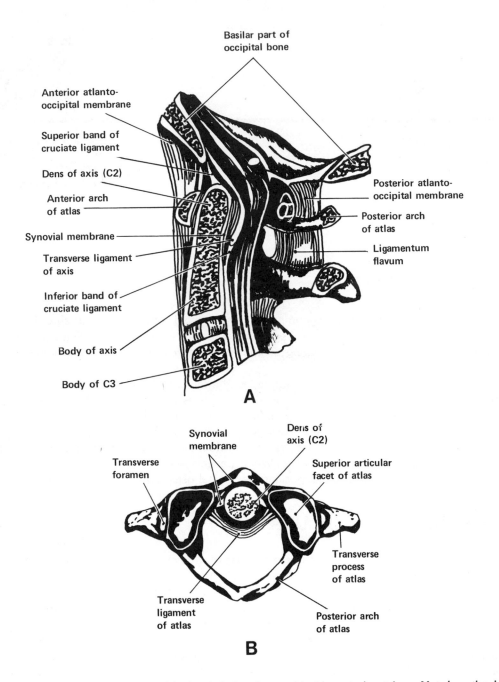

FIGURE 8. (*A*), Sagittal section of the first (atlas) and second (axis) cervical vertebrae. Note how the dens of the axis fits into the atlas. (*B*), Superior view of the articulation of the atlas and the dens of the axis. The transverse ligament of the atlas maintains the aligment of the dens. Inflammatory infiltration of this ligament and subsequent weakening can result in C1-2 subluxation and impingement of the dens on the spinal cord. (From Polly, H. F., and Hunder, G. G.: *Physical Examination of the Joints*, ed. 2. W. B. Saunders, Philadelphia, 1978, with permission.)

of the space is unoccupied. This extra amount of space allows considerable amount of subluxation to take place before the odontoid actually impinges on the spinal cord (Fig. 8).[3]

Patients with atlantoaxial subluxation present with pain and tenderness in the upper cervical spine with radiation of pain to the suboccipital area, aggravated by full neck flexion or extension. They may have paresthesias or Lhermitte's sign (electricity-like pain radiating into the extremities with neck flexion).[1,2] They may also have a feeling of weakness and instability.[1] Occasionally, the patients are able to feel the bones sublux, stating it feels like their head will "slip off."[2] Compression of either of the vertebral arteries may cause visual disturbances (diplopia, blurring) and lightheadedness.[3] Neurologic symptoms may vary from altered reflexes to quadriparesis. Patients with signs of cord compression are treated initially with traction and a cervical collar or brace. If the symptoms persist or increase, a halo and vest may be indicated.[2]

There are several different operative procedures for stabilization of the cervical spine. The procedure of choice depends on the severity of the subluxation and its responsiveness to reduction techniques.[2]

If the subluxation can be reduced the patient may need a cervical collar for 3 to 4 months following surgery. However, if the bones cannot be realigned, it may be necessary for the patient to wear a halo apparatus to provide adequate immobilization of the fusion.[2]

Postoperative therapy includes progressive muscle strengthening, ambulation training, and possibly dexterity and sensory re-education. Patients in collars may need assistive ADL equipment for self care to allow accommodation of the neck restriction. For example, a patient with severe shoulder limitations may not be able to comb his or her hair with the neck erect.

The halo and vest traction device can be very restrictive to a disabled person. Patients with these devices often need advice and counseling in all areas of ADL. Acquiring a comfortable sleeping position is often a major challenge. Some patients have found it helpful to place a Trueze Cervipillo between their neck and the posterior two bars for support. Devices such as reading racks can make reading a feasible and comfortable leisure activity. Patients with fused necks also find it helpful to have a comfortable chair with a swivel base at home. This provides an effortless rotational ability to participate in conversations and to view activities around the house. (Executive office chairs with the casters removed work well for this purpose and often can be purchased at a reasonable cost at used office furniture stores.)

THORACIC AND LUMBAR SPINE

In patients with spondyloarthropathies, severe dysfunctional spinal deformity can often be corrected with spinal osteotomy. Other than this procedure, surgery for the lower spine is the same as for nonrheumatic conditions.

REFERENCES

1. Simmons, E. H.: *Surgery of the spine in rheumatoid arthritis and ankylosing spondylitis.* In Cruss, R. L., and Mitchell, N. S. (eds.): *Surgery of Rheumatoid Arthritis.* J. B. Lippincott Co., Philadelphia, 1971.
2. Thomas, W. H.: *Surgical management of the rheumatoid cervical spine.* Orthop. Clin. North Am. 6(3): 793, 1975.
3. Jackson, R.: *The Cervical Syndrome,* 4th ed. Charles C Thomas, Springfield, Ill., 1977.

ADDITIONAL SOURCES

Hart, D. L., Johnson, R. M., Simmons, E. F., and Owen, J.: *Review of cervical orthoses.* Phys. Ther. 58 (7):857, 1978.

Johnson, R. M., et al.: *Cervical orthoses: A study comparing their effectiveness in restricting cervical motion in normal subjects.* J. Bone Joint Surg. 59A(3): April, 1977.

Fisher, S. V., et al.: *Cervical orthoses effect on cervical spine motion: Roetgenographic and goniometric method of study.* Arch. Phys. Med. Rehab. 58:109, 1977.

Ranawat, C. S., et al.: *Cervical spine fusion in rheumatoid arthritis.* J. Bone Joint Surg. (Am.) 61(77):1003, 1979.

17

HIP
SURGERY

The hip joint is a large joint highly dependent upon the shape of the articulation for stability, rather than ligamentous support like the knee or muscular support like the shoulder.[1]

Chronic synovitis of the hip results in increased intra-articular pressure pain and diminished cartilage. Hypertrophic synovium (pannus) gets trapped between the joint surfaces, increasing cartilage wear and limiting motion. Secondary muscle spasm and fibrosis of the capsule limit motion even further.[2] Subchondral cysts may appear and then collapse leaving irregularities in the femoral head. In severe RA, the head of the femur may push the softened acetabulum into the pelvic cavity, a condition referred to as "protrusion acetabulae."[2] In both DJD and RA, osteophyte formation occurs and can restrict motion.[2]

Flexion, adduction, and external rotation contractures are the most common deformities seen in the hip, and they can result from four factors: flexion, adduction, and external rotation of the hip is the position that reduces intra-articular pressure and provides the greatest comfort, therefore it is the position assumed at rest;[2] hip pain can produce spasm of the associated flexor and adductor muscles; patients with hip pain avoid walking or standing and all sitting activities encourage a flexion deformity; constant flexion positioning allows the strong anterior iliofemoral (Y) ligament to become contracted in a shortened position. Full hip extension may occur only when the patient does specific stretching exercises. Lying prone daily (see Chapter 30) is a valuable conservative as well as postoperative measure for maintaining or improving hip extension.[3]

In the hip, the weight-bearing forces are the primary stress factors that aggravate the synovitis in RA and wear out the cartilage in DJD.[1] It is estimated that a force equal to four times body weight is exerted at the hip joint when a person is weight bearing on one extremity, for example, during ambulation and climbing stairs. Therefore, a critical aspect of conservative management is body weight reduction and the use of ambulation aids to relieve stress to the joint.[1,2]

All health professionals should be aware that the cane or crutch should be used in the hand *opposite* the painful hip (or knee). Thus, when a person leans to use the cane, the center of gravity is shifted over the good hip, reducing the weight borne by the affected hip. If the cane is used on the painful side, body weight is shifted over the painful joint during ambulation, increasing pain and producing a more abnormal gait.[1,2]

Patients with progressive hip pain that interferes with daily activities despite proper medication and physical therapy are considered candidates for hip surgery.[3]

In the United States, the total hip replacement (THR) and the total hip surface replacement (THSR) are the two surgeries currently being performed for hip arthritis.[3] In Europe, osteotomies are done for selected patients with DJD. Synovectomies are rarely done, because of the high risk of osteonecrosis of the femoral head.[3] Additionally, synovectomies need to be done early to be effective. Most patients complaining of significant hip pain show radiographic cartilage changes.

Total hip replacement is still considered the treatment of choice, particularly for RA.[3] THR was developed in England by Sir John Charnley in 1961. It was first performed in this country in 1968. Currently, it is estimated that over 80,000 total hip replacements are performed annually in the United States.[3,4] All of the hip replacement prostheses currently being used are variations of the Charnley low-friction metal-to-plastic replacement.[3] The metal femoral head has an intramedullary fixation stem (Fig. 9). Both the stem and the acetabular component are fixed with acrylic cement. The long-term results of THR have been excellent, with 85 to 97 percent complete or almost complete pain relief.[3] The major complications are loosening of the components, which requires a second surgery, and sepsis, which requires removal of the prosthesis. In selected patients, it is now possible to perform a second THR after a period of asepsis.

Total hip surface replacement is an alternative to THR that has received increasing attention in the past few years.[5] This procedure involves capping the femoral head with a metal surface and enlarging and resurfacing the acetabulum with plastic. The surgery offers the advantage of retaining the femoral head and thus maintaining a more normal physiologic distribution of weight-bearing forces throughout the bone, and avoiding problems of loosening of the fixation stem.[3,5] At this time, it is too early to tell the long-term results of this procedure. The major risks are osteonecrosis of the femoral head under the metal cap and loosening of the acetabular component. If it proves effective, it may provide a solution for patients who currently have a high incidence of stem loosening with a THR, such as young patients with DJD.[3]

The postoperative management is the same for THR and THSR surgeries.

TOTAL HIP REPLACEMENT ARTHROPLASTY

Indications

1. Persistent debilitating hip pain associated with joint destruction and limited hip motion that does not respond to conservative forms of treatment.
2. Failure of prior hip surgery (cupt arthroplasty, hemiarthroplasty).
3. Hip arthrodesis in a poor functional position or associated with increasing back or knee pain.

Occurrence

Rheumatoid arthritis, degenerative joint disease, traumatic arthritis, rheumatoid variants (ankylosing spondylitis, psoriatic arthritis, inflammatory bowel disease, osteonecrosis, aseptic necrosis), and juvenile chronic polyarthritis.

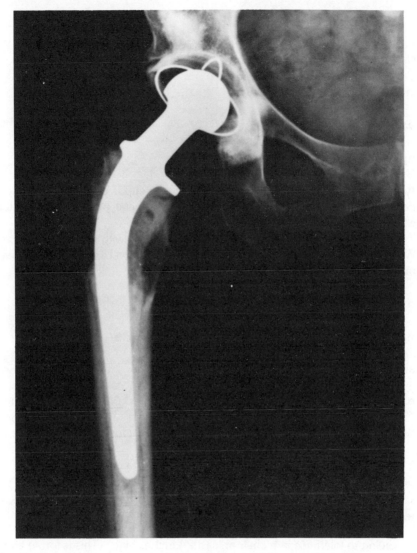

FIGURE 9. Postoperative x-ray shows placement of a total hip prosthesis. The metal femoral head articulates with a polyethylene acetublar component. Both the femoral stem and acetabular cup are cemented in place. (Courtesy of Dr. Robert Poss and the Journal of Bone and Joint Surgery.)

Functional and Surgical Goals[3,6]

Postsurgical expectations include relief of hip pain, joint stability, and increased ROM (ideally zero degrees extension and 100 degrees flexion). Restoration of hip motion improves gait and alleviates stress from the back and knees.

Surgical Prerequisites

1. Adequate bone stock for seating of the prosthesis.
2. No current sepsis anywhere else in the body.
3. Competent abductor mechanism.
4. Intact joint sensation.

Surgical Procedure

1. Approach: lateral or posterior incision.
2. Greater trochanter may or may not be removed.
3. Acetabulum remodeled: polyethylene prosthetic cup is cemented in place.
4. Femoral head is excised, shaft broached, and metal prosthesis cemented in place with methylmethacrylate (acrylic cement).
5. If greater trochanter is osteotomized, it is reattached with wire sutures.
6. When bilateral THR is indicated, a two-week interval between surgeries is recommended.[2,6]

Postoperative Physical Therapy[3,7,8,9,10,11]

For total hip replacement, average hospitalization: 2 to 3 weeks.
1. First day postoperative:
   a. Initiation of isometric strengthening exercises for knee and hip extensors (taught in the preoperative strengthening program).
   b. Instruction in proper positioning to avoid hip flexion, adduction, and internal rotation. Postoperative bed positioning varies; some facilities use a balanced suspension and traction unit for 48 hours, then at night for two weeks; other facilities use an abduction pillow.
   c. Instruction in calf-pumping exercises to prevent venous stasis.
2. Second day: Hip ROM exercises are started.
3. Fourth or fifth day: Patient begins sitting at side of the bed, feet dangling.
4. Sixth to eighth day to discharge:
   a. Begins standing.
   b. Sitting to tolerance in a chair at least 24 inches high. (This is for an average height person; it is too high for a short person.) In order that the patient can sit and rise with only 45 degrees of flexion, hip should not adduct to neutral or flex beyond 45 degrees during first preoperative week.
   c. Ambulation to tolerance with assistive equipment.
   d. If trochanter is removed, weight bearing on operated side is limited. Patients are instructed to use ambulation aids to insure partial weight bearing on the surgical hip for three months.
5. Tenth day:
   a. Exercises to increase ROM and strengthen the hip muscles are started; most patients regain sufficient motion through sitting, ambulation, and functional activities.
   b. Stationary bicycles are used to increase ROM and strength.

Postoperative Occupational Therapy[12,13,14]

(Evaluation, instruction in postoperative precautions, and issuance of an extended reach are best done preoperatively.)

1. Fifth to seventh day: Instruction in functional activities is initiated. (The type of training needed depends upon the precautions for each patient, which are determined by the position of the prosthesis, muscle tone, degree of postoperative ROM, the patient's daily activities, and the nature of the surgical procedure, that is, trochanter removed or not.) This involves training in adaptive methods or use of assistive equipment to avoid hip flexion beyond 90 degrees and hip adduction (past neutral) and internal rotation. Instruction includes training in methods for toilet, chair, tub, bed, and car transfers; stair climbing; shoe and sock dressing on the surgical extremity; adaptive methods of washing and drying the foot as well as nail care on the surgical side; and sexual positioning.

2. Precautions for at least the first three months. (Some of these precautions may be needed indefinitely, depending on the patient.) Precautions include night positioning to prevent hip flexion, adduction, and internal rotation; avoidance of excessive hip abduction with external rotation, for example, sitting cross-legged; and no hip flexion beyond 100 degrees.

After Discharge

Home program for graded strengthening of hip flexors, extensors, and abductors and to maintain ROM. Use of a stationary bicycle is encouraged.

REFERENCES

1. Singleton, M. C., and LeVeau, B.: *The hip joint: Structure, stability, and stress—A review.* Phys. Ther. 55(9):957, 1975.
2. Sledge, C. B.: *Correction of arthritic deformities in the lower extremity and spine.* In McCarty, D. J. (ed.). *Arthritis and Allied Conditions.* Lea and Febiger, Philadelphia, 1979.
3. Poss, R., and Sledge, C. B.: *Surgery of the hip in rheumatoid arthritis.* In Kelley, W. M., et al. (eds.): *Textbook of Rheumatology.* W. B. Saunders, Philadelphia, 1981.
4. Hori, R. Y., Lewis, J. L., Zimmerman, J. R., and Compere, C.: *The number of total joint replacements in the United States.* Clin. Orthop. 132:46, 1978.
5. Amstutz, H. C., Graff Radford, A., Gruen, T. A., and Clarke, I. C.: *Thaires surface replacements: A review of the first 100 cases.* Clin. Orthop. 134:2, 1978.
6. Jergensen, H. E., Poss, R., and Sledge, C. B.: *Bilateral total hip and knee replacement in adults with RA: Evaluation of function.* Clin. Orthop. 137:120, Nov-Dec 1978.
7. Richardson, R. W.: *Physical therapy management of patients undergoing total hip replacement.* Phys. Ther. 55(9):984, 1975.
8. Wiesman, H. J., Simon, S. R., Ewald, F., Thomas, W. H., and Sledge, C. B.: *Total hip replacement with and without osteotomy of the greater trochanter: Clinical and biomechanical comparisons in the same patients.* J. Bone Joint Surg. 60A:203, 1978.
9. McCann, V. H., Phillips, C. A., and Quigley, T. R.: *Preoperative and postoperative management: The role of the allied health professionals.* Orthop. Clin. North Am. 6:881, 1975.
10. Thielen, P. L., and Mueller, K. H.: *Immediate postoperative management of patients with total hip replacement.* Phys. Ther. 53(9):949, 1973.
11. Myers, M. H., McNelly, D. B., and Nelson, K.: *Total hip replacement: A team effort.* Am. J.

Nurs. 78(9):1485-1488. (Description of the nursing and PT program at Rancho Los Amigos Hospital.)

12. Seeger, M., and Fisher, L.: *OT for total hip replacement—Patient use of assistive devices.* Am. J. O. T., (In press) (Detailed description of THR program at UCLA and survery of patient use of assistive equipment.)

13. Todd, R. C., Lightowler, C. D. R., and Harris, J.: *Low friction arthroplasty of the hip joint and sexual activity.* Acta Orthop. Scand. 44(6):690, 1973.

14. *You and Your New Hip.* Patient booklet clearly describing postoperative functional precautions, developed by the occupational therapy department at University Hospitals of Cleveland, 2065 Adelbert Road, Cleveland, Ohio 44106. (Excellent patient education aid.)

18

KNEE SURGERY

The knee joint is a frequent site of involvement in all of the rheumatic diseases.

In rheumatoid arthritis, the most common consequence of chronic synovitis is knee flexion contractures. Unfortunately, many contractures develop because patients have not received appropriate instruction, splinting, or physical therapy early enough. When the knee is inflamed, a position of slight flexion provides the greatest comfort. Patients sleep with pillows under their knees for comfort and then cannot regain extension after the inflammation subsides. It is also theorized that pain and tension of the capsule cause a reflex spasm of the knee flexor muscles and inhibition of the extensors, which encourages a flexed position.[1,2] A flexion contracture greater than 15 degrees impairs functional ability by decreasing quadriceps efficiency and increases the energy cost of ambulation. If possible, knee flexion contractures greater than 30 degrees should be reduced through serial casting, traction, and exercise prior to surgery. If a contracture is nonresponsive to traction, due to shortening of the muscles and posterior capsule, a posterior lateral soft tissue release may be performed.[3,4]

For patients with persistent synovitis and beginning flexion deformity, but minimal cartilage changes, a synovectomy is a feasible short term solution for relieving pain and forestalling joint damage. The benefits of synovectomy typically are from one to three years but can last longer in some patients.[5]

In the moderate stages of RA, synovitis erodes all of the articulating surfaces equally, causing a symmetric reduction in the height of the joint. The loss of height creates laxity in the supporting ligaments and knee instability. With progression and severity of the disease, asymmetric erosions and collapse of the cartilage can occur, producing valgus; however, varus rotational deformities and posterior subluxation of the tibia are also seen.[4]

For either moderate or late destruction, the total knee replacement is considered the treatment of choice. The TKR is designed to restore height to the joint so the ligaments can be at appropriate tension to provide stability. If valgus or varus deformity is present, the tibial components can be adjusted to correct angulation. Rotation deformity or posterior subluxation requires additional soft tissue reconstruction.[3,4]

There have been over 300 different prostheses designed in the past 30 years. Currently, the most successful replacements fall into two categories:[4,7]

1. Nonconstrained: The tibia and femoral components resurface the joint and provide height. They have gliding contact and are dependent upon the ligamentous integrity for stabil-

ity (Fig. 10). The Unicondylar, Modular, Polycentric, and Duocondylar prostheses are in this category.

   2. Semiconstrained: These provide greater stability because of their highly congruent surfaces and a tibial peg or protrusion that fits loosely into the femoral component compensating for the damaged cruciate ligaments. The Geometric, Freeman-Swanson (ICLH), Variable Axis, and Total Condylar prostheses are in this category.

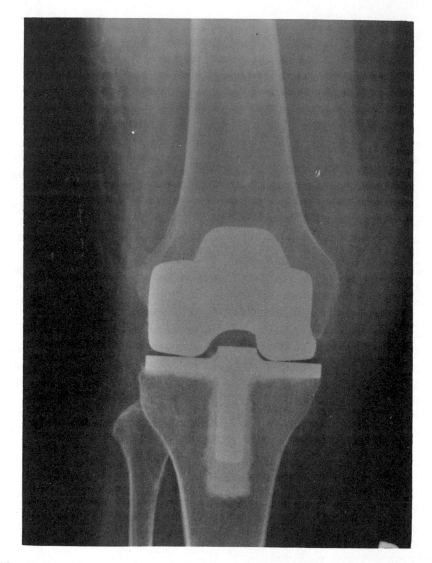

FIGURE 10.   Postoperative x-ray of a nonconstrained total knee arthroplasty. The femoral component is all metal and secured with cement. The tibial component is metal with a 6 mm-thick polyethylene surface to articulate with the femoral component. The angle of this film does not clearly show the plastic tibial surface and gives the impression that the two metal surfaces are touching. (Courtesy of Dr. Robert Poss and the Journal of Bone and Joint Surgery.)

There have been several attempts to develop a full hinge prosthesis that would provide full stability for the severely destroyed joint. The all metal hinges (Wallidius, Shiers, Guepar) are no longer used owing to a high rate of infection and loosening and the consequence of an arthrodesed or totally unstable knee in the event of failure. New metal-to-plastic hinges are being developed on an experimental basis.[4,7]

The problems encountered in DJD of the knee are very different from those seen in RA. In DJD, the cartilage destruction is often unilateral, involving one compartment of the knee, and typically produces a varus deformity. These patients often have monoarticular involvement and are more active than patients with RA and, therefore, place greater demands on the surgical repair.[3]

Surgical options for the patient with DJD include:

1. Débridement. This includes removing osteophytes, degenerated menisci, and loose cartilage bodies; shaving degenerated cartilage; and drilling eburnated bone. This procedure can provide satisfactory pain relief, particularly in younger patients.[3]
2. Osteotomy. For patients with unicompartmental destruction and varus deformity, a thin wedge of bone is removed from the tibia beneath the unaffected compartment to shift weight-bearing forces to the unaffected lateral side. It is effective for mild (10 degrees) varus and valgus deformities. For marked valgus deformity, a femoral osteotomy or a unicompartmental arthroplasty is often used.[3]
3. Total knee replacement. This is indicated for patients with persistent pain and decreased ROM who are *not* candidates for an osteotomy or débridement procedure.[3]

KNEE SYNOVECTOMY

Indications

Persistent painful synovial mass with intermittent or constant effusion that has not responded to at least 4 to 6 months of adequate medical treatment.

Occurrence

Primarily rheumatoid arthritis and rheumatoid variants.

Surgical and Functional Goals

1. Relief of pain.
2. Increase in active ROM of knee from zero degrees to at least 90 degrees of flexion.
3. Delay in the progression of joint destruction.[4]

Surgical Prerequisites

1. Absence of cartilage destruction on preoperative x-ray studies.
2. Flexion contracture less than 15 degrees.
3. Ligamentous stability.

4. Competent quadriceps mechanism.
5. Motivation to participate in an extensive postsurgical rehabilitation program. No presurgical depression.

Surgical Procedure

1. Approach: Anteromedial.
2. The deep fascia and capsule are incised.
3. As much synovium as possible is excised. Most surgeons remove both menisci.

Postoperative Physical Therapy

Average hospitalization: 2 to 3 weeks.
Isometric quadriceps-strengthing exercises are started preoperatively.
1. First to fifth day:
   a. Isometric quadriceps-strengthening exercises are re-established and assisted straight leg-raising exercises are initiated.
   b. Posterior plaster resting splints are worn when the patient is at rest throughout the postoperative period.
2. Fifth to tenth day:
   a. Active-assisted ROM exercises may be added to the program.
   b. Resistive isometric quadriceps-strengthening exercises are started when the quadriceps are a grade 3.5 on a 5 point scale (fair plus).
   c. Ambulation guideline: Patient can be ambulatory in posterior plaster splint with crutches or a walker as soon after surgery as pain permits. Weight bearing without the splint depends on the amount of pain and the strength of the quadriceps muscles.
3. Tenth to fourteenth day: Joint manipulation under anesthesia is considered if the expected amount of flexion has not been achieved.[4]

Postoperative Occupational Therapy

When patient is ready for weight bearing, instruction in joint protection techniques and use of assistive equipment can be started if indicated. (See Chapter 26, Joint Protection and Energy Conservation Instruction, and Chapter 27, Assistive Equipment.)

TOTAL KNEE REPLACEMENT ARTHROPLASTY
(With Non-Hinge Prosthesis)

Indications

Persistent debilitating pain associated with joint destruction or limited joint motion.[7]

Occurrence

Rheumatoid arthritis, degenerative joint disease, and other arthropathies such as trauma, gout, or hemophilia.[7]

Surgical and Functional Goals

Ideally, this surgery will result in relief of pain, joint stability, and range of motion from zero to 90 degrees.

Surgical Prerequisites[7]

1. Intact extensor mechanism.
2. Ligamentous stability. (Completely unstable joints require a hinge prosthesis.)
3. Intact joint sensation (not for neuropathic joints).
4. Flexion contractures should be less than 15 degrees. (Contractures between 15 and 40 degrees should be considered for serial casting prior to surgery.)
5. Adequate bone stock on which to seat the prosthesis.
6. Motivation to participating in an extensive postsurgical rehabilitation program. Absence of marked clinical depression.

Surgical Procedure

1. Approach: anteromedial incision.
2. Synovectomy, if active synovitis is present.
3. Resection of bone ends and cementing of components in place.
4. Repair of capsule and quadriceps mechanism.

Postoperative Physical Therapy[3,4,7,8]

Average hospitalization: 2 to 3 weeks.
1. First to third day:
   a. Initial immobilization—Compression dressing, posterior plaster leg splint.
   b. Isometric quadriceps exercises and straight leg-raising exercises (taught to patient in preoperative strengthening program) are initiated.
   c. Instruction in transfer methods.
2. Fourth to eighth day:
   a. Posterior splint or cast removed.
   b. Gentle, active, and active-assisted flexion and extension ROM exercises are started.
   c. Quadriceps- and hamstring-strengthening program is started.
3. One to three weeks: Ambulation is initiated, depending on type of prosthesis, degree of leg control, pain, and other factors.

4. Posterior leg splints are indicated for at least 3 months at night to maintain full extension.

Postoperative Occupational Therapy

The most difficult task for patients following a TKR is lower extremity dressing and hygiene on the surgical extremity because of limited knee flexion. Patients with monoarticular arthritis are generally independent in functional activities by the second week, since they can substitute hip mobility for limited knee range of motion. Patients with polyarticular involvement may need aids such as an extended shoe horn, sock donner, elastic shoe laces, and extended handle sponge, to allow independence in these activities until full knee mobility is achieved. At the time of discharge, the patient should have at least 90 degrees of flexion (120 degrees of flexion is needed to meet ambulation and transfer requirements).

When the patient begins ambulation, the following program is initiated.
1. Evaluation of lower extremity dressing skills, equipment issued as needed.
2. Review of methods for partial weight bearing (PWB) during activities of daily living, particularly: tub transfer, kitchen, and housework activities. Patient will be PWB for approximately 6 weeks.
3. Instruction in joint protection methods.
4. Instruction in proper positioning at night and during leisure activities.

Ideally, the patient should be independent in ADL, with or without assistive devices at the time of discharge.

REFERENCES

1. Choen, L. A., and Cohen, M. L.: *Arthrokinetic reflex of the knee.* Am. J. Physiol. 184:433, 1956.
2. deAndrade, J. R., Grant, C., and Dixon, A. St. J.: *Joint distension and reflex muscle inhibition in the knee.* J. Bone Joint Surg. 47A:313, 1965.
3. Sledge, C. B.: *Correction of arthritic deformities in the lower extremity and spine.* In McCarty, D. J. (ed.): *Arthritis and Allied Conditions.* Lea and Febiger, Philadelphia, 1978.
4. Insall, J.: *Reconstructive surgery and rehabilitation of the knee.* In Kelley, W. M., et al. (eds.): *Textbook of Rheumatology.* W. B. Saunders, Philadelphia, 1981.
5. Gschwend, N.: *Synovectomy.* In Kelley, W. M., et al. (eds.): *Textbook of Rheumatology,* Vol. II. W. B. Saunders, Philadelphia, 1981.
6. Laurin, C. A., et al.: *Long-term results of synovectomy of the knee in rheumatoid patients.* J. Bone Joint Surg. 56(Am):521, 1974.
7. Kettelkamp, D. B., and Leach, R. B. (eds.): *Clinical Orthopaedics and Related Research: Symposium on Total Knee Replacement.* 94:2, Jul–Aug, 1973. (Review of all major knee replacement surgeries).
8. Manske, P. R., and Gleeson, P.: *Rehabilitation program following polycentric total knee arthroplasty.* Phys. Ther. 57:915, 1977.

19

FOOT AND ANKLE SURGERY

Rheumatoid arthritis involves the foot as frequently as it does the hand. It is common for RA to affect the metatarsophalangeal (MTP) and subtalar and talonavicular joints. Less frequently it may involve the true ankle joint. Although sometimes clinically this distribution is difficult to appreciate because patients unfamiliar with ankle anatomy mistakenly describe subtalar (hindfoot) synovitis as ankle pain.[1,2]

Initially synovitis creates swelling and pain in the MTP joints and possibly the distal digital joints. Patients often describe the pressure on the ball of the foot as walking on marbles. During ambulation, particularly during the toe push off phase, the MTP joints bear the full weight of the body in a dorsiflexed position. The kinematics of push off cause stretch of the plantar capsule and supporting ligaments, resulting in dorsal subluxation of the MTP joints.[2] Another dynamic force that occurs during the early phases of synovitis is spasm of the intrinsic muscles and the extrinsic digital flexor muscles.[1] All of these factors combine to create an imbalance deformity of the toes, referred to as cock-up toe deformity. The complete deformity consists of MTP dorsiflexion, PIP flexion, and DIP hyperextension. Occasionally, patients do not develop hyperextension of the DIP joint and the deformity is referred to as a hammer toe. Additionally, chronic MTP joint synovitis stretches the transverse ligaments resulting in widening of the forefoot referred to as splayed forefoot.[3]

The hindfoot includes the talus and calcaneus bones and the joints between these bones and the midtarsal bones. The subtalar (subastragalar) joint is the articulation between the talus and the calcaneus bones.[2,6] It is a critical joint and is responsible for inversion and eversion of the foot. (Flexion and extension takes place in the ankle joint.) The signs and symptoms of subtalar joint synovitis and subluxation include pain with passive inversion and eversion; greater than 5 degrees of valgus between the heel and tibia upon weight bearing, measured on the posterior surface (children with arthritis often develop varus deformity); and peroneal spasm elicited with brisk passive inversion, while the foot is dangling in mid-air.[1]

When synovitis stretches the capsule and ligaments of the subtalar and talonavicular joints, the natural tendency of the talus to glide forward, downward, and medially is increased. Subsequent pressure on the calcaneus and plantar-calcaneonavicular (or spring) ligament typically results in hindfoot pronation and flattening of the longitudinal arch. Erosion of the subtentaculum tali (a process on the calcaneus that provides medial support to the talus) results in marked displacement of the talus and severe pronation of the foot.[1]

Ambulation with the hindfoot in supination necessitates medial pressure against the large toe and contributes to a hallux valgus deformity of the first MTP joint and additionally alters the weight-bearing forces on the knee.[5]

Advances in foot orthotic materials and fabrication methods over the past few years have had a significant impact on management of the rheumatoid foot. The incorporation of a comprehensive foot orthotics program at the Robert B. Brigham Hospital resulted in a 30 percent decrease in foot surgeries.[3]

Surgery for rheumatoid foot involvement can be described by location: forefoot, hindfoot, and ankle. Treatment for midfoot synovitis is usually accomplished with conservative measures.[1]

COMMON SURGERIES FOR FOREFOOT INVOLVEMENT

MTP RESECTION ARTHROPLASTY WITH SILASTIC IMPLANT

This operation is for the first MTP joint and soft tissue correction of cock-up toe deformities. It combines several procedures and is the most common surgery for classic severe rheumatoid foot involvement.[2] This surgery relieves pain by eliminating the MTP joint and corrects hallux valgus and toe deformities, alleviating pressure areas on the dorsum of the PIP joints and plantar surface of the foot. The correction of deformities improves the appearance of the foot and may enable the patient to wear normal style shoes. The main disadvantage of the surgery is that it compromises the push off ability of the toes. The first MTP implant preserves the length and stability of the first MTP for weight bearing.[1]

This operation is reserved for severe foot deformities and is often done on both feet during the same surgery.[1] Correction of toe contractures may require manipulation of the digits and Kirschner wire fixation.[1]

Postoperative Management

Three weeks of continuous splinting are followed by three weeks of night splinting using a hallux valgus splint to maintain neutral alignment of the first MTP joint.[1] Generally, commercial splints can be used or adapted. Occasionally, it is necessary to make custom splints.[3,4] The patient begins ambulation to tolerance on the third or fourth day following surgery and wears a wooden sole postoperative sandal for approximately 6 weeks.[1] Plastazote liners can increase the comfort of these sandals. The average hospitalization for this surgery is about ten days.

METATARSAL OSTEOTOMY

When MTP subluxation results in a cock-up toe deformity that is easily reducible by pressing on the metatarsal head, the deformity can be corrected by a simple dorsal metatarsal osteotomy.[1] This is indicated for isolated MTP involvement in patients with nonerosive joint disease.[1] This surgery relieves pain from pressure on prominent MTP heads and associated callus is eliminated and prevents development of a fixed deformity.[1]

HALLUX VALGUS CORRECTION

There are several operative procedures for this problem. The Keller procedure is widely used and involves resection of the proximal third of the proximal phalanx and the medial prominence of the metatarsal head.[1] Fusion of the first MTP in dorsiflexion is often advised to maintain the stability of the great toe for ambulation.[1] The postoperative splinting program is the same as described under resection arthroplasty.

HALLUX RIGIDUS CORRECTION

Occasionally, osteophyte formation around the first MTP joint will block dorsiflexion, creating rigidity in the toe. This condition is painful, restricts the push off ability of the foot, and causes compensatory stress to the IP joint of the great toe. This condition is most commonly seen in DJD but can also occur in RA.[1]

For the younger active patient with DJD, a simple débridement and removal of the spurs is the procedure of choice. For the patient with RA or the older patient with DJD, an excision arthroplasty with Silastic implant is recommended.[1]

Postoperatively, active-assistive exercises are started as soon as symptoms permit. Ambulation is resumed to tolerance. Splinting is generally not indicated.[1]

COMMON SURGERIES FOR HINDFOOT INVOLVEMENT

TRIPLE ARTHRODESIS

In the early stages, subtalar joint and hindfoot involvement can often be managed effectively with a heel cup orthosis, which restricts inversion and eversion of the foot.[1,4] If disability persists despite conservative measures or if the deformity cannot be reduced passively, a triple arthrodesis is often recommended.[1] This procedure effects a fusion between the talus and calcaneus, the calcaneus and cuboid, and the talus and navicular bones. When successful, this procedure provides a pain-free stable hindfoot; however, it is a difficult surgery in patients with rheumatoid arthritis because of the softness of the bone.[2] If there is severe ankle involvement, it may be necessary to perform a total ankle arthroplasty after the arthrodesis has healed, before pain-free functional ambulation is possible.[1]

Postoperative management involves 12 weeks of cast immobilization followed by use of a heel cup or foot-ankle molded orthosis for 6 to 12 weeks until the bone union is solid.[1]

TALONAVICULAR ARTHRODESIS

In some patients, the talonavicular joint may be the only joint in the hindfoot with significant involvement. For these patients, a single arthrodesis of the talonavicular joint is recommended.[1]

Postoperative management includes immobilization in a posterior splint for several days until swelling subsides, followed by cast immobilization for 10 to 12 weeks.[1]

COMMON SURGERIES FOR ANKLE INVOLVEMENT

The two operations commonly performed for arthritis of the ankle are arthrodesis and total ankle replacement.[1] Currently, the arthrodesis is recommended for the younger active patient with DJD or traumatic arthritis who has sufficient mobility in the hindfoot to compensate for rigidity in the ankle, or patients with gross instability and uncorrectable hindfoot deformity. A total ankle arthroplasty is the procedure of choice for patients with limited mobility in the hindfoot either from ankylosis or arthrodesis; patients with RA, a stable ankle, and mild to moderate hindfoot involvement; and the older patient with DJD with limited ambulation requirements.

Postoperative management for an ankle arthrodesis requires 12 to 20 weeks of case immobilization. For the total joint replacement, active and passive ROM is started approximately 3 to 5 days postoperatively. Ambulation begins on the seventh to tenth day, as tolerated.[1] Partial weight bearing is continued until the patient has gained sufficient strength to insure stability.

REFERENCES

1. Thomas, W. H.: *Reconstructive surgery and rehabilitation of the ankle and foot.* In Kelley, W. M., et al. (eds.): *Textbook of Rheumatology.* W. B. Saunders, Philadelphia, 1981.
2. Giannestras, N.: *Foot Disorders; Medical and Surgical Management,* ed. 2. Lea and Febiger, Philadelphia, 1973.
3. Wood, B.: *The painful foot.* In Kelley, W. M., et al. (eds.): *Textbook of Rheumatology.* W. B. Saunders, Philadelphia, 1981.
4. Inman, V. T., and DuVries, H. L: *Surgery of the Foot,* ed. 3. C. V. Mosby, St. Louis, 1973.
5. Inman, V. T.: *Hallux valgus: A review of etiologic factors.* Orthop. Clin. North Am. 5(1):59, 1974.

ADDITIONAL SOURCES

Inman, V. T.: The Joints of the Ankle. Williams & Wilkins, Baltimore, 1976.
Moseley, H. F.: *Traumatic Disorders of the Ankle and Foot.* CIBA Symposia Vol. 17, No. 1, 1965. CIBA Pharmaceutical Co., Summit, New Jersey, 07901. (Presented 1980. Excellent resource for anatomic drawings of the foot.)
Tillmann, K.: *The Rheumatoid Foot: Diagnosis, Pathomechanics, and Treatment.* PSG Publishing, Littleton, MA, 1979.
Zamosky, I., and Licht, S.: *Shoes and their modification.* Orthotics Etcetera, New Haven, 1966, pp. 402-432.

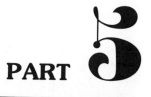

PART

EVALUATION TECHNIQUES

20

EVALUATION OF MEDICAL HISTORY AND SYMPTOMS

Each occupational therapy clinic has its own system for obtaining the patient's medical and social history. Some therapists conduct a specific interview, while others include the data in the evaluation of activities of daily living (ADL). A sample of a form that includes the medical history with the ADL assessment is included at the end of Chapter 24, Evaluation of Activities of Daily Living.

This chapter reviews medical information that is applicable to patients with rheumatic disease and pertinent to planning an effective treatment program.

Diagnosis and Onset

As a means of determining the patient's level of disease sophistication, it is helpful when recording the patient's diagnosis to ask the patient his or her diagnosis before recording it from the referral. It is important to ask the patient the dates of onset of both *disability* and *disease*. Because these dates frequently differ, this information provides a clearer picture of how the disease has affected the patient's lifestyle. For example, a patient may have knee pain years before it limits his or her ability to walk or to work.

Joints Affected

Determine which joints are currently involved and which joints were involved in prior exacerbations and the nature of the involvement, that is, pain, swelling, warmth, catching, limited ROM, or deformity. The patient should identify the joint involved. Frequently, a patient will state that he or she has arthritis all over, but further inquiry may actually reveal a report of joints not involved. This situation often occurs with patients who have RA of the peripheral joints but not of the axial or central joints. These patients feel as if the pain is all over, but when you interview them closely, you find that they may not have any pain in the back, sternum, or jaw. Some patients with RA will not have involvement of the large peripheral joints, for example, hips and shoulders. The typical or most common joints affected with each disease are discussed in Part 2.

Medication

Note the name and dosage of the medication and the frequency and regularity of the patient's intake. It is important to determine when medications have been taken prior to a physical evaluation, such as range of motion (ROM) or grip strength, since a decrease of medication on a given day can significantly affect objective assessments. Is the patient taking a fast-acting medication or a slow-acting medication? Did the patient take an extra analgesic (pain killer) before the therapy interview?

If a patient speaks of an increase in symptoms, the source of the complaint may lie in altered or reduced medication rather than true exacerbation of the disease. The effect of specific medications is reviewed in Chapter 12, Drug Therapy.

Presence of Systemic Manifestations

Percentage of good versus bad days

Patients with intermittent or episodic arthritis often report that they have good days during which they can do all activities independently and bad days during which they cannot work or do housework. If it becomes difficult during the interview to assess the patient's functional ability, it is helpful to have the patient estimate the approximate number of days per month during which he or she has more problems than usual from the arthritis. This can be computed into an approximate percentage, if desired. In addition to a clearer picture of the patient's life-style and disability status, this information can provide a convenient quantitative means of relaying information to the physician or other therapist. For example, if the patient has 3 to 4 bad days a week, this is equal to being disabled approximately 50 percent of the time. Even though this person's arthritis is not constant, he or she would have difficulty maintaining a house or working full time. The need for work simplification and assistive devices is much greater for a patient with 50 percent disability compared with the need in a patient who may be limited only one day a week (14 percent).

Morning Stiffness

Morning stiffness is a term used to describe the prolonged generalized stiffness that occurs in association with the inflammatory polyarthritides (especially RA and AS) upon awakening. The stiffness tends to be generalized and may last for several hours and is indicative of systemic involvement. This contrasts with the stiffness of DJD that occurs only in involved joints after inactivity and that disappears within one-half hour after moving the involved joint.

Morning stiffness is an objective indicator of the degree of disease activity present.[1,2] Patients with uncontrolled or untreated RA may have up to 5 hours of generalized stiffness in the morning. As the disease becomes controlled by medications or becomes less active, the duration of morning stiffness decreases and may only be 15 to 30 minutes long. Patients may have some degree of stiffness all day. This is usually due to swelling or inflammation of the joints. Morning stiffness is a distinct feeling of excessive stiffness that wears off at a given point. Patients will often describe the situation thus: "My morning stiffness wears off about 10:00 AM; then I have my regular stiffness the rest of the day."

Severity

Determining how morning stiffness interferes with or influences functional ability also needs consideration. Many patients feel stiff but are able to get around and to perform self-care functions, while others are totally dependent during periods of morning stiffness.

The ability to assess the duration effectively can facilitate OT treatment planning. Many patients are quite disabled by morning stiffness. If the patient has 3 to 5 hours of morning stiffness, he or she may need assistive devices to increase independence during this period. Consequently, functional ability may need to be assessed when morning stiffness is present and later in the afternoon after it has subsided.

Duration

The duration of morning stiffness is a common rheumatologic assessment tool. It is calculated from the time the patient wakes up until the stiffness wears off. It is recorded in number of hours.[1]

Every patient with arthritis seems to have his or her own routine for limbering up in the morning. This needs to be taken into account when interviewing the patient. Some patients have established a pattern of waking up, taking medications, and then going back to sleep for a couple of hours until the stiffness wears off. Simply asking patients what time they get up and what time the stiffness wears off may not reveal the extra two hours of stiffness described in the above example.

The following questions are suggested for determining the patient's *duration of morning stiffness*:

Are your joints usually stiff in the morning when you awaken?

What time do you usually awaken?

What time do you usually get out of bed?

Does the stiffness wear off? About what time? Or, What time does the *morning* stiffness wear off and do you have the regular stiffness?

It is also helpful to ask: Which joints are stiff in the morning? If patients describe stiffness only in specific or isolated joints, then this is probably due to swelling and not generalized systemic morning stiffness.

Endurance

Easy fatigability is one of the complications of all systemic diseases. It is further enhanced by chronic loss of sleep, decreased muscle tone and strength, and psychological factors such as depression. (Methods for evaluating depression are discussed in Chapter 2.) Fatigue associated with systemic disease varies with the time of day, whereas fatigue associated with depression tends to be more constant. Early afternoon fatigue is such a consistent finding that physicians frequently use the elapsed time between arising in the morning and onset of fatigue as a parameter of disease status.

Assessment of the patient's energy patterns provides a basis for determining the need for and extent of instruction in energy conservation methods. Energy patterns include what time of day fatigue occurs, its duration, and how the patient handles it (e.g., short naps or continuation of work in spite of fatigue). The average time for onset of fatigue in patients with chronic systemic diseases is about 4 hours after first arising in the morning. Awareness of the patient's energy pattern is also important when scheduling therapy appointments.

AMERICAN RHEUMATISM ASSOCIATION (ARA) FUNCTIONAL CLASSIFICATION[3,4]

This general classification system was specifically designed for patients with rheumatoid arthritis but, because it is so general, it can be used with other rheumatic diseases.

Class I Complete functional capacity with ability to carry on all usual duties without handicaps.

Class II Functional capacity adequate to conduct normal activities despite handicap of discomfort or limited mobility of one or more joints.

Class III Functional capacity adequate to perform only a few or none of the duties of the patient's usual occupation or of self care.

Class IV Largely or wholly incapacitated with patient bedridden or confined to wheelchair, permitting little or no self care.

This classification is limited, in so far as it is general and can reflect only gross changes in the patient's progression or regression. However, it is often helpful in providing a quick overall gestalt of the patient's status.

REFERENCES

1. McCarty, D. J.: *Clinical assessment of arthritis.* In McCarty, D. J. (ed.): *Arthritis and Allied Conditions.* Lea and Febiger, Philadelphia, 1979, pp. 131–149.
2. Polley, H. F., and Hunder, G. G.: *Rheumatologic Interviewing and Physical Examination of the Joints,* ed. 2. W. B. Saunders, Philadelphia, 1978.
3. *Primer on the Rheumatic Diseases.* Am. Rheumatism Assoc., The Arthritis Foundation, New York, ed. 7. Reprinted from J. A. M. A. 224, No. 5, Suppl., 1973, p. 140.
4. Steinbrocker, O., Traeger, C. G., and Batterman, R. C.: *Therapuetic criteria in rheumatoid arthritis.* J. A. M. A. 140:659, 1949.

21

HAND PATHODYNAMICS AND ASSESSMENT

The key to effective management of the arthritic hand is early identification of pathodynamics that can cause secondary limitations and the prevention of those secondary limitations. It is generally not possible to prevent the primary disease, but the consequences of disease can often be controlled or reduced.

For example, it may not be possible to prevent tendon adhesions in the wrist due to tenosynovitis, but with early detection, it is often possible to prevent digital joint contractures secondary to the restricted tendon function. Another example is joint stiffness secondary to digital flexor tenosynovitis. Again, it is not possible to prevent the tenosynovitis, but it is possible to prevent stiffness or restore joint motion, if stiffness results from flexor tenosynovitis. These are just two of many deformities that can be prevented with early detection and intervention. In order to detect early manifestations of disease and thereby have an opportunity for early intervention; a systematic and thorough hand assessment must be carried out.

Comprehensive hand assessment and treatment offers a major contribution to rheumatologic rehabilitation. The occupational therapist with a knowledge of hand anatomy, skill in functional analysis, and the ability to determine splinting and joint protection interventions is in a unique position to provide this service. (Figure 11 shows normal hand structures.) This chapter will review the assessment criteria for determining the status of anatomic structures and the common manifestations of arthritis in the hand. There is an emphasis on the pathology that can be altered by treatment and on secondary limitations that can be prevented.

This chapter can be used in sections to review specific phenomena, or it can be used in its totality as a description of a comprehensive hand evaluation program. It incorporates the hand assessment guidelines developed by the occupational therapy department at the Robert B. Brigham Hospital in 1978. The hand assessment form was developed to facilitate documentation and data retrieval and is included at the end of this chapter as an example of how these complex data can be organized in a medical record format. The grouping of arthritis manifestations on this form was based on the natural sequence of evaluation by the staff therapists. The same grouping or sequence is used in this chapter to review assessment criteria. Thus, arthritis manifestations are discussed in the following order: joint and soft tissue involvement, common hand deformities, muscle involvement, tendon involvement, skin and vascular involvement, and neurologic involvement.

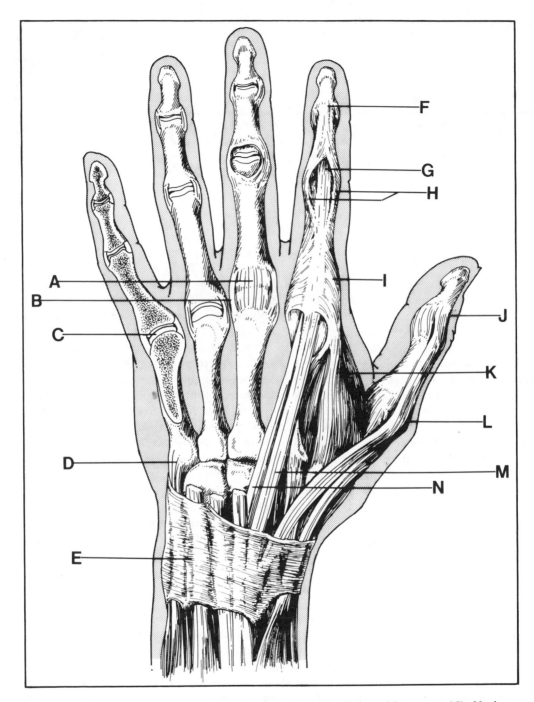

FIGURE 11. Normal hand structures. (*A*), Joint capsule; (*B*), Collateral ligaments; (*C*), Hyaline cartilage; (*D*), Insertion of the extensor carpi ulnaris tendon; (*E*), Dorsal retinaculum; (*F*), Distal attachment of the extensor communis tendon; (*G*), Central slip of the extensor communis tendon; (*H*), Lateral bands of the extensor communis tendon; (*I*), Extensor hood mechanism; (*J*), Insertion of the extensor pollicis longus tendon; (*K*), First dorsal interosseous muscle; (*L*), Insertion of the extensor pollicis brevis tendon; (*M*), Extensor communis tendon; (*N*), Extensor indicis proprius tendon. (Adapted from Gatter, R. A., and Andrews, R.: *Articular and Periarticular Diseases of the Wrist and Hand.* Merck, Sharp, and Dohme, West Point, Pa., 1972.)

CONSIDERATIONS PRIOR TO HAND ASSESSMENT

Medications

The type of medication and dosage pattern used by the patient can significantly affect objective measurements and the accuracy of longitudinal assessments. The effect of the patient's medication regimen on functional ability should be determined prior to performing a hand assessment. Most patients can describe the effects the medication has on their mobility, pain, stiffness, and function.

Fast-acting medications can create a day-to-day variability in performance. Slow-acting medications (remission-inducing drugs; see Chapter 12) can influence longitudinal assessments, i.e., re-assessments that may occur over a 1- to 3-month period. For example, some patients who take aspirin or another NSAID every 4 hours have greater stiffness at the end of the 4-hour cycle than 30 minutes after taking the medication. Patients on steroid medication every other day can have marked fluctuations in mobility, depending on what day of the cycle it is at the time of assessment. Also, some patients take an extra analgesic on "bad days," which can affect mobility and strength measures.

See Chapter 12, Drug Therapy, for additional information on classification of medication, side effects, and references.

Neck, Shoulder, Elbow, and Forearm Involvement

There are several conditions in the proximal upper extremity that can cause deformity in the hand or alter hand function in some manner. When there is a marked or noticeable condition present, relevant information is usually conveyed in the referral to occupational therapy and included in the assessment. However, there may be minor conditions or disabilities that may have occurred in the past that can influence a detailed hand assessment and the treatment plan but that the physician did not consider important enough to note on the referral form. Additionally, in some clinics, the patient's chart, history, or assessment by the physician is not available at the time of the patient's therapy session. It therefore becomes the responsibility of each therapist to be knowledgeable of conditions in the neck and upper extremity that can influence hand function. Assessment of the proximal upper extremity prior to performing the hand assessment helps safeguard against accidental omission of one of these contributing factors and can provide information that may explain pathology seen in the hand.

In clinics in which the occupational therapist treats all upper extremity disorders, it is reasonable to perform an in-depth musculoskeletal evaluation of the neck and upper extremity prior to the hand assessment for arthritis. In clinics in which the physical therapist treats the neck and proximal extremity, it is more reasonable for the occupational therapist to perform a cursory proximal assessment and then refer the patient to physical therapy for a detailed assessment if significant problems are detected.

Methods for conducting a detailed musculoskeletal evaluation are available in several excellent texts.[1,2,3,4] The most common proximal conditions that can mimic localized hand problems and confound the hand assessment for arthritis are included here.

1. Cervical arthritis (RA or DJD) producing nerve root compression. This can result in paresthesias and sensory loss along associated dermatomes and motor loss along nerve root patterns.[5] For example, compression at C-6 level can cause sensory loss on the volar aspect of

the thumb, which may be confused with carpal tunnel syndrome. Sensory loss usually occurs before motor loss.

Patients with neck pain or stiffness may be candidates for instruction in joint protection techniques and a cervical pillow. (See Chapters 26 and 30.)

2. Shoulder pain secondary to synovitis or bursitis frequently refers pain down the extremity, usually along the lateral border to the midarm or midforearm level. Occasionally it can extend into the palm.[6] In one clinical experience, the patient related the pain in her palm to newly made wrist splints; however, there were no evident pressure areas. After several splint adjustments had been made, it was determined that the pain was referred from shoulder synovitis. It is also possible for certain internal organs such as the gallbladder to refer pain *to* the shoulder. In these cases, the patient may complain of shoulder pain but have no clinical shoulder findings.[6] Shoulder pain may limit the kind of exercises used for the hand, for example, isometric towel-loop exercises.

3. Shoulder-hand syndrome. This can occur in patients with arthritis. In the early stages it can be very mild. When this occurs, it typically results in diffuse unilateral hand pain that does not correlate with joint or tendon involvement. (This condition can also be bilateral.) Shoulder-hand syndromes can result in flexion deformities of the digits.[7] Occasionally, a patient with arthritis presents with residual contractures from a shoulder-hand syndrome or reflex dystrophy that resolved several years prior to the arthritis.[1]

4. Elbow synovitis commonly causes ulnar nerve entrapment, resulting in paresthesias, sensory loss, and eventually weakness in the ulnar innervated muscles distal to the forearm.[8] Weakness in two-point pinch and mild clawing of the ring and little fingers are easily detected clinical signs. Although rare, it is possible for elbow synovitis to cause compression (volar to elbow) of the posterior interosseous branch of the radial nerve, resulting in weakness of the thumb and finger extensors.[9] (A detailed review of other nerve entrapment syndromes is given on pages 247 through 257.)

5. Forearm rotation can be limited by synovitis at either the distal or proximal radioulnar joint or both.[1] The patient generally feels pain in the joint that is causing the limitation at the end of the rotation.

6. Tennis elbow (lateral epicondylitis) and golfer's elbow (medial epicondylitis) are common conditions. They are believed to result from occupational strain on the tendoperiosteal junction of the respective lateral or medial muscles. These conditions often occur unrelated to their namesake sports. The characteristic symptom is pain over the lateral epicondyle when resistance is applied to the wrist extensors and pain over the medial epicondyle when resistance is applied to the wrist flexors.[10,11]

History of Hand Surgery or Trauma

Mallet finger and boutonniere, swan neck, and angulation deformities can result from trauma. Contributing factors in the patient's history should be ruled out before deformities are attributed to arthritis. It is also helpful to specifically ask the patient about prior surgery or hand therapy. Many patients forget to mention these issues, which can influence a treatment plan.

ASSESSMENT OF JOINT AND SOFT TISSUE INVOLVEMENT

The following parameters are applicable to the wrist and individual digital joints.

Pain

Pain is a major symptom of both synovitis and degenerative joint disease. Therefore the assessment of pain provides information about the severity of these two conditions. For synovitis, joint pain during rest (when the joint is not moving) indicates severe or acute inflammation, and the pain is a result of increased intra-articular pressure.[1] Pain during motion but not at rest indicates active but less acute inflammation. Patients with mild synovitis may only have pain with lateral-medial compression of the joint, i.e., they will report no pain with active motion, but when gentle compression is applied they identify pain in the involved joints.[1] In most cases, applying lateral-medial pressure is sufficient (Fig. 12). A more discriminating procedure in the PIP and DIP joints is to apply medial-lateral pressure with one hand and then anterior-posterior pressure with the other hand. Extremely mild synovitis will be evident when this additional pressure is applied.[1] (Care must be taken not to apply pressure over a tender area such as an osteophyte.) Mild synovitis identified with compression is common in patients in whom medications are controlling the disease. Joint protection methods may be appropriate for joints with mild synovitis; however, it is more difficult for the patient to perceive the benefits of the techniques if there is no pain with active motion.

Pain from DJD typically occurs with motion or weight bearing. In the absence of inflammation, the exact source of this pain is often unclear. One possibility is that heat secondary to friction or microfracture in the subchondral bone stimulates the pain receptors surrounding the

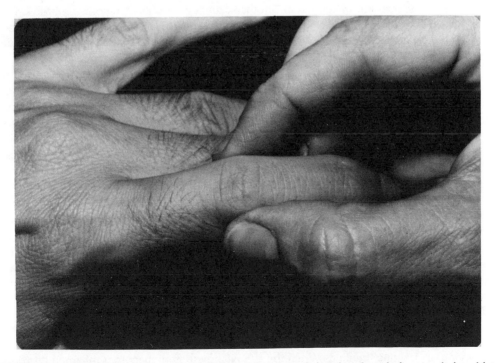

FIGURE 12. Palpation for mild synovitis. Support the patient's hand and apply firm medial and lateral compression as shown. When synovitis is present, tenderness will be elicited with this maneuver. Compare with a noninvolved joint, if possible.

blood vessels in the subchondral bone. It is also possible for joint distortion or mechanical derangement to alter the intra-articular pressure significantly enough to trigger nociceptive nerves in the capsule.

Often a mild inflammatory process is the source of pain in DJD. Frequently, the degenerative process, cartilage debris, or the formation of bony cysts can create local synovial irritation or inflammation and the joint will become painful at rest or may actually swell.

Pain can also inhibit muscle function.[12,13] Pain may be sudden, for example, when acute knee or wrist pain inhibits supporting muscles and the joint gives way. It may also be subtle and only reduce rather than completely stop muscle function. This may manifest as a sense of subjective weakness; for example, the patient will report that his or her hands are weak because he or she can no longer open jars or apply hard pressure. It is possible for true muscle weakness to be present with this same symptom, but for patients with painful hands, pain inhibition of muscle strength is the most common cause of this problem. Whenever a patient reports weakness it is important to determine if there is true muscle weakness, which will be clearly evident on a group or individual manual muscle test, or if pain during the activity is impairing muscle performance. If pain is the limiting factor, the treatment is often joint protection instruction to eliminate the pain during the activity. If muscle weakness is present, strengthening exercises are indicated.

Often this problem initially becomes evident during a grip strength test. For example, if a woman patient records a 20-lb grip and denies any pain in her fingers, wrist, or upper extremity during the test, it is likely that her grip is diminished due to muscle weakness. (A group muscle test is indicated; however, it may not provide additional information because it is less sensitive than an objective grip gauge.) If in another situation, a patient records a 20-lb grip but reports pain in her fingers or wrist during the test, a manual group muscle test is indicated. If the patient scores normal or 5 out of 5 on this test it is likely that the diminished grip is due to pain inhibition during the grip test rather than true muscle weakness.

Whenever muscle strength is evaluated it is important to document the presence of pain during the test, for pain invariably affects muscle performance.

Pain is usually identified as articular or periarticular (external to the joint). When it is periarticular, it is helpful to localize it to anatomic structures; for example, pain over the first dorsal interosseous muscle.

It is often very difficult for some patients to distinguish between pain and joint stiffness. If a patient reports pain that is disproportionate to the degree of joint involvement, careful interviewing may reveal that the patient is interpreting stiffness as pain.

There have been multiple attempts to quantitate pain, primarily to provide objective measurements of drug effectiveness.[14,15] Having patients grade or indicate their pain on a visual analog scale (a line marked with increments ranging from mild to severe) has proven to be one of the most effective measures.[14] Mechanical devices that quantitate the pressure required to elicit pain (dolorimeter) have also been used.[16] These devices are useful in research but are not practical or helpful in a clinical hand assessment designed for treatment planning.

Synovitis

The synovial tissue is responsible for producing synovial fluid, which lubricates the joint, and for removing or draining the fluid. When the synovial membrane becomes inflamed it produces excessive amounts of fluid. The drainage mechanism becomes ineffective and the fluid becomes trapped in the joint capsule (an effusion). The swelling conforms to the shape of the capsule and is referred to as fusiform swelling (Fig. 13). (Fusiform means spindle-shaped, i.e., larger in the center and tapered on the ends.)[1] In rheumatology, fusiform swelling is a specific term, indicating synovitis or inflammation confined to the capsule. In the early stages of synovitis, the swelling is soft and fluctuant and is often described as boggy. The synovium is still thin and the joint is essentially full of fluid. As the synovitis becomes chronic, the synovial membrane proliferates and becomes thicker. The tissue may grow from 3 to 20 or more cells in depth. If the inflammation is not controlled by medication, pannus tissue begins to develop and fill the joint.[1] Pannus is a combination of synovial and granulation tissue. As the joint becomes filled with tissue it starts feeling firm rather than boggy, when compressed or palpated.[1] In the advanced stages, the synovium may herniate dorsally through the joint capsule and can present as a hard, focal mass and is often mistaken for a subcutaneous rheumatoid nodule.[17]

The signs of inflammation are swelling, warmth, redness, or discoloration; and the symptoms are pain and decreased motion.[1] Typically, the severity of inflammation is described as acute, denoting a hot, swollen, painful joint with marked limitation of motion; or active or subacute, denoting a warm, swollen joint, with less than acute inflammation. (The term active is redundant in this instance, since all synovitis is active.) Chronic and chronic-active are terms used to describe low-grade synovitis that persists over time. These joints are warm and swollen, and generally this synovitis is present despite an optimal medication regimen.[15] The joints typically involved in early rheumatoid arthritis are shown in Figure 14.

Clinical examples of descriptions of synovitis include: boggy swelling, localized to the MCP joints; fusiform swelling of the PIP joints; synovial herniation over the dorsum of right and middle finger PIP joints; and active synovitis in all MCP joints and wrist.

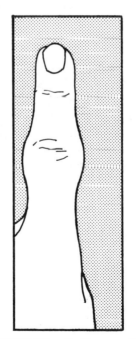

FIGURE 13. Fusiform swelling.

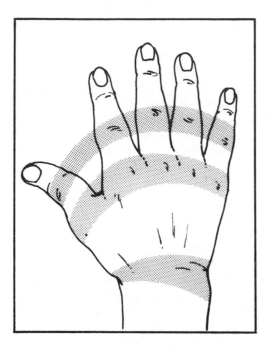

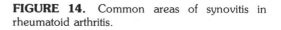

FIGURE 14. Common areas of synovitis in rheumatoid arthritis.

Swelling

Any type of enlargement can be referred to as swelling. In rheumatology, articular swelling most frequently refers to synovitis, but occasionally it is used to designate bony enlargement such as Heberden's nodes. Diffuse swelling throughout an area may be referred to as periarticular.

Patients with severe or acute rheumatoid arthritis can develop various patterns of diffuse edema in the hand. Periarticular swelling may be around the inflamed joints or throughout the dorsum of the hand.[1] The lymphatic system drains towards the dorsum of the hand, and it is theorized that interference with lymphatic drainage could be a factor contributing to diffuse dorsal edema.[18,19] Positioning at rest with the wrist flexed can also impair lymphatic return.[19] Bilateral diffuse swelling of the hands and feet should be brought to the attention of the referring physician, because it may occur with other types of systemic involvement such as congestive heart failure or renal failure.

Patients with psoriatic arthritis or one of the other spondyloarthropathies often develop a characteristic firm swelling throughout the entire digit referred to as sausage swelling (Fig. 15). This diffuse swelling is attributed to a combination of acute PIP (and possibly MCP and DIP) joint synovitis and severe flexor digital tenosynovitis. It is not known why people with psoriatic arthritis develop a diffuse edema in response to these conditions and patients with rheumatoid arthritis do not.[20]

One method for determining the degree of swelling is to compare the skinfolds of the edematous hand with the nonedematous hand. The skinfolds will be diminished if there is swelling. If the swelling is unilateral, it is helpful to compare side views of the digit with the con-

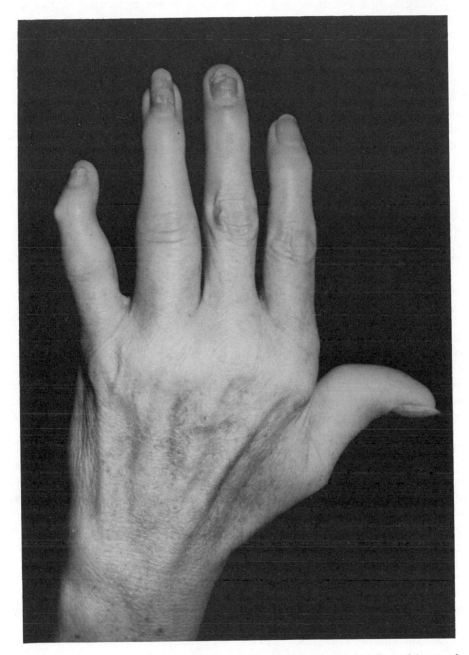

FIGURE 15. This woman has psoriatic arthritis with characteristic sausage swelling of the ring finger and classic psoriatic nail changes. Also, note the mild dorsal wrist swelling, the marked mallet deformity of the little finger, beginning mallet deformity of the index finger, and the enlargement of the thumb, typical of flexor tenosynovitis.

tralateral digit by placing the palms together. Swelling of the digits can be quantitated by measuring the circumference of the fingers using a regular tape measure, a circumference arthrometer, or a jeweler's ring sizer.[19] The measurement can be taken over the PIP joint or over the proximal phalanx depending on whether the goal is to document synovitis or diffuse swelling. It is important that the measurement process be consistent and that the measurement device does not constrict or compress the swollen area.

If there is a need to quantitate edema throughout the entire hand, a circumference measure is not sufficient. The most effective means for measuring the total hand is by using water volume displacement, that is, submerging the hand in a tank containing a precise amount of water (a volumeter) and measuring the water displaced in a graduated cylinder.[19] This process is not commonly used with arthritis patients, but it can be very useful on certain occasions for documenting the effectiveness of treatment to reduce edema.

Subcutaneous (Rheumatoid) Nodules

These nodules are discrete tissue masses present under the skin and occasionally in the skin and are composed of fibrous and granulomatous tissue.[1] A subcutaneous nodule is one form of rheumatoid nodule that can occur in RA. These nodules can be any size, and it is not unusual to find them as large as 4 cm in diameter at the elbow. They can be freely movable or fixed to other structures. Generally, they are not painful but can become tender if irritated by pressure.[17,21]

Subcutaneous nodules are commonly found over bony prominences exposed to pressure, for example, along the ulnar ridge of the forearm just distal to the olecranon process or the ulnar edge of the hand and wrist (Fig. 16). Occasionally they occur on the dorsum of the finger joints and less commonly on the palmar surface of the hand.[1] Nodules may arise over the bony prominence created by a subluxed joint, typically the thumb IP joint. (They also occur in other areas of the body, such as over the ischial tuberosities, occipital bone of the skull, and in the Achilles tendon of the heel.) There is a rare condition called rheumatoid nodulosis, in which patients develop multiple nodules and have a positive RA factor and do not have a mild arthritis.[22]

Some nodules appear to occur in response to pressure (microtrauma) or are aggravated and enlarged by pressure. However, others can occur in nonpressure areas.[21] Nodules that are related to pressure will diminish in size (or disappear) if the pressure source is eliminated. Nodules on the palmar surface of the hand appear to be particularly sensitive to pressure forces.

Subcutaneous nodules are associated with seropositive rheumatoid arthritis, and their presence indicates a more severe disease course.[1,21] Since subcutaneous nodules have a prognostic significance, it is important that they be appropriately defined. In the hand, synovial hypertrophy or herniation is often mistaken as a nodule.[17] Also, Heberden's nodes are due to bony proliferation and are completely unrelated to rheumatoid nodules. (In rheumatology, nodes and nodules are not interchangeable terms.)

To document a nodule, it is helpful to note consistency, sensitivity to pain, size, number, fixation, and location; for example, "Patient has a single, fully movable, nontender nodule about 0.5 cm in diameter, overlying the dorsum of the ring PIP joint." Size can also be related in terms of a common object, for example, pea size, or golf ball size, or by diameter.

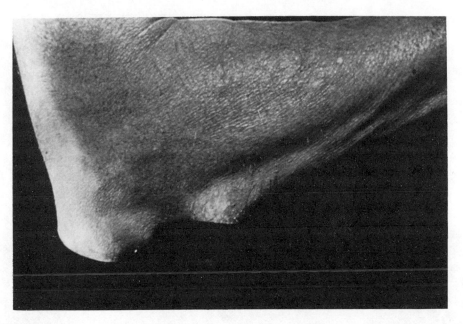

FIGURE 16. Subcutaneous rheumatoid nodules are most commonly seen over the olecranon and ulnar border of the forearm. They can also occur over the dorsum of the knuckles and in the palm. They are often but not always associated with pressure irritation. They can occur over other regions of the body, e.g., occipital skull, Achilles tendon, ischial tuberosity, and foot. (From the ARA slide collection.)

Synovial Cysts and Ganglion

This is a soft enlarged mass (cyst) under the skin, usually found overlying tendon sheaths. It is most commonly found over the dorsum of the wrist but can be found overlying any synovial joint.

A dorsal wrist ganglion is a synovial cyst that arises from the portion of the joint capsule that attaches to the scapholunate ligament. Dorsal ganglions can be primary and occur in people without any other form of arthritis. They may be asymptomatic or very tender during functional activities.[23]

Since it is often difficult to distinguish between ganglions, cysts, tumors, or synovium, it is preferable for the therapist to describe the location and size of the swelling or mass; for example, "Flattened, puffy enlargement over the dorsum of the wrist (about 3 cm in diamter)."

Osteophytes (Heberden's Nodes, Bouchard's Nodes)

Degenerative joint disease (osteoarthritis) involves two major processes: degeneration of the cartilage, and bone proliferation around the margin of the joint. In the digits, this bone growth takes the form of osteophytes. When osteophytes occur at the DIP joint they are referred to as Heberden's nodes; at the PIP joint they are referred to as Bouchard's nodes (Fig. 17). Osteophytes are also common around the thumb CMC joint. They rarely occur at the MCP joint level.[24]

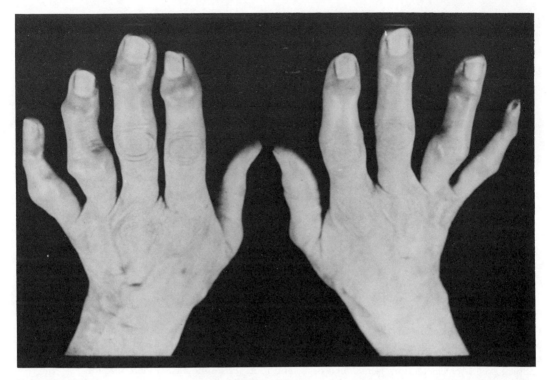

FIGURE 17. Osteophyte formation in the PIP joints (Bouchard's nodes) and DIP joints (Heberden's nodes) are characteristic of primary DJD. These bony protuberances are hard to the touch and asymmetric, compared with synovitis, which is symmetric and boggy. Generally these nodes are nonpainful and noninflammatory. Occasionally patients like the one pictured here will have painful localized inflammatory episodes. Note the redness or discoloration over the DIP joints secondary to inflammation. She also has an angulation deformity of the right middle finger DIP joint and a mallet deformity of the right little finger. (From the Arthritis Teaching Slide Collection, Arthritis Health Professions Association, Arthritis Foundation, with permission.)

The presence of these osteophytes is diagnostic of DJD. The ability to assess osteophytes correctly can be a valuable aid to the therapist for treatment planning because osteophytes are a sign that the cartilage is damaged. Many patients have both DJD and RA. Often the limitations in the joints with DJD are greater than or disproportionate to the other joints and to the degree of inflammation present. The ability to determine the presence of DJD (indicated by osteophytes) allows the therapist to determine if the limitation is due to DJD or RA and to plan treatment appropriately.

Thumb CMC Joint Arthritis

In the DIP and PIP joints, DJD is generally easily recognizable by the presence of osteophytes. However, detection of early DJD in the thumb CMC joint is often more difficult, since the structure of the joint and the overlying muscles prevents palpation or visualization of osteophyte formation.

Evaluation of DJD of the CMC joint requires a separate assessment for several reasons. First, this joint may be the first joint to become symptomatic in DJD. Patients with no previous history of arthritis may seek medical care for the sole complaint of CMC pain. This symptom can be quite limiting since the thumb accounts for 45 percent of hand function.[26] Second, this condition is often confused with de Quervain's tenosynovitis, particularly when the DJD causes inflammation of the CMC joint with pain radiating into the wrist or forearm. These two conditions need to be differentiated, since their evaluation, treatment, and prognosis are completely different. Third, x-ray evidence of DJD does *not* necessarily correlate with clinical symptoms. Patients can have minimal to absent x-ray changes and debilitating pain or the reverse—severe x-ray changes and no pain. It is not uncommon for some patients to progress to marked subluxation without pain.

The most common symptom of DJD is pain with motion owing to cartilage damage or osteophyte formation. Occasionally, the DJD process or functional stress causes irritation of the joint and local inflammation occurs.[25] Pain may then become present at rest and radiate distally along the metacarpal or proximally into the wrist. With progression and osteophyte formation, the joint can sublux giving a squared off appearance to the joint. Squaring of the CMC joint is considered indicative of DJD.[27]

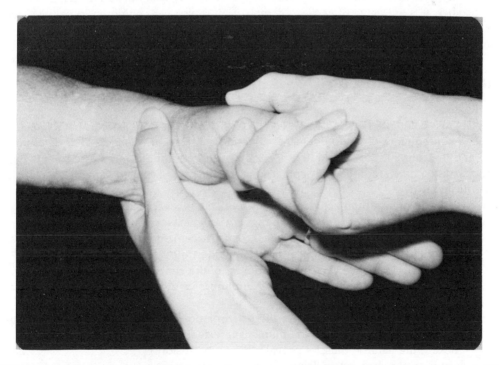

FIGURE 18. The grind test to determine cartilage damage (degenerative arthritis) of the thumb CMC joint is performed by stabilizing the patient's hand with the examiner's thumb over the CMC joint, then grasping the thumb metacarpal bone and gently approximating and rotating the metacarpal bone in the CMC joint. The test is positive if pain or crepitus occurs in the CMC joint. In DJD, crepitus is indicative of cartilage damage.

Procedure: (Fig. 18) The grind test is a specific procedure for localizing pain to the CMC joint.[1,27] Method: Stabilize the patient's hand with your thumb over the CMC joint to palpate crepitus or subluxation. Then grasp the patient's metacarpal bone and approximate the joint; that is, press the head of the metacarpal into the trapezium then gently rotate the metacarpal in the joint. The test is positive for CMC involvement if the maneuver elicits pain or crepitus.

Splinting to immobilize the CMC joint is very effective for relieving symptoms and thus improving function.[27] Splints for this condition are discussed in Chapter 25. Splints are considered the treatment of choice for patients with short-term or sporadic episodes of pain or pain related only to a specific task, such as writing or driving. Splints are also useful for patients who do not want surgery. Once the pain becomes unrelenting or nonresponsive to splinting, some form of arthroplasty should be considered.[27] (See Chapter 13, Hand, Wrist, and Forearm Surgery.)

Crepitation

Crepitation refers to a grating, crunching, or popping sensation (or sound) that occurs during joint or tendon motion; it can be heard and felt (audible and palpable).[1] The cause or source can be bony, synovial, tendinous, or bursal. If it is caused by roughened articular surfaces rubbing together, it is indicative of cartilage damage.[28] It is also very common to palpate crepitus over the volar aspect of the digit during flexor tenosynovitis. Crepitus is present if it can be heard or felt and is further documented by its location and/or the motion that elicited it.

Range of Motion Lag

Lag refers to a difference between active and passive ROM. It is not a specific pathologic condition but a consequence of tendon damage, adhesions, or muscle weakness. The determination of lag and the causal factor should be a specific focus of an arthritis hand assessment. Each of the factors listed here are discussed separately in this chapter. Types of lag and possible causal factors include:

Passive extension greater than active extension (evaluate extensor structures):

1. At the wrist: rupture or weakness of the wrist extensors.
2. At the MCP joint: rupture, weakness, or displacement of the finger extensors; rarely, it is due to dorsal tenosynovitis blocking tendon motion.
3. At the PIP joint: overstretching or rupture of the central slip.
4. At the DIP joint: partial or complete rupture of the distal attachment of the extensor communis tendon.
5. At the thumb IP joint: rupture; the extensor pollicis longus tendon at the wrist can reduce IP extension when the thumb is in extension. (When the thumb MCP joint is flexed, the intrinsic muscles provide IP joint extension.)

Passive flexion greater than active flexion (evaluate flexor structures):

1. Flexor tenosynovitis at the wrist or digit level.
2. Flexor tendon rupture.
3. Trigger finger (nodule catching on the pulley mechanism).

Tenodesis, Extrinsic Tendon Tightness

Technically, the term tenodesis* means fixation of a tendon at a new point. For example, a tendon transfer involves a surgical tenodesis. Clinically, tenodesis action or motion refers to aberrant motion in the digit joints due to tightness or tethering of a tendon at a proximal location. The excursion of the tendon can become limited owing to the proximal end of a ruptured tendon becoming adherent to an adjacent tendon; swelling and tenosynovitis in the carpal tunnel, blocking flexor tendon motion; and adherence of the long finger extensors or flexors at the wrist. (In cases of hand trauma, the tendon can become limited because of scarring at any point along its course.)

For a tight tendon to create tenodesis action, it must cross over two or more joints. Consequently, this results in the motion of the distal joint(s) varying, depending on the position of the proximal joint. This process is also referred to as extrinsic tightness, a preferable term since it connotes an abnormal process and avoids confusion with normal tenodesis (full wrist extension elicits finger flexion and full flexion elicits finger extension) and with desirable tenodesis created by positioning or surgery.

Examples of extrinsic tendon tightness are:

1. Binding of the flexor tendons in the carpal tunnel can result in lack of PIP joint extension when the wrist is in neutral but full PIP joint extension when the wrist is flexed. (If the condition is severe, MCP joint motion will also be altered.) Upon cursory evaluation, it may appear as if the patient has PIP joint flexion contractures. If the PIP joints straighten with the wrist or MCP joints in different positions, the problem is in the tendons, not in the PIP joints. (Evaluation and treatment for flexor tenosynovitis is discussed under a separate section in this chapter.)

2. The distal ends of a ruptured extensor tendon can become adherent to an adjacent tendon or structure on the dorsum of the hand in a manner that reduces tendon excursion. In this case, PIP and DIP joint motion can vary depending on the position of the MCP joint. When the MCP joint is flexed, the PIP joint will lack full active or passive flexion; when the PIP joint is fully flexed, the MCP joint will lack flexion.[29] In other words, the new length of the tendon is only long enough to go around one bend or corner at a time.

3. Tendons can also become limited owing to adhesions following surgery.

Evaluation: The test for extrinsic tightness refers to assessing distal joint motion with the proximal joint in different positions. It is positive if the position of the proximal joint influences the range of motion of the distal joint.[29]

Measuring ROM when tenodesis is present: To determine the effectiveness of treatment for this type of tendon problem it is necessary to document ROM of the joints distal to the tendon fixation both pre-treatment and post-treatment. There are two methods for doing this. Method I: (This is the most accurate method for patients with polyarthritis.) Stabilize the proximal joints in neutral (zero degrees), e.g., the wrist and MCP joints; then measure the maximal motion possible at the PIP joint. (The DIP joint should be measured if it is affected.) Method II: Position the proximal joint, e.g., the wrist, in full flexion or extension and measure the maximal

---

*Tenodesis is a tendon problem. It is included in the joint assessment section because it can influence joint ROM evaluation and is easily assessed at the time of joint measurement.

motion of the distal joint, e.g., MCP and PIP joints. The motion measured depends on which tendon is tight. This method can be reliable in patients with normal proximal joints, e.g., in hand trauma patients.

Subluxation and Dislocation

Subluxation describes any degree of malalignment between normal and dislocated. Dislocation occurs when the articular surfaces are no longer in functional contact (Figs. 19 and 20).

In the MCP joint, the proximal phalanx slips volar or ulnar and volar on the metacarpal head. Evaluate by palpating over the dorsum of the joint. When the joint is in neutral, an abnormal step can be felt between the two bones if it is subluxed[1] (Fig. 21).

Subluxation is common in the radiocarpal joint (Fig. 22), the radioulnar joint, and the MCP joints. In the PIP and DIP joints, volar subluxation is rare. Typically, the joint is described in terms of the contracture or deformity pattern, such as swan neck. Occasionally, bone erosions or osteophytes cause lateral deviation of the PIP or DIP joints. In the thumb, volar subluxation of the distal phalanx and CMC joint is common.[30]

Subluxation can be described in the following manner: *mild:* palpable subluxation, no interference with function, full extension possible; *moderate:* visible subluxation limits range slightly, may or may not interfere with function; *severe:* gross malalignment of articulating bones; there is definite interference with ROM but articulating surfaces are still in functional contact.

Ligamentous Instability (Laxity)

In the digits, the collateral ligaments are the structures that prevent excessive lateral motion (see Fig. 11). The digital collateral ligaments reinforce the joint capsule on either side of the joint. Each is composed of two sections: the cord portion that extends from the dorsal lateral side of the proximal bone to the volar lateral side of the distal bone, and the accessory section that attaches into the volar plate (Fig. 23). Chronic synovitis can result in stretching or lengthening of the collateral ligaments and abnormal lateral motion.[31,32]

The evaluation procedures are different for the MCP joint, compared with the PIP and DIP joints, because the shape of the metacarpal head alters the length of the ligaments. In the MCP joints, the cord portion predominates in determining mobility and stability of the joint. In the PIP and DIP joints, the cord and accessory portions appear to play a more equal role.

In the MCP joint, the collateral ligaments have a variable length, depending on the position of the joint. When the joint is flexed, the full length of the wide portion of the collateral liga-

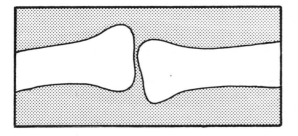

FIGURE 19. Subluxation of two digit bones.

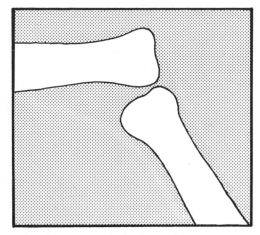

FIGURE 20. Dislocation occurs when the bones are no longer in functional contact.

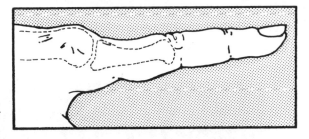

FIGURE 21. Metacarpophalangeal volar subluxation.

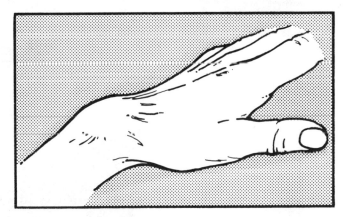

FIGURE 22. Volar wrist subluxation.

ment is required to accommodate the wide volar aspect of the lateral condyles of the metacarpal head.[31,33] When the joint is in extension, the full length is not required, and this section of the ligament is slack. This allows greater lateral mobility in extension. Consequently, *to evaluate the integrity of the collateral ligament in the MCP joint, it is necessary to position the joint in full passive flexion,* so the ligament is at full length and there is minimal lateral motion (Fig. 24).

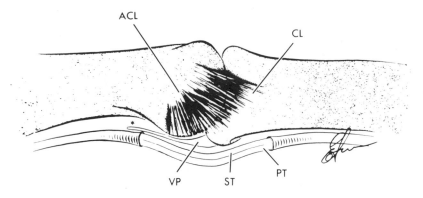

FIGURE 23.   This lateral view of the proximal interphalangeal joint shows the collateral ligament (CL), cord portion, and the accessory collateral ligament (ACL) attaching the middle phalanx and volar plate (VP). The flexor tendon sheath containing the superficialis tendon (ST) and the profundus tendon (PT) is closely attached to the periosteum of the phalanges and volar plate. The asterisk notes the recess between the volar plate and phalanx. The collateral ligaments are similar in the DIP joints. (From Wilson, R. L., and Carter, M. S.: *Joint injuries in the hands.* In Hunter, J. M., et al.: *Rehabilitation of the Hand.* C. V. Mosby, St. Louis, 1978, with permission.)

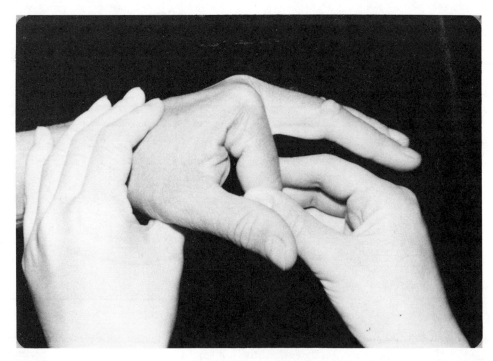

FIGURE 24.   The collateral ligaments of the MCP joint are lax in extension and stretched their full length in flexion. To test the integrity of the collateral ligaments of the MCP joint, position the joint in full flexion and move the phalanx from side to side. Excessive lateral motion in this position is indicative of damage to the collateral ligaments.

The metacarpal bone should be stabilized and the proximal bone moved from side to side. This positioning also applies to the thumb MP joint. The PIP and DIP joints receive equal support from both sections of the ligament. When the joint is in extension, the cord portion of the collateral ligament is slack and the accessory ligament is taut. When the joint is flexed, the reverse occurs—the collateral ligament becomes taut and the accessory ligament is slack.[34]

This dual ligament structure insures stability in any position, but unfortunately it also makes the PIP joints very prone to stiffness during immobilization. When the joint is splinted in extension, the collateral ligament tends to become fibrosed in a shortened position; and when the joint is splinted in flexion, the accessory collateral ligament can become contracted in a shortened position. Either ligament can prevent mobility.[35]

In arthritis, laxity tends to occur simultaneously in both ligaments, and testing the PIP and DIP joints in extension is sufficient. In cases of traumatic injury, only one ligament may be torn, and it is necessary to test the integrity of the cord portion of the collateral ligament with the joint in flexion and the accessory portion with the joint in nearly full extension. Nearly full extension centers the middle phalanx over the proximal phalanx, creating maximal tension on the accessory ligament.[35]

Normal joint stability is highly variable. Normal for a specific person can be determined by comparing the digit being evaluated with an unaffected contralateral joint, when possible.

Excessive anteroposterior motion without lateral excess indicates laxity of the capsule and volar plate, rather than the collateral ligaments.

Laxity can be described as *slight,* approximately 5 to 10 degrees in excess of normal; *moderate,* approximately 10 to 20 degrees in excess; and *severe,* approximately 20 degrees in excess.

Mutilans Deformity (Opera Glass Hand, La Main Lorgnette)

Mutilans refers to severe bone resorption of the bone ends. The bone resorbs into the body, shortening the bone and leaving the joint completely unstable. This process most commonly occurs at the MCP and PIP joints and the radiocarpal and radioulnar joints. In severe cases, the entire carpus can be resorbed. Mutilans is a devastating deformity and severely limits functional ability.[36]

The fingers appear shortened because of loss of phalangeal and/or metacarpal bone. Loose overlying skin and tissue become folded, producing a telescoping appearance. The fingers tend to feel soft or fleshy. Joints are unstable and floppy as a result of resorption.[36] Severity is described in terms of instability, resorption, and degree of shortening.

The only treatment for mutilans is surgical. Arthrodesis arrests the resorption process and preserves the length of the digit, but this can be done only in the early stages of mutilans (Fig. 25).[36] This procedure is preferable to reconstructive surgery, using bone grafts to restore length.

Joint Contractures

Contracture is a term used to describe a fixed or more permanent limitation in joint motion, rather than a temporary limitation caused by pain, edema, or inflammation. A *flexion contracture* limits or prevents full extension. (The term assumes that the limitation is on the flexor surface.) Consequently, an *extension contracture* limits or prevents full flexion.

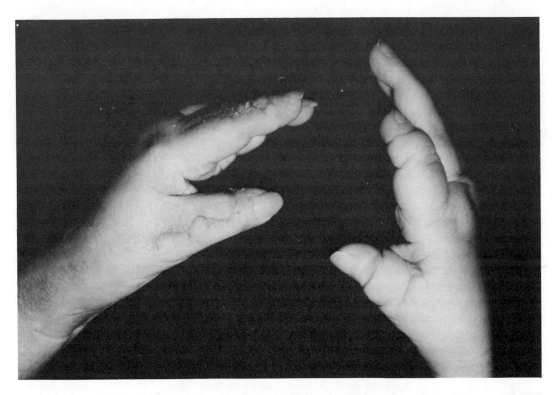

FIGURE 25. This woman has severe bilateral mutilans deformity of the thumb and index fingers. Resorption of the bone ends results in shortening of the digits and instability of the joints, impairing prehension skills. In the left hand the length and stability of the thumb and index finger have been restored by means of a bone graft and arthrodesis. Surgical fusion can prevent progress of bone resorption if performed early. Note the loss of length of the right index finger compared with the middle finger and the telescoping appearance of the shortened digits created by redundant skin.

In the presence of rheumatic disease, contractures can result from any of the following:

1. Synovial hypertrophy can block motion and lead to secondary fibrosis. Also, synovitis with very little swelling (dry form) can result in fibrosis of the capsule and supporting structures.
2. Ineffective tendon motion (ROM lag). If a patient does not actively (or passively) utilize full available joint motion daily, permanent contractures of the capsule and ligaments can develop.
3. Shortening of the collateral ligaments due to chronic positioning or inappropriate splinting. (See section on ligamentous instability.)
4. Periarticular edema causes compression of the joint structures, leading to adhesions in a tight or shortened position.
5. Subluxation can block motion creating a fixed limitation, e.g., radioulnar subluxation can prevent supination.
6. Osteophyte formation can block motion and eventually lead to ankylosis.
7. Muscle weakness. When muscle strength is 3.5/5 (fair plus) or less, the muscle is no

longer able to balance antagonistic forces, resulting in chronic positioning that leads to contractures, e.g., adduction contractures of the thumb are common sequelae if the abductor pollicis brevis becomes weak due to carpal tunnel syndrome.

8. Skin tightness occasionally appears to be a causal factor, but it is usually secondary to joint or muscle limitations. In scleroderma (systemic sclerosis) limitations are due to fibrosis of all the soft tissues.

The importance of chronic or habitual positioning cannot be emphasized enough. In the treatment of hand trauma, a condition called extensor habitus is frequently seen. Classically, it involves complete stiffness of the entire index finger, secondary to minor trauma. This condition occurs when a patient keeps the index finger in an extended position to avoid pain or allow healing. The patient begins to use the middle finger habitually for prehension. The index finger gradually becomes stiff and immobile, solely owing to this unconscious positioning process. Interestingly, upon taking the initial history, these patients often report that their finger became stiff overnight. Later, when the process is explained, the patient recalls gradual changes. Fortunately, this form of contracture can be readily resolved if treated early. This same physiologic process can occur in patients with rheumatic diseases in a more subtle form. Patients with an unstable or painful DIP joint or isolated synovitis of a PIP joint may avoid using that finger. Patients with advanced carpal tunnel syndrome and a diminished two-point discrimination (7 mm or more) often start using their ulnar fingers instead of the median fingers for prehension. Altered patterns of functional use should be considered as a possible causal factor in digits with inordinate stiffness.

Contractures are usually described by the degree of limitation; for example, left elbow has a 40-degree flexion contracture; (patient cannot straighten elbow to neutral).

Ankylosis

When a joint becomes immobile, it is referred to as ankylosed. The fixation can be fibrous, that is, due to growth of fibrous tissue around the joint; or it can be bony, resulting from ossification within or around the joint (Figs. 26 and 27).[37] (The term arthrodesis describes a surgical fusion.)

Fibrous ankylosis is the most common in rheumatoid arthritis. Since the limitation is due to changes in the soft tissue, there may or may not be slight motion present in this type of ankylosis. In bony ankylosis, there is no motion. This form is more common in psoriatic arthritis and juvenile chronic polyarthritis.[37,38]

Complete fibrous ankylosis can only be distinguished from bony ankylosis by roentgenography.[37] Therefore, for documentation purposes, it is best to describe the joint as ankylosed or describe the amount of motion available and the angle of fixation; for example, left

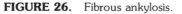

FIGURE 26. Fibrous ankylosis.

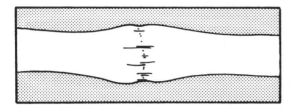

FIGURE 27. Bony ankylosis.

middle finger PIP joint is essentially ankylosed (has a jog of motion) in 45 degrees of flexion; or right wrist is ankylosed in 20 degrees of flexion; left wrist has a jog of motion in neutral.

Tuft Resorption

This is a condition in which the tuft of the distal phalanx becomes resorbed. Seen in systemic sclerosis, it causes distinct shortening of the distal phalanx and nail.[39]

Evaluate by comparing length of finger with contralateral digit, if unaffected. Describe severity in terms of loss of digit length; for example, distal shortening of index and ring fingers. The length of loss, e.g., 1 cm, can be measured and compared with a normal contralateral digit.

COMMON HAND AND WRIST DEFORMITIES

Radiocarpal Joint Subluxation

The carpal bones may slide volarward, dorsalward, or ulnarward on the distal radius, or they may sublux in both planes simultaneously.[30]

VOLAR SUBLUXATION AND DISLOCATION. Chronic synovitis of the wrist joint weakens the supporting ligaments about the wrist. Loss of ligamentous support combined with the normal 10 to 15 degrees of volar inclination of the distal radius results in volar slippage of the carpal bones on the radius (Fig. 28). This volar subluxation may be further enhanced by volar displacement of the extensor carpi ulnaris tendon. Once displaced volarly the extensor carpi ulnaris loses its effectiveness as an extensor and creates an additional flexor force on the carpus. The carpus may dislocate completely beneath the radius if erosion of the volar lip of the distal radius occurs.

ULNAR SUBLUXATION AND DISLOCATION (Radial Deviation Deformity). Chronic synovitis of the wrist leads to loss of radial ligamentous support and destruction of the triangular fibrocartilage on the ulnar side of the wrist. Loss of radial and ulnar support allows the carpus to slide down the distal radius, which has a normal incline toward the ulna. It is most common for the proximal carpal bones to *sublux ulnarward* and for the distal carpal bones to rotate in a radial direction, resulting in the hand being *radially deviated on the forearm*. This condition often contributes to ulnar drift of the MCP joints (Fig. 29). Less frequently, the distal carpal bones do not rotate, and the hand may appear ulnarly deviated on the forearm.[40] This is a favorable consequence, since it creates less stress on the MCP joints.

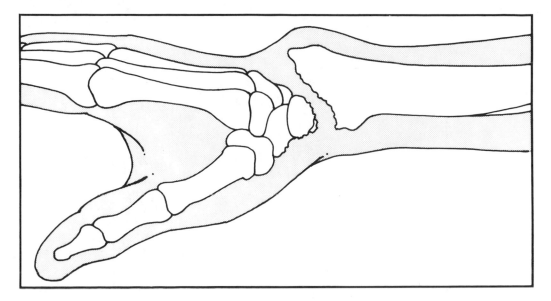

FIGURE 28. Volar subluxation of the carpus on the radius as a result of erosive synovitis of the radiocarpal joint.

If erosive synovitis continues, the carpus may eventually slide completely off the radius and dislocate on the ulnar side of the forearm, at a marked 90-degree angle, resulting in a right angle wrist deformity.

Distal Radioulnar Joint Subluxation

In rheumatoid arthritis, the distal radioulnar joint is often one of the first sites of wrist disease. Weakening of the supporting ligaments results in dorsal subluxation of the ulna on the radius, which creates a prominence on the dorsal aspect of the wrist (Fig. 30). If subluxation is severe, it can limit supination and wrist extension.[40,41]

To evaluate dorsal subluxation of the ulna on the radius: Face the patient and stabilize the head of the radius with a lateral pinch grip. With the opposite hand, move the ulna head in a dorsovolar plane. Excessive motion indicates subluxation. Caution is needed in documentation, since the normal degree of laxity is highly variable; compare with the other wrist if normal. This procedure is referred to as the piano key test or sign.[30]

Metacarpophalangeal Ulnar Drift and Volar Subluxation

The term drift refers to an abnormal amount of deviation. Ulnar drift is most common in adult rheumatoid arthritis. Radial drift rarely occurs in adults but is frequently seen in children with arthritis.[42]

Ulnar drift (Fig. 31) occurs because of the interrelationship of several factors including anatomic structure of the hand, which favors ulnar deviation; functional patterns of use and the

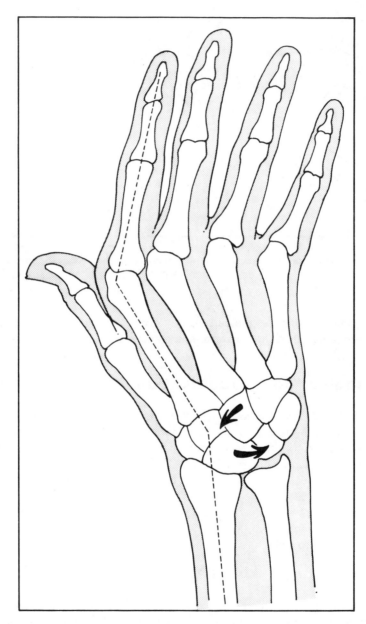

FIGURE 29. Relationship between wrist and metacarpophalangeal joint deformity. In this drawing, the proximal end of the carpus has subluxed in an ulnar direction rotating the hand radially on the forearm. This requires ulnar deviation of metacarpophalangeal joints to bring the index finger in line with the radius. The resulting articular alignment indicated by the dotted line produced the term zig-zag effect.

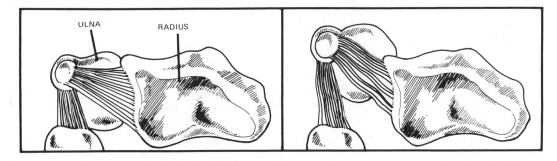

FIGURE 30. Distal radioulnar joint. *Left*, Normal alignment showing intact ligaments between the ulna, radius, and carpal bones; *Right*, Laxity of the supporting ligaments allows dorsal subluxation of the ulna.

influence of the flexor tendons during prehension; presence of chronic synovitis; and the position of the wrist, which is the keystone of the hand.

ANATOMIC STRUCTURE OF THE HAND

In the normal hand, both at rest and during motion, the phalanges are on an ulnar incline in relation to the metacarpals. This incline occurs because all the structural components favor the ulnar direction: the shape of the bones, placement and length of the collateral ligaments, and insertion of the intrinsic muscles. In addition, the flexor tendons cross the MCP joint from an ulnar angle. This in itself does not appear to produce ulnar motion at the joint because of the restraining power of the proximal annular ligaments (fibrous portion of the flexor sheath). However, when this ligament is weakened by synovitis, it loses its restraining power and the

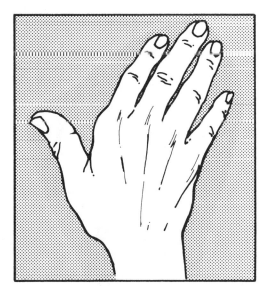

FIGURE 31. Metacarpophalangeal ulnar drift.

anatomic alignment of the flexor tendons creates a strong ulnar component for drift deformity, particularly for the index and middle fingers (Fig. 32).[43,44]

FUNCTIONAL USE OF THE HAND

All functional activities that involve MCP flexion, especially power pinch and grasp, increase the ulnar forces across the MCP joint (Fig. 32). (See section later in this chapter regarding functional components of the hand.)[44,45]

When the flexor tendon sheath is damaged by chronic synovitis, the flexor tendon is allowed to pull across the MCP joint in an exaggerated volar-ulnar direction during power

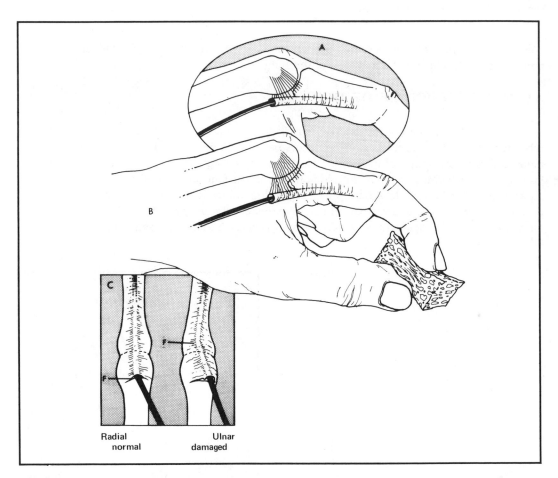

Radial   Ulnar
normal   damaged

FIGURE 32. Influence of the long flexors in metacarpophalangeal drift deformity. (*A*), MCP joint with normal ligamentous stability. (*B*), The flexor tendons bowstring across the joint and elongate the supporting fibers during power pinch (or grasp), resulting in volar subluxation of the proximal phalanx. This can occur only when the fibers are weakened by chronic synovitis. (*C*), Volar view of the MCP joint showing that, with damage to the supporting fibers, the fulcrum of force (F) from the flexor tendon changes, placing the ulnar pull on the proximal phalanx.

pinch and grasp. In addition, the ulnar interossei demonstrate a power dominance over the radial interossei during functional use.[45]

The forces imposed on the MCP joint during prehension have been analyzed by Smith and his colleagues.[45] They determined that for every unit of force exerted during palmar (2 point) pinch, six units of force are required by the long finger flexors and three units of force are displaced over the MCP joint. Thus, if a person uses a 5-pound pinch to open a container, 15 pounds of force are exerted on the MCP joint. It is this understanding of flexor forces that forms the theoretical basis for joint protection instruction for the MCP joints.[45]

CHRONIC SYNOVITIS

The main cause of ulnar drift deformity is chronic MCP joint synovitis. Single limited acute bouts of MCP synovitis for the most part do not cause permanent deformity. Early synovitis appears to affect the joint in three ways. First, the inflammatory process, often referred to as inflammatory infiltration, damages and weakens the capsule and supporting ligaments.[46] Second, chronic intra-articular swelling, caused by synovial effusion and hypertrophy, stretches the supporting joint structures and reduces their restraining power against ulnar forces, thus allowing the tendons to pull across the joint in a manner that enhances ulnar drift and volar subluxation. Third, pain and stretch of the joint capsule are hypothesized to cause reflex muscle spasm (muscular splinting) of the lumbricals and interossei.[47]

POSITION OF THE WRIST

In functional positions the index finger is in line with the radius. This requires the wrist to be in about 5 to 10 degrees of ulnar deviation. If the wrist becomes radially deviated with loss of ulnar ROM (the most common early wrist deformity in rheumatoid arthritis), the fingers deviate ulnarly to bring the index finger back into line with the radius. This theory or process is commonly referred to as the zig-zag effect (see Fig. 29).[40]

The position of the wrist can have such a strong influence that some patients (with RA of the wrist and MCP synovitis) who develop an ulnar deviation deformity of the wrist can go on to develop a mild radial drift (instead of ulnar drift) of the MCP joints. In clinical practice patients with a natural ulnar deviation deformity of the wrist seem to have less MCP ulnar drift than patients with a radial deviation deformity of the wrist (the most common form). Occasionally, a patient will position his or her wrist radially to make ulnar deviated fingers appear straighter. These patients may appear to have wrist deformity, but a detailed assessment reveals an absence of wrist pain and radiographic changes.

ULNAR DRIFT IN LATE STAGES

In advanced stages of ulnar drift, synovium may herniate through the radial transverse fibers of the extensor hood and the extensor communis tendons may slip ulnarward between metacarpal heads, giving the extensor tendon a mechanical advantage in an ulnar direction; however, these conditions usually occur after ulnar drift is established.[48]

EVALUATION: Severity is determined by the degrees of drift present. Methods for measuring ulnar drift vary across the country. One of the most effective methods is to measure the angle between the phalanx and metacarpal joint *during active extension, without active correction.* (The measurement method is described in detail in Chapter 22, Evaluation of Range of Motion.) When evaluating ulnar drift, it is important to keep in mind that the index finger normally has about 10 to 20 degrees of ulnar deviation during active extension.[17] Asking the patient to actively correct the drift provides additional information regarding the integrity of the joint structures.

Severity can be described as follows: *for the index finger,* slight (20 to 30 degrees); moderate (30 to 50 degrees); severe (50 degrees or more); and *for the other digits:* slight (0 to 10 degrees); moderate (10 to 30 degrees); severe (30 degrees or more).[49]

Swan Neck Deformity

The crooked shape of this deformity may or may not remind you of a swan's neck; however, it impressed someone in this manner and the name has been retained ever since.

The complete swan neck deformity consists of three components: PIP joint hyperextension; DIP joint flexion; and MCP joint flexion.

Most deformities result from damage to a single joint. The swan neck deformity can occur secondary to synovitis at either the MCP, PIP, or DIP joint. It can also result from trauma in the nonarthritic patient.

The normal extensor mechanism is shown in Figure 33 for comparison with Figures 34, 35, and 36, which demonstrate the imbalance that can result from synovitis at each of the digit joints.

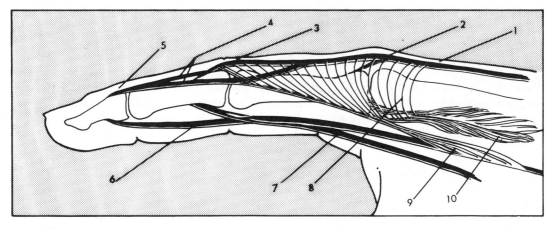

FIGURE 33. Normal finger extensor mechanism. (*1*), Extensor communis (EC) tendon; (*2*), EC insertion to proximal phalanx; (*3*), EC insertion to middle phalanx (forms the central slip); (*4*), Fibers from the EC separate to form the lateral bands; (*5*), EC insertion to distal phalanx; (*6*), Profundus tendon; (*7*), Superficialis tendon; (*8*), Extensor hood fibers; (*9*), Lumbrical muscle, originates from the profundus tendon; (*10*), Interosseous muscle with dual insertion, one part into the hood fibers and one part into the proximal phalanx.

INITIAL INVOLVEMENT AT MCP JOINT (Fig. 34)

This is the most frequent etiology for swan neck deformity in rheumatoid arthritis. Chronic synovitis in the MCP joints is hypothesized to cause reflex intrinsic muscle spasm and eventual muscle contracture.[47] The arrows in Figure 34 indicate the direction of pull that the intrinsic muscles produce on the extensor mechanism.

Contracture of the intrinsic muscles in association with natural hypermobility of the PIP joint (or PIP synovitis stretching the volar capsule) can lead to flexion of the MCP joints and hyperextension of the PIP joints.[50]

INITIAL INVOLVEMENT AT PIP JOINT (Fig. 35)

Synovitis of the PIP joint most frequently results in a flexion contracture or a boutonniere deformity. Less frequently, chronic synovitis of the PIP joint can cause stretching of the volar

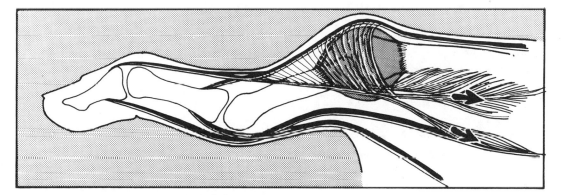

FIGURE 34. Swan neck deformity with initial synovitis at the metacarpophalangeal joint. This is the most common cause of swan neck deformity in RA.

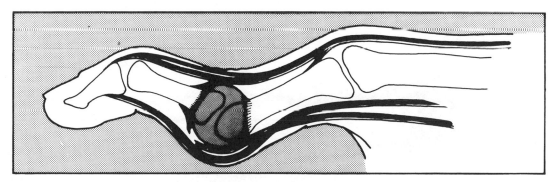

FIGURE 35. Swan neck deformity with initial synovitis at the proximal interphalangeal joint.

capsule and the dorsal migration of lateral bands. Hyperextension of the PIP joint creates tension on the profundus tendon, flexing the DIP joint.[50]

Synovitis of the PIP joint may also lead to rupture of the flexor digitorum sublimus insertion, which predisposes the PIP joint to swan neck deformity. This is the common cause of swan neck deformity in severe RA.[50]

INITIAL INVOLVEMENT AT DIP JOINT (Fig. 36)

Chronic synovitis of DIP joint (most commonly seen in psoriatic arthritis and JRA) can cause stretching or rupture of the insertion of the extensor tendon into the base of the distal phalanx.

As the DIP joint is pulled into flexion by the flexor digitorum profundus tendon, the PIP joint hyperextends because of the resultant imbalance.[50]

It is also possible for patients with DJD to develop a mallet deformity when osteophyte formation ruptures the distal attachment of the extensor communis, consequently leading to a swan neck deformity.

LATE STAGES

In the late stages, intrinsic contracture, stretching of the volar PIP capsule, collateral ligament shortening, tight skin, and tension on the profundus tendon become an integral part of most swan neck deformities regardless of the initiating source.[50]

OTHER ETIOLOGIES

Approximately 10 percent of the general population has natural hyperextensibility of the PIP joint that creates a swan neck appearance upon active extension. Occasionally, a patient with arthritis will have a swan neck deformity from a prior traumatic injury. Traumatic swan neck injuries primarily result from rupture of the extensor attachment at the DIP joint, rupture of the volar plate of the PIP joint and dorsal dislocation of the PIP joint, or an imbalance created by laceration, excision, or transfer of a flexor superficialis tendon.[35]

The swan neck deformity involves a pattern of MCP joint flexion, PIP joint hyperextension, and DIP joint flexion. *Severity is determined by loss of PIP joint flexion.*[49] It can be

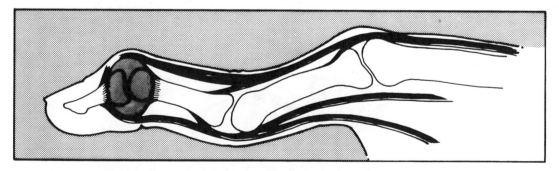

FIGURE 36. Swan neck deformity with initial synovitis at the distal interphalangeal joint.

described as (approximate guidelines): mild, 15 degrees hyperextension to 90 degrees flexion or more; moderate, 25 degrees hyperextension to 70 degrees flexion; and severe, 30 degrees hyperextension to 40 degrees flexion or less.[49] (Measure PIP flexion with the MCP joint flexed to rule out the effects of intrinsic tightness.) It is the loss of PIP joint flexion that reduces functional ability.

For surgical correction, the swan neck deformity can be divided into four categories. These categories are described in detail in Chapter 13, Hand, Wrist, and Forearm Surgery.

Boutonniere Deformity (Fig. 37)

Boutonniere is a French word for buttonhole. The term is used to describe this deformity because the lateral bands separate, like a buttonhole, allowing the joint to protrude between them.

Initially, the deformity involves a flexion deformity of the PIP joint and hyperextension of the DIP joint. However, with chronicity, the PIP joint becomes a fixed contracture necessitating hyperextension of the MCP joint to achieve grasp.[51]

The boutonniere is the most difficult deformity to treat conservatively. Part of the reason is that by the time the lateral bands have displaced sufficiently to create a boutonniere, significant stretching of the supporting fibers has already taken place. There have been informal reports of reduction of early boutonniere deformities with splints. This is an area that needs more exploration and documentation.

CHRONIC SYNOVITIS (Fig. 37(A))

The boutonniere deformity differs from the swan neck deformity in that the primary etiology is in the PIP joint. The inflammatory process damages the extensor structures to the PIP joint and

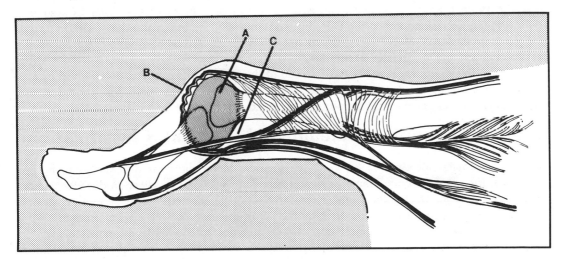

FIGURE 37. Boutonniere deformity. (*A*), Chronic synovitis; (*B*), Lengthening of the central slip; (*C*), Volar displacement of the lateral bands.

weakens their attachments. Synovial hypertrophy distends the dorsal capsule mechanically, thus stretching or displacing the extensor structures.[51]

LENGTHENING OF THE CENTRAL SLIP (Fig. 37(B))

Rupture or lengthening of the central slip attachment of the extensor communis tendon limits its effectiveness as an extensor for the middle phalanx.[51]

VOLAR DISPLACEMENT OF THE LATERAL BANDS (Fig. 37(C))

Weakening and synovial distention of the transverse fibers that connect the lateral bands to the central slip allow the lateral bands to displace in a lateral-volar direction. This limits the ability of the interossei and lumbricals to extend the PIP joint. In addition, this process increases the mechanical advantage of the extensor mechanism for extending the DIP joint, thereby creating a hyperextension deformity of the DIP joint. With severe deformity, the lateral bands can be displaced volarward to the axis of the PIP joint and thus become an active flexor mechanism to the joint.[51] Compare alignment of structures in Figure 37 with normal alignment in Figure 33.

The deformity involves a pattern of PIP flexion, DIP hyperextension, and in the late stages, MCP hyperextension. *Severity is determined by loss of active PIP joint extension.*[49] It can be described as mild, loss of 5 to 10 degrees; moderate, loss of 10 to 30 degrees; and severe, loss of approximately 30 degrees or more.

Mallet Finger Deformity (Fig. 38)

This deformity involves flexion only of the DIP joint due to partial or complete rupture of the distal attachment of the EC tendon. In degenerative joint disease, osteophyte formation can stretch the extensor tendon reducing its effectiveness for DIP joint extension, or cartilage loss can result in a collapse of the distal phalanx into flexion. In inflammatory joint disease, particularly psoriatic arthritis, synovitis causes lengthening or rupture of the distal EC tendon, removing the extension force to the DIP joint and thus allowing the profundus insertion to pull the joint into flexion.[49] Mallet finger deformity can also be caused by trauma to the distal extensor mechanism that is unrelated to arthritis.[35]

Since this deformity involves flexion only of the DIP joint, *severity is determined by loss of DIP extension.* Involvement can be described as mild, partial active extension; moderate, no active extension, but joint is mobile; and severe, fixed DIP contracture in flexion.[49]

Thumb Deformities — Rheumatoid (Nalebuff Classification)

Thumb deformities are referred to by several names. Many clinicians describe them by appearance, for example, boutonniere or swan neck. The Nalebuff Classification describes deformities according to which joint is initially or most seriously affected.[52] This system provides a reference for analyzing and documenting thumb involvement. Since this system is based on the site of initial involvement, it is most appropriate for early to moderate thumb deformity. In severe end-stage deformity, it may not be possible to determine the initial site of involvement or to use this four-point system. Thumbs that defy classification are documented by descrip-

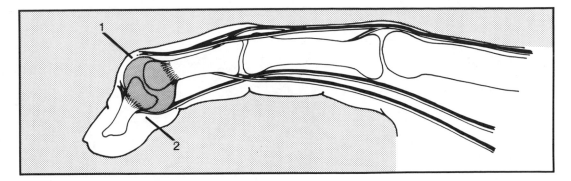

FIGURE 38. Mallet finger deformity secondary to synovitis. (1), Rupture of the extensor tendon to the distal joint; (2), Attachment of the profundus tendon.

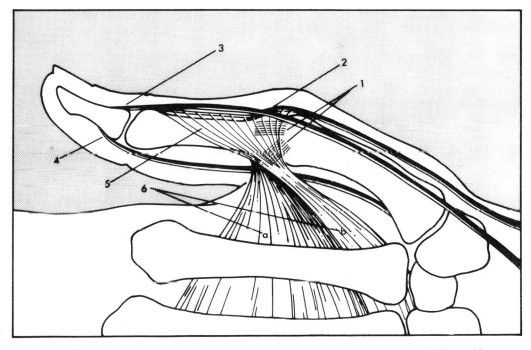

FIGURE 39. Dorsal-ulnar view of normal extensor mechanism of the thumb. (1), Collateral ligaments; (2), Extensor pollicis brevis tendon (inserts into the extensor hood fibers and the base of the proximal phalanx); (3), Extensor pollicis longus (inserts into the base of the distal phalanx and is attached to the hood mechanism; (4), Flexor pollicis longus tendon; (5), Extensor hood fibers; (6), Adductor pollicis in which the transverse fibers (a) attach to the proximal phalanx and the oblique fibers (b) attach into the hood mechanism and assist in interphalanageal extension (on the radial side, the abductor brevis inserts into the radial hood fibers).

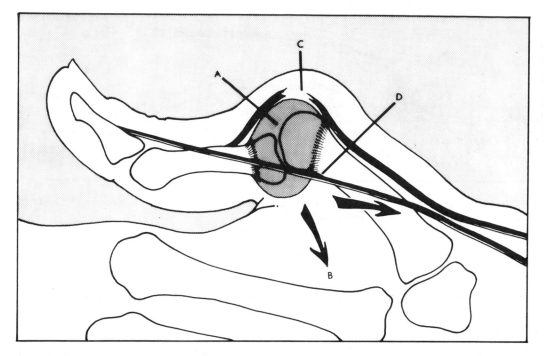

FIGURE 40. Thumb deformity: Nalebuff classification Type I. (A), Chronic synovitis of the metacarpophalangeal joint; (B), Intrinsic muscle tightness; (C), Attenuation of the extensor pollicis brevis tendon; (D), Ulnovolar displacement of the extensor pollicis longus. Pull of muscle shown by arrows.

tion. Figure 39 illustrates the normal extensor mechanism of the thumb for comparison with Figures 40, 41, and 42. Figure 43 summarizes the development of these deformities.

TYPE I—FLEXION OF MCP JOINT WITH HYPEREXTENSION OF IP JOINT (NO CMC JOINT LIMITATIONS) (Fig. 40)

This is the most frequently seen deformity in rheumatoid arthritis. This deformity starts with chronic synovitis of the MCP joint, resulting in the following events.

1. Stretching of the joint capsule and collateral ligaments.
2. Stretching of the dorsal hood mechanism thus reducing the effectiveness of the extensor pollicis brevis and creating an extrinsic minus condition.
3. The extensor pollicis longus tendon, which normally passes directly over the MCP joint, may be displaced ulnarward, creating a flexor force for the MCP joint and a hyperextension force for the IP joint.[52]

It is also theorized that pain and distention of the joint capsule can elicit a reflex spasm of the intrinsic muscles of the thumb, resulting in an intrinsic plus posture of MCP flexion and IP hyperextension.[47] However, in many hands it appears that an extrinsic minus condition contributes to the MCP flexion deformity and that the thumb intrinsic muscles become shortened secondary to the chronic flexion posture.[52]

HAND FUNCTION DURING PINCH ACTIVITY. The dynamics of Type I deformities result in flexion of the MCP joint and hyperextension of the IP joint. Pinch during functional activities adds another strong dynamic force to this process that further increases deformity. In order to approximate the pad of the thumb in pinch and grasp activities the patient needs to abduct the thumb and consequently develops an abduction posture.

In its most severe form, the deformity consists of fixed contractures of both joints with subluxation resulting in 90 degrees of IP hyperextension and 90 degrees of MCP joint flexion, referred to as 90-90 thumb.[52]

Severity is determined by the loss of active MCP joint extension and the degree of IP joint instability. It may be described as mild, loss of 5 to 20 degrees of active MCP joint extension; moderate, loss of 20 to 40 degrees; and severe, loss of 40 degrees or more.

TYPE II—CMC JOINT SUBLUXATION (ADDUCTION) WITH IP JOINT HYPEREXTENSION (Fig. 41)

Thumb deformities resulting from initial involvement of the CMC joint are far less common in RA than those resulting from MCP synovitis (Type I). In Type II, thumb synovitis of the CMC joint stretches the joint capsule, allowing the joint to sublux or dislocate in adduction. This adducted posture results in secondary shortening of the adductor pollicis muscle.[52]

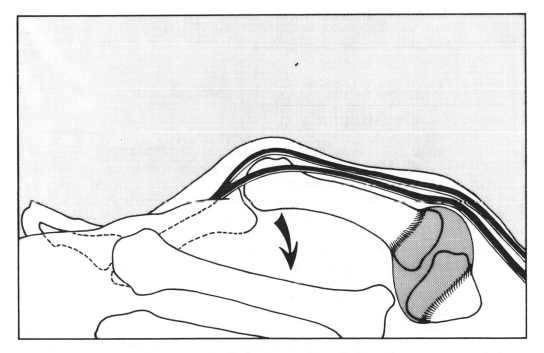

FIGURE 41. Thumb deformity: Nalebuff classification Type II. (A), Chronic synovitis of the carpometacarpal joint; (B), Intrinsic muscle tightness.

During hand function, the patient actively attempts to clear the thumb from the palm. If there is a natural laxity (or laxity resulting from synovitis) of the IP joint, it will go into hyperextension, creating a Type II thumb. If the MCP joint is the most lax, it will hyperextend to clear the palm, creating a Type III thumb.[52]

Severity is determined by the loss of active MCP extension, as in Type I, and the degree of CMC limitation present.

TYPE III—CMC JOINT SUBLUXATION (ADDUCTION) WITH MCP JOINT HYPEREXTENSION (Fig. 42)

This type of thumb deformity is more common in RA than a Type II thumb. It is also a common sequela to DJD of the CMC joint.

The initial dynamics of this deformity are the same as in Type II deformity. MCP joint hyperextension develops as the patient attempts to abduct the contracted first metacarpal bone.[52]

Severity is determined by the loss of active MCP flexion and the degree of CMC limitation present.

TYPE IV—MCP LATERAL DEVIATION WITH CMC JOINT ADDUCTION

This deformity occurs with the least frequency. Initially, it involves synovitis of the MCP joints with attenuation of the capsule and ulnar collateral ligaments. The MCP joint develops lateral instability and the first metacarpal drifts into adduction.[17]

Severity is determined by the degree of lateral deviation present and the extent of the adduction contracture. (See Figure 5 in Chapter 13.)

Figure 43 presents a summary of thumb deformities.

MUSCLE INVOLVEMENT

Intrinsic Muscle Atrophy

Assessment of intrinsic muscle atrophy is done to determine median and ulnar nerve involvement and to help define the extent of the disease on the peripheral structures.

When there is neurologic impairment, the degree of atrophy correlates with muscle weakness, i.e., the greater the atrophy, the weaker the muscle. Atrophy of thenar muscles is indicative of median nerve entrapment (carpal tunnel syndrome).[53] Atrophy of the hypothenar muscles may possibly be due to ulnar nerve entrapment.[8]

Atrophy can also occur secondary to disuse and systemic rheumatic disease. In the absence of neurologic impairment the degree of atrophy does not necessarily correlate with weakness. It is possible to have severe atrophy and muscle strength at the grade 4 or 5 level. When atrophy is present, it is important first to evaluate for neurologic involvement and second to assess for functional strength.

Diffuse atrophy of the intrinsic muscles (interossei and lumbricals) is indicative of the chronicity and severity of the disease. It is determined by the visual assessment of the first dorsal interosseous muscle. If there is atrophy of this muscle, it can be assumed that the other interossei have diminished in size also.

Severity is generally described as slight or marked.

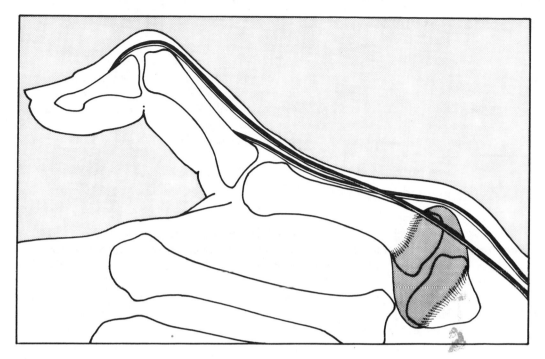

FIGURE 42. Thumb deformity: Nalebuff classification Type III.

TYPE I	TYPE II	TYPE III
M.P. FLEXION ↓ I.P. HYPEREXTENSION METACARPAL ABDUCTION	CARPOMETACARPAL SUBLUXATION ↓ METACARPAL ADDUCTION	
	I.P. HYPEREXTENSION M.P. FLEXION	M.P. HYPEREXTENSION I.P. FLEXION

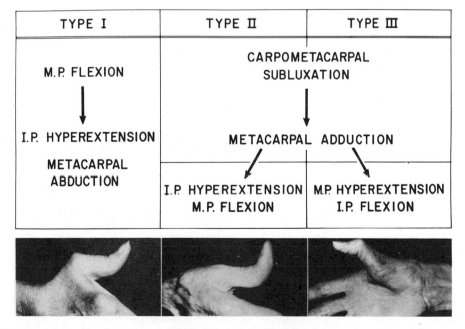

FIGURE 43. Common rheumatoid thumb deformities. Type I is the most common deformity seen in RA, followed by Type III. Although Type II is seen infrequently in RA, it is a common sequela of DJD of the CMC joint. (From Nalebuff, E. Λ.: Bull. Hosp. Joint Dis. 29:119, 1968.)

Intrinsic Muscle Weakness

Muscle weakness can occur due to peripheral nerve entrapment, cervical radiculopathy, and disuse.[8] All of the muscle can be affected. If there is a neurologic deficit, an individual muscle examination should be performed. In a routine arthritis hand assessment, it is generally sufficient to test selected muscles in order to screen for neurologic impairment or disuse weakness. Testing of the abductor pollicis brevis, dorsal and volar interossei, and the abductor digiti quinti can be done quickly and easily, and it can provide information about key ulnar and median innervated muscles.

ABDUCTOR POLLICIS BREVIS

This muscle should be checked in all arthritis hand assessments since weakness is often indicative of carpal tunnel syndrome. It is an important muscle and provides abduction for grasping objects.[1] Patients with chronic weakness of this muscle often develop thumb adduction contractures.

Testing method: Support the patient's hand in supination and stabilize the ulnar metacarpals and wrist. Have the patient abduct the thumb volar to the index finger and perpendicular to the palm. Apply resistance to the radial side of the thumb proximal phalanx. Grade according to a standard muscle strength evaluation.[54,55,56]

DORSAL AND VOLAR INTEROSSEI

The interossei are prime MCP joint flexors. In some patients strengthening of the interossei can help compensate for extrinsic finger flexors that are not working effectively owing to tenosynovitis, attenuation, or contractures.

Testing method, dorsal interossei: Have the patient place his or her hand (palm down) on the table, and abduct the fingers. Stabilize the MCP joints. For the first and third muscles, apply resistance (to the proximal phalanx) to the radial side of the index and the ulnar side of the middle finger. For the second and fourth muscles, apply resistance to the ulnar side of the ring finger and the radial side of the middle finger. Volar interossei: Have the patient tightly adduct the fingers, with MCP and PIP joints in extension, and the hand supported in midair, not on the table (to minimize flexor muscle substitution). During active adduction, attempt to abduct the patient's little finger and then the index finger. The resistance or abduction should be applied in a manner that allows the digit to snap. The muscles are graded on the following scale: 5/5 if the digit snaps back strongly, 4/5 if it snaps weakly, 3/5 if it adducts but cannot resist abduction, 2/5 if it partially adducts, and 1/5 for trace motion.

ABDUCTOR DIGITI QUINTI

Have the patient place his or her hand on the table and actively abduct the little finger. Apply resistance to the ulnar border of the proximal phalanx.[55] This can be done during the testing of the volar interossei.

Intrinsic Muscle Tightness

For patients with beginning swan neck deformities, intrinsic muscle tightness can be a major deforming force.[17,31]

Shortening or tightness of the intrinsic muscles contributes to hand limitations in the following ways: (1) it can be a deforming causal factor for swan neck deformity; (2) by itself, it can reduce dexterity; (3) it can contribute to flexion deformity of the MCP joints; and (4) if severe, it can limit the patient's ability to grasp large objects by prohibiting PIP and DIP flexion while the MCP joints are in extension.

It is recommended that intrinsic muscle length be evaluated on all patients with inflammatory arthritis of the hands. It is theorized that pain and swelling in the MCP joints elicit a reflex spasm of the associated interossei muscles.[49] If this spasm is prolonged, the muscles can become contracted in a shortened position.[17] It is also possible for the intrinsic muscles to become contracted secondary to chronic flexion positioning of the MCP joints. Only a position of MCP extension and PIP flexion requires full excursion of the interossei muscles. Patients with painful MCP joints may not experience this position for months or even years.

Rationale for the test for intrinsic muscle tightness: The function of the interossei muscles is flexion of the MCP joints and extension of the PIP joints (Fig. 44).[31] When a person actively maintains a position of MCP joint flexion and PIP extension, the interossei muscles are contracting and are in their shortest position. Consequently, the opposite position (Fig. 45), MCP extension and PIP joint flexion, places the interossei muscles on stretch, and they have to extend their full length to allow this positioning. If a person's intrinsic muscles are tight or shortened they will not be able to fully flex the PIP joint while the MCP joint is in full extension (Fig. 46).[17] In fact, they will have greater PIP flexion with the MCP joint flexed than with the MCP joint extended. A patient has to have nearly full PIP flexion to be able to perform the test.

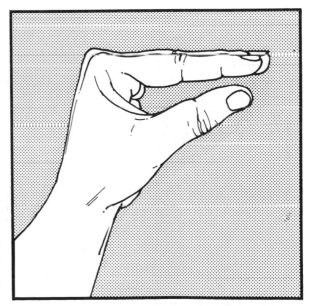

FIGURE 44. Intrinsic plus position. The interossei and lumbricals act together to provide PIP extension when the MCP joints are flexed. In this position they are actively contracted and at their shortest length. This position should be avoided in swan neck deformity.

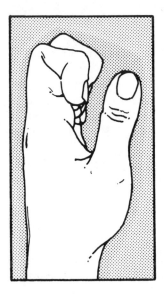

FIGURE 45. Normal intrinsic muscles stretched full length.

If a patient has MCP ulnar drift the standard test may not demonstrate tightness in the ulnar intrinsics. For these patients the test should be done with the digit radially deviated so the MCP joint is in neutral deviation during testing (except for the index finger, which should be in 20 degrees of ulnar deviation).

Procedure:

1. This test must be done with passive motion. The patient has to be able to relax and not actively move the hand during the procedure.
2. Place the MCP joint in comfortable midrange. (Each finger must be done separately.)

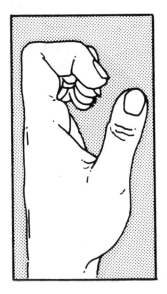

FIGURE 46. Tight intrinsic muscles—do not allow full proximal interphalangeal flexion.

3. Passively and gently flex the PIP joint as fully as possible. (Note ROM.)
4. Passively extend the MCP joint to neutral (zero extension).
5. Repeat passive PIP flexion. (Note ROM.) A loss of PIP flexion when the MCP joint is extended is indicative of intrinsic tightness.

The objective of this procedure is to determine if there is a difference in PIP joint range of motion when the MCP joint is flexed, compared with when it is extended.[31]

Intrinsic tightness can be described in the following manner: *negative,* PIP joint flexion is the same with MCP flexion or MCP extension; *minimal shortening,* tightness is palpable or there is less than 10 degrees change in PIP joint ROM; *marked shortening,* there is greater than 10 degrees difference in PIP joint ROM. Intrinsic tightness is documented in the degrees of difference of PIP joint motion, e.g., 15 degrees tightness. (The criteria for goniometric measurement of the PIP joint in patients with arthritis are described in Chapter 22, Evaluation of Range of Motion.)

TENDON INVOLVEMENT

Tenosynovitis

In the hand, the tendons pass through a synovial lined sheath at four locations: the volar aspect of the wrist; the volar aspect of the fingers; the length of the flexor pollicis longus sheath; and the dorsum of the wrist (Fig. 47).[18] The purpose of the sheath is to facilitate lubrication and gliding of the tendons, particularly where the tendons slide over several bones. The sheaths have a double wall construction, and inflammation of the synovial lining results in excessive fluid being trapped within the walls of the sheath. If the inflammation becomes chronic, synovial tissue will proliferate. Tenosynovitis impedes the gliding of tendons and, through an enzymatic process, directly attacks the tendons reducing their integrity.[17]

Tenosynovitis differs from joint synovitis in two ways. First, in most cases, there is no warmth present; and second, there may not be any pain associated with it. The only indicative signs may be swelling and possibly impaired tendon function.

VOLAR WRIST TENOSYNOVITIS

The signs and symptoms of volar wrist tenosynovitis can include one or all of the following:
1. Swelling over the volar aspect of the wrist.
2. Carpal tunnel syndrome (median nerve entrapment).
3. Decreased excursion of the profundus and/or superficialis tendons affecting all four digits. This can result in decreased active finger flexion or decreased passive finger extension and tenodesis motion in the fingers.[57]
4. Pain and warmth may or may not be present.

Evaluation method:
1. Support the patient's wrist in neutral and palpate the volar aspect of the wrist just proximal to the palm. In patients with early disease, distention or visible swelling of this area is indicative of volar wrist tenosynovitis.
2. Evaluate for carpal tunnel syndrome (see page 248).
3. To determine the excursion capability of flexor tendons, gently and passively extend the patient's fingers and wrist (Fig. 48). If the flexor tendons are not extending fully,

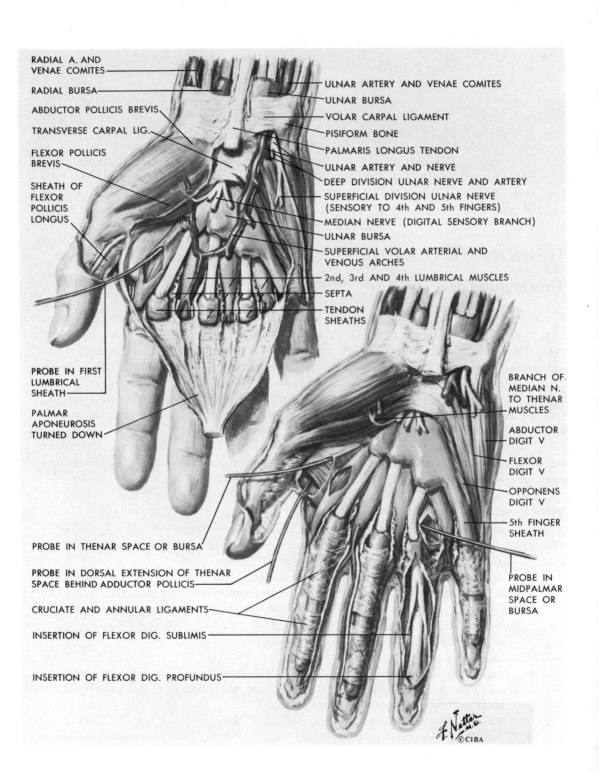

RADIAL A. AND VENAE COMITES

RADIAL BURSA

ABDUCTOR POLLICIS BREVIS

TRANSVERSE CARPAL LIG.

FLEXOR POLLICIS BREVIS

SHEATH OF FLEXOR POLLICIS LONGUS

ULNAR ARTERY AND VENAE COMITES

ULNAR BURSA

VOLAR CARPAL LIGAMENT

PISIFORM BONE

PALMARIS LONGUS TENDON

ULNAR ARTERY AND NERVE

DEEP DIVISION ULNAR NERVE AND ARTERY

SUPERFICIAL DIVISION ULNAR NERVE (SENSORY TO 4th AND 5th FINGERS)

MEDIAN NERVE (DIGITAL SENSORY BRANCH)

ULNAR BURSA

SUPERFICIAL VOLAR ARTERIAL AND VENOUS ARCHES

2nd, 3rd AND 4th LUMBRICAL MUSCLES

SEPTA

TENDON SHEATHS

PROBE IN FIRST LUMBRICAL SHEATH

PALMAR APONEUROSIS TURNED DOWN

BRANCH OF MEDIAN N. TO THENAR MUSCLES

ABDUCTOR DIGIT V

FLEXOR DIGIT V

OPPONENS DIGIT V

5th FINGER SHEATH

PROBE IN THENAR SPACE OR BURSA

PROBE IN DORSAL EXTENSION OF THENAR SPACE BEHIND ADDUCTOR POLLICIS

CRUCIATE AND ANNULAR LIGAMENTS

INSERTION OF FLEXOR DIG. SUBLIMIS

INSERTION OF FLEXOR DIG. PROFUNDUS

PROBE IN MIDPALMAR SPACE OR BURSA

F. Netter M.D.
©CIBA

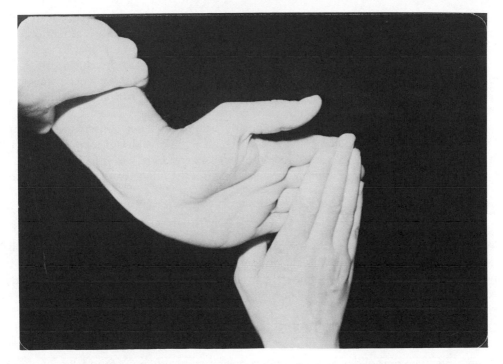

FIGURE 48. Flexor tenosynovitis at the wrist can cause limitations of the flexor tendons. Here the therapist is gently, passively extending the patient's wrist and fingers to determine if the flexor tendons can complete full excursion. If the tendons were blocked the patient would not be able to fully extend the wrist and digits at the same time. This patient has normal excursion.

there will be a difference in PIP or MCP joint extension when the wrist is extended compared with when the wrist is flexed, i.e., tenodesis motion.

4. It is often difficult to determine if a patient has pain associated with the tenosynovitis, since most patients with RA also have painful radiocarpal or radioulnar synovitis.[57]

When tendon excursion is reduced, generally all four digits are affected. However, it is possible for only three or two digits to be involved. If the limitation is only in a single digit, it is probably due to digital rather than wrist tenosynovitis.[57]

If there is a decrease in active finger flexion, it is important to rule out extensor tendon tightness as a cause.

FIGURE 47. Flexor sheaths at four levels: wrist, thumb, palm, and digits. In the digits the annular ligaments (pulleys) are the transverse fibers that encircle the flexor sheath and maintain the alignment of the flexor tendons. These fibers are strong and close fitting; nodules or thickened areas on the tendon can catch on these annular fibers. In this illustration the flexor sheaths are filled with air to demonstrate that they are a closed space. This emphasizes how the sheaths would expand if they were filled with synovial fluid during flexor tenosynovitis. Normally the sheaths are close-fitting to the tendons. Palpation for digital flexor tenosynovitis is most effective over the cruciate (cross) fibers, since they are weaker than the annular fibers and allow swelling to protrude. (Copyright 1969 CIBA Pharmaceutical Co., Division of CIBA-Geigy Corp. Reprinted with permission from Clinical Symposia, illustrated by Frank H. Netter, M.D. All right reserved.)

Severity can be related either to the degree of swelling or to the interference with tendon functioning. Some patients have a minimal amount of swelling but severe loss of tendon excursion, while others can have severe swelling but full tendon excursion.

If tendon excursion is limited and left untreated, permanent contractures will develop (Fig. 49). This condition should be treated as early as possible. The most effective conservative measures are ice compresses and intrasynovial steroid injections (not at the same time). If neither of these measures is successful, surgery is indicated.

To document tendon limitations, particularly before and after conservative treatment, the following methods are recommended. Measure MCP, PIP, and DIP joint ROM with the wrist in neutral; or record the maximal degree of wrist extension at which full MCP, DIP, and PIP joint extension is possible. Either method will rule out the influence of tenodesis motion.

PALMAR TENOSYNOVITIS

Severe hypertrophy of the tenosynovium can distend the sheath into the palm as well as fill the entire length of the sheath of the fifth digit tendons, which is often continuous between the wrist and digit level. Early tenosynovitis in the palmar region is difficult to detect because of overlying muscle and fascia. It is only palpable after marked hypertrophy has occurred.

DIGITAL FLEXOR TENOSYNOVITIS

The signs and symptoms of digital flexor tenosynovitis can include any of the following:[57]
1. Swelling along the volar aspect of the digit (Fig. 50).
2. Decreased excursion of the flexor tendons, resulting in decreased active flexion or decreased passive extension.
3. Trigger finger due to tenosynovium (or nodule) catching on the pulleys (annular ligaments: see Figure 47).
4. Pain or warmth may or may not be present.

Evaluation method:
1. Tendon sheath effusions are first evident over the volar aspect of the proximal phalanx.[1] Palpate this area with the digit in extension. Swelling, fullness, or tension in this area is indicative of tenosynovitis. When possible, compare swelling with uninvolved contralateral digits. Moderate or severe tenosynovitis can also be palpated over the volar aspect of the middle phalanx.
2. If tenosynovitis is not readily palpable, stabilize the patient's MCP joints in extension and have him or her actively flex the PIP and DIP joints. Palpate over the volar aspect of the proximal phalanx. This procedure may allow a minimal effusion to be detected.

Tenosynovitis is considered slight if it is palpable but does not limit finger flexion or tendon excursion; moderate if there is some joint or tendon limitation; and severe if there is marked limitation in motion.

Treatment is similar to that for wrist tenosynovitis. Ice compresses and steroid injections are the recommended conservative measures. From personal experience, splinting can be very effective in those cases in which there is a great deal of warmth and pain. It has not proven ef-

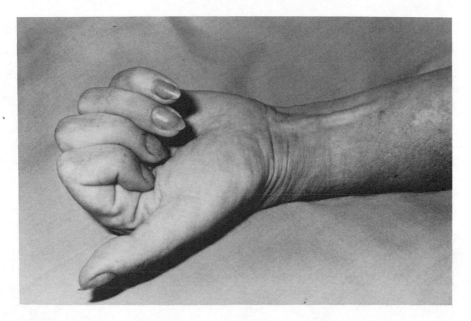

FIGURE 49.   This young woman presented with a carpal tunnel syndrome. The hand evaluation reveal-ed a flexion lag in the middle, ring, and little fingers indicating the profundus tendons were not gliding freely through the carpal tunnel. This suggested flexor tenosynovitis in the wrist, despite the absence of wrist pain or warmth. Her symptoms were alleviated and ROM restored following a tenosynovial steroid injection and wrist splinting for two weeks.

fective in cases without these two symptoms, and in a few cases splinting has increased stiff-ness.

The flexor pollicis longus tendon has its own synovial sheath that is continuous from the IP joint to approximately 3 cm proximal of the wrist (see Figure 47).[18] Tenosynovitis of this ten-don can be nonpainful, with the effusion easily detected over the volar aspect of the proximal phalanx, or it can be painful and difficult to detect if inflammation is in the region beneath the thenar muscles. Sometimes resistance applied to IP joint flexion can elicit pain along the ten-don, distinguishing tendon involvement from CMC joint pain, which can also radiate into the thenar eminence. During palpation of this tendon, keep in mind that there are two small sesamoid bones over the volar aspect of the MP joint. These can often be misinterpreted as nodules.

DORSAL WRIST TENOSYNOVITIS

Each extensor tendon passes through a separate tendon sheath over the dorsal aspect of the wrist. As the tendons pass beneath the dorsal retinacular ligament, they are divided into six compartments (Fig. 51). Tenosynovitis can occur in a single compartment or in all six compart-ments at one time (Fig. 52).[18] Since the skin over the dorsum of the wrist is thin, effusions tend to feel puffy and are readily detectable; they often clearly delineate the length of the sheath.

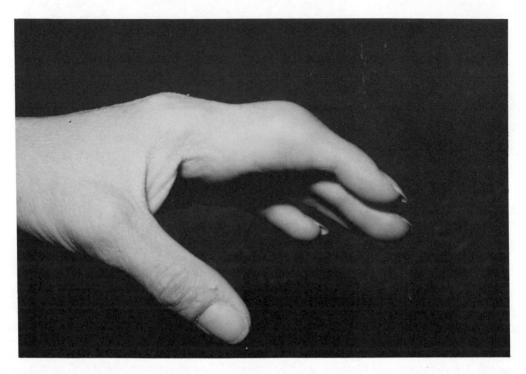

FIGURE 50. This is an example of severe digital flexor tenosynovitis and hypertrophy. Digital swelling due to flexor tenosynovitis is most evident when viewed from the lateral aspect.

Synovitis of the radiocarpal and intercarpal joints can also cause swelling in this area. Joint synovitis is firm to the touch and is usually warm and painful.

Inflammation of the first compartment, which contains the abductor pollicis longus and the extensor pollicis brevis, is referred to as de Quervain's disease.[58] Unlike other areas of tenosynovitis, inflammation of the first compartment is almost always painful. Since this is a common condition, which frequently is primary and unrelated to arthritis, it is discussed in a separate section below.

The incidence of pain in dorsal tenosynovitis varies. The first compartment is usually painful; the sixth compartment, containing the extensor carpi ulnaris, is frequently painful; and compartments two through five are rarely painful. It is theorized that the first and sixth compartments have more pain because of their close approximation to the superficial branch of the radial nerve and dorsal cutaneous branch of the ulnar nerve, respectively. When the tenosynovitis is painful, splinting can be very effective for reducing pain and inflammation. When there is no pain, it is very difficult to get patients to wear wrist splints. A full hand splint would be required to provide rest for the tendons in compartments three, four, and five. This would be impractical, particularly for patients without any symptoms. The value of splinting for painless tenosynovitis needs much more investigation. For some patients splinting can increase stiffness and swelling by eliminating muscle action as a mechanism for venous and lymphatic return. For conservative management, ice is more effective than heat in reducing swelling and pain.

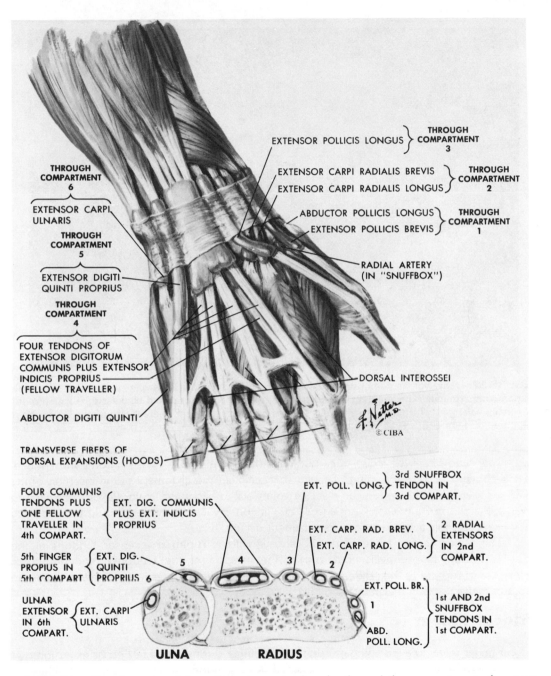

FIGURE 51. This illustration defines the extensor tendon sheaths and the compartments they pass through. The sheaths, in this drawing, are filled with air to demonstrate that they are a closed structure and their expansiveness if filled with tenosynovial fluid. Tenosynovitis may afflict a single compartment or all compartments. Since the dorsal covering is thin, swelling is readily detected and conforms to the length of the sheath. (Copyright 1969 CIBA Pharmaceutical Co., Division CIBA-Geigy Corp. Reprinted with permission from Clinical Symposia, illustrated by Frank H. Netter, M. D. All rights reserved.)

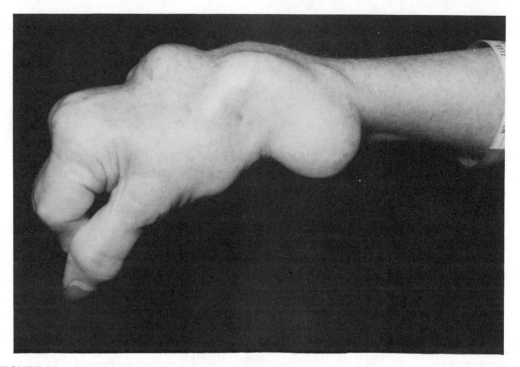

FIGURE 52.   This woman demonstrates the extreme of dorsal tenosynovitis with involvement of multiple tendon compartments. The apparent enlargement of the MCP joints is created by volar subluxation of the proximal phalanges, which also gives the digits a shortened appearance. There is also marked synovitis of the thumb IP joint and a Type IV thumb deformity.

Tenosynovitis of the extensor carpi ulnaris (ECU) tendon in the sixth compartment is of special concern. If the supporting ligaments that maintain the alignment of the insertion of the ECU are stretched, the tendon can displace volarward to become a major flexor force causing volar subluxation of the wrist (see page 231). All conservative measures should be employed early to protect this tendon, before displacement occurs.

The major consequence of dorsal tenosynovitis is ruptured extensor tendons at the wrist.[59] Chronic tenosynovitis compromises the integrity of the tendons, rendering them vulnerable to rupture as they slide over sharp or subluxed wrist bones.[59] (Evaluation of tendon ruptures is discussed in a separate section.)

Trigger Finger

Trigger finger refers to a snapping or catching of a finger during active flexion or extension owing to a nodule, tenosynovium, or a thickened flexor tendon becoming trapped at either the proximal, middle, or distal flexor pulley (Fig. 53).[58]

A network of fibrous bands (annular and cruciate ligaments) covers the flexor tendon sheath. These bands are thickest directly over the volar aspect of the MCP, PIP, and DIP joints (annular ligaments).[18] This strong thickened portion or band is referred to as a pulley. (This

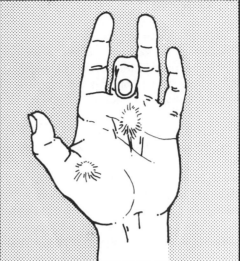

FIGURE 53. Trigger finger: common palpation sites.

pulley functions similar to a mechanical pulley, which maintains the position of a rope but allows it to slide.) The pulley hugs the tendon to the joint during flexion. If a pulley were cut, the flexor tendons would bowstring across the joint.[60]

A nodule or tenosynovial build-up on a tendon can get caught on any one of the three pulleys during either flexion or extension. Clinically this presents in one of the following ways: a slight catch or snap during motion; inconsistency in the degree of active motion; and inability to actively extend or flex a digit completely.

In the early stages, it is usually annoying but not painful. As the lump becomes larger the catching can be quite painful. Triggering can occur in one or more digits. It occurs most frequently at the MCP joints of the fingers and thumb, followed by the DIP joints and thumb IP joint; rarely does it occur at the DIP joints.[58]

Evaluation procedure:
1. First, ask the patient if his or her fingers ever catch or stay closed when opening or closing the hand. Most patients are aware of this problem if it is present.
2. Determine if it occurs rarely, occasionally, or consistently; if there is any pain associated with it; and if it interferes with function.
3. Palpate for a nodule over the flexor pulleys.[58]

Severity can be described as minimal, inconsistent, painless triggering during active ROM; moderate, constant triggering during active ROM or intermittent but painful triggering; severe, prevents full active flexion or extension or is severely painful.

There is no specific OT treatment for triggering. If the condition interferes with function or is painful, the patient should be advised to see a physician. Many patients do not mention the problem to their doctor because they believe the only solution is surgery. It is often encouraging for them to find out that the initial treatment of choice is an intrasynovial steroid injection.[58,60]

de Quervain's Tenosynovitis

This is tenosynovitis of the first dorsal wrist compartment, which encloses the abductor pollicis longus and the extensor pollicis brevis tendons. This condition is common and frequently occurs in people without arthritis secondary to trauma or occupational stress.[58]

Signs and symptoms include pain over the first compartment and thumb with active or passive motion; swelling; and decreased thumb ROM secondary to pain. Warmth may or may not be present.

Evaluation procedure:

The Finkelstein Test.[1] The original version of this test is to have the patient make a fist, with the fingers holding the thumb in flexion, then to deviate the wrist ulnarward. This method is too painful for patients with arthritis. Therefore, the following adapted version is recommended. Passively and gently fully flex the patient's thumb and have the patient identify pain areas; then gently deviate the wrist ulnarward, keeping the thumb flexed (Fig. 54).

The test is positive if the maneuver elicits pain over the first compartment, possibly radiating to the first metacarpal bone. The test may elicit pain localized to the thumb IP or MCP joints or to the wrist joints, but this is usually indicative of joint involvement, not tenosynovitis.

When de Quervain's tenosynovitis is secondary to trauma or functional use, it is generally responsive to splinting or a combination of steroid injection and splinting. The ideal splint is a radial gutter wrist splint with an extension to immobilize the thumb MCP joint. This type of splint allows patients to make a fist and use their thumb IP for prehension. The splint prevents excursion of the extensor pollicis brevis and abductor pollicis longus tendons, yet allows the patient to continue working. If de Quervain's syndrome becomes chronic and is nonresponsive to splinting, injections, and activity modification, then surgical tenosynovectomy may be indicated.

Tendon Ruptures

The most frequent cause of tendon rupture is a combination of tenosynovitis diminishing the strength and integrity of the tendons (attenuation) and attrition over rough subluxed bones or bone spurs. Occasionally the tenosynovium can cause sufficient pressure to compromise the blood supply to the tendon, creating ischemic areas.[59]

Ruptures of the finger extensors are usually found over the distal end of the ulna (Fig. 55). The extensor pollicis longus tendon commonly ruptures at Lister's tubercle, where it turns radially to the thumb. The flexor tendons most frequently rupture over the scaphoid carpal bone. However, they can rupture at the palm or digit level.[59]

Because of the manner in which the extensor tendons slide over the carpal bones, rupture of the dorsal tendons is more common than rupture of the flexor tendons. The extensor digiti quinti (EDQ) is generally the first tendon to rupture. Interestingly, this muscle, which is of little functional importance, is the key tendon to evaluate in an arthritis hand assessment.[59] If this tendon is ruptured, the extensor communis tendons are in danger of attrition also. Patients with partial or complete rupture of the EDQ are candidates for a dorsal tenosynovectomy to protect the other extensor tendons from attrition. In many cases, it is necessary to use a wrist splint to protect the remaining tendons until surgery can be scheduled. Rupture of the EDQ does not impair function, and since it is rarely noticed by patients, it requires a specific testing procedure.

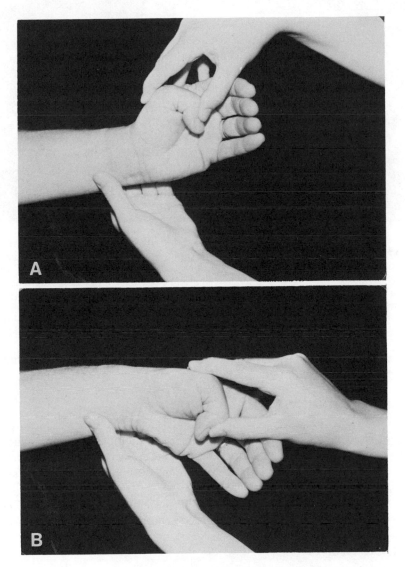

FIGURE 54. Finkelstein test (adapted for patients with arthritis) for de Quervain's tenosynovitis. (*A*), Support the patient's wrist in neutral, gently passively flex the thumb, and note any pain. (*B*), Then deviate the wrist ulnarward, while maintaining thumb flexion. This maneuver places the tendons in the first wrist compartment, i.e., the extensor pollicis brevis and the abductor pollicis longus on stretch. The test is considered positive if the maneuver elicits pain directly over the first compartment (see Figure 51). Joint pain is not characteristic of tenosynovitis and may indicate arthritis. *Caution:* Try this procedure on several normal hands before trying it on a patient. The mechanics of the maneuver can create discomfort in normal hands.

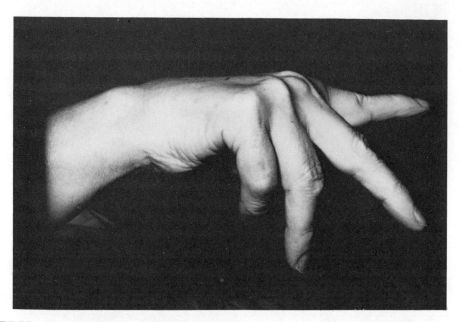

FIGURE 55. Extensor tendons are typically ruptured at the wrist level owing to attrition by the eroded and roughened end of the ulna. This woman has complete rupture of the extensor digitorum quinti tendon and the extensor communis tendons to the little, ring, and middle fingers, as evidenced by the inability to fully extend the MCP joints of these fingers and the inability to palpate tendon function during active extension. Partial extension of the middle finger is possible due to intertendinous connections to the index finger. The extensor communis tendon to the index finger and the indicis proprius tendon are intact.

The following tendons have the highest incidence of rupture. They are listed in order of greatest frequency.[59]

EXTENSOR DIGITI QUINTI (EDQ)

Test procedure: Hold the MCP joints of the ring, middle, and index fingers in flexion to prevent function of the extensor communis tendon. Have the patient actively extend the little finger. Inability to actively extend the little finger MCP joint in this position indicates damage to the EDQ tendon (Fig. 55).

Considerations: It is necessary to rule out displacement of the extensor tendons as a cause for loss of MCP extension. PIP joint extension is accomplished by the intrinsic muscles.[59]

EXTENSOR COMMUNIS (EC)

Rupture of this tendon occurs most frequently to the little and ring fingers. If there is a rupture, the patient will be unable to actively extend the associated MCP joint. The indicis proprius provides extension to the index finger (Fig. 55).

Considerations: The EC tendons may displace into the ulnar MCP valleys and lose their mechanical advantage for extension. Rule out tendon displacement by positioning the MCP joints in extension. If the patient can maintain extension, once positioned, the tendons are intact. Palpate for tendon function over the dorsum of the hand during active extension. Inability to actively extend the little finger MCP joint indicates possible rupture of the fifth EC as well as the EDQ (Fig. 55).[59] Although rare, it is possible to have paralysis of the thumb extensors due to entrapment of the posterior interosseous branch of the radial nerve.[9]

EXTENSOR POLLICIS LONGUS (EPL)

Rupture of this tendon results in decreased active thumb IP joint extension (when the MP joint is extended) and possible decreased active MCP extension (Fig. 56).[59]

Considerations: The abductor pollicis brevis, adductor pollicis, and the flexor pollicis brevis (superficial head) also extend the IP joint of the thumb through their attachment to the dorsal expansion. Their pull on the IP joint is strongest when the MCP joint is flexed. To determine an EPL rupture, evaluate active thumb IP extension with the thumb MCP stabilized in extension.

FLEXOR POLLICIS LONGUS (FPL)

Rupture of this tendon results in loss of active thumb IP flexion and decreased ability for pinch. To determine if there is a partial rupture, test IP flexion with the thumb MCP and CMC joints stabilized in extension. This places the tendon on tension and allows slight motion to be detected.[59]

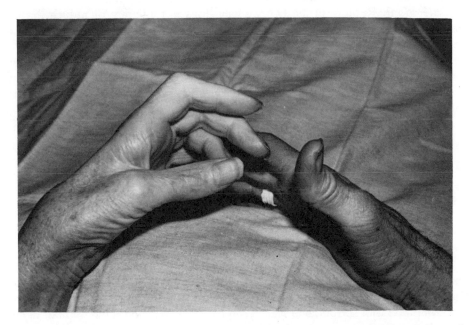

FIGURE 56. The extensor pollicis longus tendon is ruptured in this woman's left hand. To evaluate for EPL rupture it is advisable to palpate for tendon function. Observation of IP joint motion alone is not sufficient, since the thumb intrinsic muscles are also capable of extending the IP joint.

Considerations: A tendon nodule catching on the IP and MCP flexor pulley can also prevent thumb IP flexion. A rare condition that can impair FPL function is entrapment of the anterior interosseous nerve in the forearm. (See section on nerve entrapment.)

FLEXOR DIGITORUM PROFUNDUS

Rupture of this tendon occurs primarily in the index finger. Rupture results in absent or diminished active DIP joint flexion, and the patient may lose the ability for tip-to-tip pinch.[59]

To evaluate tendon function, elicit active DIP joint flexion while stabilizing the PIP and MCP joints in extension.

Considerations: The ruptured distal tendon end may become adhered to other flexor tendons, resulting in partial active flexion with the digit in extension. If this occurs there would be an absence of active flexion with the digit flexed.[59] A flexor tendon nodule can block profundus tendon excursion and imitate a rupture. This phenomenon can be ruled out by palpating for a nodule and observing the resting digital posture. If the tendon is ruptured, the finger will assume a more extended position than the other digits.[59]

FLEXOR DIGITORUM SUPERFICIALIS (FDS)

Fortunately, rupture of the FDS is uncommon.[59] However, when it occurs, it is often in conjunction with rupture of the FDP tendon, to the index finger.

Evaluation: Stabilize all of the digits in full extension (to rule out profundus function), except the digit to be assessed. Have the patient actively flex the PIP joint.

Considerations: Rupture of the FDS usually does not interfere or reduce the patient's functional ability. However, the proximal end of the ruptured tendon may retract and become adherent to the profundus tendon and consequently limit profundus excursion. In the presence of severe digital flexor tenosynovitis, hand function may be improved by surgical removal of the FDS (or one slip of the FDS) to provide more room for the profundus tendon to slide effectively. To evaluate the superficialis tendon in the little finger it may be necessary to apply additional stabilization of the proximal phalanx in extension and adduction, while having the patient attempt active flexion, since many patients do not have independent function of the superficialis tendon in the little finger.

SKIN AND VASCULAR INVOLVEMENT

Skin Changes

There are characteristic skin lesions associated with systemic sclerosis (and mixed connective tissue disease), psoriatic arthritis, systemic lupus, dermatomyositis, and chronic juvenile polyarthritis.[61] These are discussed in detail in the chapters on each disease in Part II.

The following terms are often used to describe skin rashes in medical documentation.[61]

Macule: A circumscribed area of alternation of normal skin color. It is neither raised nor depressed compared with surrounding skin. It can be of any size and is the result of pigmentary or vascular abnormality.

Papule: A solid lesion, most of which is elevated above the skin.

Plaque: A lesion that is elevated above the skin with a relatively large surface area. It is formed by a confluence of papules.

Evanescent: This is used to describe a rash that appears and disappears over a short period of time, i.e., within hours or a day. This is characteristic of the rash seen with chronic juvenile polyarthritis.

Skin Ulcerations

Skin breakdown typically can occur in three ways.

1. In systemic sclerosis, fingertip ulcerations are common and extremely painful. Also, the skin may break down over calcium deposits.[39]
2. In RA, the skin may break down over bony prominences created by joint subluxation, such as over the dorsum of a severely flexed PIP joint. Nodules over the dorsum of the PIP joints are particularly vulnerable to trauma.
3. In hands with severe deformity or contractures, the skin can become macerated between the digits owing to the difficulty in washing and drying the hands thoroughly in these areas.

Drug Reactions

Skin rashes are a common consequence of gold therapy, antimalarials (Plaquenil), and penicillamine.[61] In all cases, the rash is highly variable and can have any appearance; there is no characteristic pattern. All rashes that cannot be explained should be reported to the physician.

Chronic use of systemic steroids can result in atrophic skin changes. The skin feels dry and smooth; there is decreased height in the dorsal joint folds and atrophy of the fingertip pulp. The skin appears thin and delicate and is sometimes referred to as tissue paper skin.[61]

Skin Tightness

This occurs primarily in systemic sclerosis. If the skin is tight in the hands, it is usually difficult to pinch the skin over the dorsum of the middle and proximal phalanges.[39]

Vasculitis

Patients with RA can develop an arteritis of the small digital arteries. This can result in a peripheral neuropathy, nailfold infarcts, ulcers, and digital gangrene.[61] When it develops, vasculitis usually becomes the primary diagnosis. Therapy is generally minimal. Custom splints are often helpful for protecting ulcerated areas.

Telangiectasia

These are small reddish spots in the skin that result from a chronic dilatation of the capillaries.[61] They are indicative of the vascular changes that are taking place internally as well as cutaneously. They are most common in systemic sclerosis but occasionally can occur in rheumatoid arthritis.

Palmar Erythema

In patients with systemic diseases, the thenar and hypothenar eminences appear red, with discrete small red irregular-shaped blotches. This erythema is evidence of the vascular systemic involvement of the disease.[1]

Purpura

This refers to a spontaneous hemorrhage into the skin. The appearance varies with the type of purpura, and the color of the lesion varies from red to purple to brownish-yellow, as it dissipates.[61]

Purpura can occur in several disorders, including Henoch-Schönlein (anaphylactoid) purpura, erythema nodosum, severe RA, thrombocytopenia (low platelets), and in certain drug reactions.

Purpura can be purely cutaneous, or it can be indicative of hemorrhage in the internal organs. The term ecchymosis has the same definition as purpura but is generally used to describe a singular bruise or skin hemorrhages resulting from trauma.

Keratoderma Blennorrhagica

This is the characteristic skin lesion that occurs with Reiter's syndrome. The skin changes most frequently involve the acral (peripheral) regions, especially the soles, toes, and fingers, but can occur anywhere on the body. The lesions begin as vesicles (small blisters) on an erythematous base, progress to sterile pustules, and evolve to manifest keratotic scale. Psoriasis-like lesions can also appear in Reiter's syndrome.[61]

Temperature Changes and Sweating

Systemic diseases can alter vasomotor and sudomotor stability, resulting in hands that feel cold and clammy with increased sweating. Owing to these changes, the hand may feel very soft to the touch.[61]

Raynaud's Phenomenon

In this disorder, vasoconstriction causes blanching or cyanosis of the skin, with subsequent erythema upon vasodilation. The vasoconstriction can be in response to exposure to cold, emotional stress, or to dependent positioning of the arm to the side; or it can appear spontaneously. The color changes may be limited to the tip of a finger or encompass the entire hand.[62]

Raynaud's phenomenon most commonly occurs with systemic sclerosis, mixed connective tissue disease, and systemic lupus erythematosus. It is uncommon in rheumatoid arthritis. It can also be idiopathic and unrelated to rheumatic disease.[62]

The only clinical sign of Raynaud's phenomenon may be the white, blue, or red color changes in the skin, or there may be symptoms of pain and paresthesias.[62]

To evaluate, first ask the patient if he or she has noticed color changes in the hand, i.e., turning red, white, or blue. Most patients are aware of these changes when they occur. Second, determine the extent of the changes—whether or not it is painful and how the symptoms interfere with functional ability. Also, can the patient identify any causal factors or measures that relieve the symptoms? Smoking habits should also be addressed. Patients with Raynaud's phenomenon should not smoke or use nicotine, a vasoconstrictor.[62] (See Chapter 5 for treatment.)

Severity may be described in the following manner: *mild,* patient is aware of skin changes but does not experience any discomfort or functional loss; *moderate,* changes are uncomfortable but are of short duration and do not interfere with functional use; *severe,* skin changes are painful and may last 10 minutes or longer and functional ability of the hand is limited during attacks.

Documentation should include a description of the skin changes, their severity, and location.

NEUROLOGIC INVOLVEMENT

The most common or widely recognized neurologic conditions that can occur secondary to arthritis will be reviewed in this section. All of these conditions can result from other causes such as trauma or occupational use and are covered in detail in the neurologic and orthopedic surgery literature. Practical guidelines for sensory evaluation are discussed at the end of this section.

Cervical Radiculopathy or Nerve Root Compression Syndrome

This condition can result from osteophyte formation or from cervical subluxation. Initial symptoms typically include pain, paresthesias, and sensory loss in the upper extremity and hand along dermatome patterns, followed by motor weakness of the affected associated muscles.

Cervical nerve root compression should be the first differential diagnosis considered when sensory deficits in the hand are not consistent with typical median or ulnar nerve loss. For example, sensory loss isolated to the thumb can be due to C-6 compression.[5,6,63]

Entrapment Neuropathies

These conditions refer to direct compression of peripheral nerves from edema, synovitis, synovial hypertrophy, or trauma.

In association with arthritis, the median nerve is the most commonly affected, the ulnar nerve is next in frequency, and radial nerve entrapment is uncommon but not rare.[8]

Entrapment can occur at various sites, resulting in both sensory and motor impairment distal to the lesion.

Median Nerve Entrapment

The median nerve can be compressed at the wrist or in the forearm.

CARPAL TUNNEL SYNDROME (CTS) WRIST LEVEL (FIG. 57)

This is the most common entrapment syndrome seen in association with arthritis.[8] Evaluation for CTS should be a part of every arthritis hand evaluation.

The carpal tunnel is bordered on three sides by the carpal bones. The volar side or roof is formed by the strong transverse carpal ligament. This narrow, rigid passageway contains nine flexor tendons and their sheaths, blood vessels, and the median nerve. (See Figure 47.) Any swelling in the tendon sheaths or thickening of the tendons or bones can cause compression of the nerve.[53]

The position of the wrist can expand or decrease the space of the carpal tunnel, thereby diminishing or increasing symptoms accordingly. The space in the tunnel is maximized when the radius and the scaphoid are in neutral alignment. When these two bones are in neutral, the second metacarpal is in approximately 10 degrees of extension, using standard goniometric placement. (When the second metacarpal is at zero degrees extension, the scaphoid is in 10 degrees of flexion.) Any position other than 10 to 15 degrees of wrist extension reduces the carpal tunnel space.

All patients with rheumatoid arthritis are at high risk for developing CTS. Therefore, it is recommended that all wrist or hand splints made for patients with rheumatoid arthritis be in 10 degrees wrist extension. The main exception to this would be patients who are rapidly losing wrist extension and developing wrist flexion contractures. For these patients, the treatment of choice may be to maintain wrist extension by positioning in their maximal extension (which may be very limited).

The classic early symptoms of CTS include wrist pain or paresthesias in the fingers occurring only at night.[53] This pattern is attributed to prolonged positioning in either flexion or extension at night and nocturnal hand swelling that occurs in everyone when not actively using the hand. Occasionally patients report the symptoms occur only during certain functional activities such as driving, using a telephone, and so forth.

Splinting the wrist in 10 degrees of extension can be a very effective treatment for early CTS or for patients who have symptoms only at night. Once motor loss occurs, splinting may reduce discomfort but generally it will not alleviate or reverse symptoms. Surgery is indicated to release the transverse carpal ligament.[8]

There are two specific test procedures commonly used to diagnose CTS. The Tinel Test: percussion over the median nerve at the wrist, which lies just lateral to the palmaris longus tendon. The test is positive if the maneuver elicits paresthesias along the median distribution. Second, the Phalen test: passive flexion of the wrist for one minute. The test is positive if the maneuver reproduces the symptoms.[53] If flexion is painful, a reverse Phalen test, holding the wrist in extension, can be done. These assessments are helpful in locating the site of the compression. The most reliable clinical assessment is a clear accurate history, identification of altered sudomotor function (sweating), a sensory evaluation for two-point discrimination, and an individual muscle test if motor loss is suspected.

Muscles affected: abductor pollicis brevis, opponens pollicis, flexor pollicis brevis (superficial head), and the first and second lumbricals.[8]

Sensation affected: palmar surface of the thumb, index, and middle fingers, and the lateral half of the ring finger.[8]

Muscles to monitor: the abductor pollicis brevis is the key muscle to evaluate, since it can be easily isolated and is the first to be affected.

Symptoms: The sole symptom may be wrist pain at night. The pain may radiate into the palm or occasionally up the forearm. Paresthesias or numbness along the median distribution (with or without pain) may be present. Numbness in all digits may mean the ulnar nerve is also involved.[53]

MEDIAN NERVE ENTRAPMENT IN THE PROXIMAL FOREARM

Although uncommon, it is possible for the median nerve to be compressed by fibrous bands at several levels as the nerve passes through the pronator teres and under the flexor superficialis arch (Fig. 58).[64]

Symptoms of proximal compression include paresthesias in the median innervated fingers; pain in the proximal forearm, increased by resistance to pronation, with occasional radiation to the upper arm; clumsy use of the hand with decreased grip or prehension skill; and tenderness over the pronator teres muscle.[64]

Johnson, Spinner, and Shrewsbury[64] in a report of 71 cases of proximal entrapment identified the following clinical pattern: (1) tenderness, firmness, or enlargement of the pronator teres muscles; (2) a positive Tinel's sign on percussion of the pronator teres muscle; (3) no weakness of the median innervated muscles (no significant conduction defect); (4) marked increase in paresthesias in the affected fingers during resistance to pronation with the elbow flexed and an increase in paresthesias when the elbow is gradually extended localizes the lesion to the pronator teres; (5) paresthesias or pain following resistance to elbow flexion and forearm supination identifies entrapment by the lacertus fibrosus of the biceps tendon; (6) a reproduction of paresthesias in the median innervated fingers upon independent flexion of the flexor superficialis of the middle finger localizes the entrapment to the fibrous arcade of the flexor superficialis; and (7) reproduction of symptomatology with a tourniquet above diastolic pressure on the upper arm. Additionally, these patients may have a negative Phalen test and their symptoms are generally not responsive to splinting of the wrist.[64]

In rheumatoid arthritis, the high incidence of flexor tenosynovitis makes wrist entrapment the most likely source for sensory disturbances in the median innervated digits. Proximal entrapment should be considered in patients with no apparent wrist involvement; early or mild symptoms that do not increase at night (due to positioning); a negative Phalen's test; or in cases that do not respond to conservative measures.

ANTERIOR INTEROSSEOUS NERVE (AIN) SYNDROME

The anterior interosseous nerve is a motor branch of the median nerve (Fig. 58). Entrapment of this nerve can occur in the forearm; however, it is rare. Typically patients present with nonspecific pain in the forearm or elbow and weakness of the flexor pollicis longus muscle, resulting in a characteristic pinch, (Fig. 59). Testing further reveals weakness of the flexor profundus to the index and occasionally the middle fingers.

In addition to the AIN syndrome several other conditions can cause weakness or inability to flex the thumb IP joint and index DIP joint. These conditions include partial or complete rupture of the FPL or FDP at the wrist; flexor tenosynovitis; tendon nodules in the digital or palm sheath; and proximal median nerve compression above the AIN. The presence of tenodesis motion can help rule out the possibility of tendon rupture.

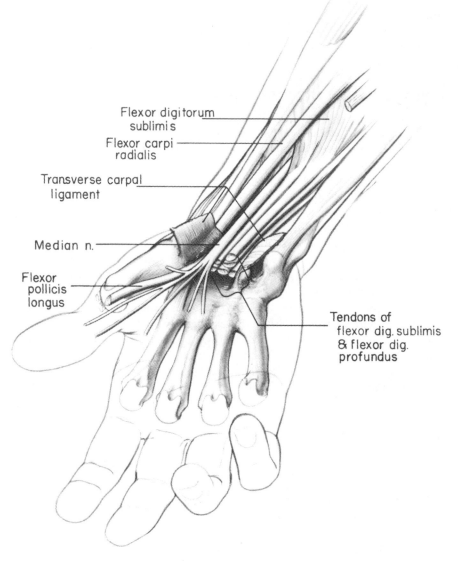

Flexor digitorum
sublimis

Flexor carpi
radialis

Transverse carpal
ligament

Median n.

Flexor
pollicis
longus

Tendons of
flexor dig. sublimis
& flexor dig.
profundus

FIGURE 57.   This shows reflection of the transverse carpal ligament to reveal passage of the median nerve and nine flexor tendons through the narrow carpal tunnel. Note the rigid bony floor and sides of the tunnel formed by the carpal bones. (From Liveson, J. A., and Spielholz, N. I.: *Peripheral Neurology*. F. A. Davis, Philadelphia, 1979, with permission. Illustration by Hugh Thomas.)

FIGURE 58.   This shows the course of the median nerve and its anterior interosseous branch. Entrapment of the median nerve in the forearm is uncommon but should be considered in patients with median nerve paresthesias, a negative Phalen's test, and no apparent wrist involvement. (From Liveson, J. A., and Spielholz, N. I.: *Peripheral Neurology*. F. A. Davis, Philadelphia, 1979, with permission.)

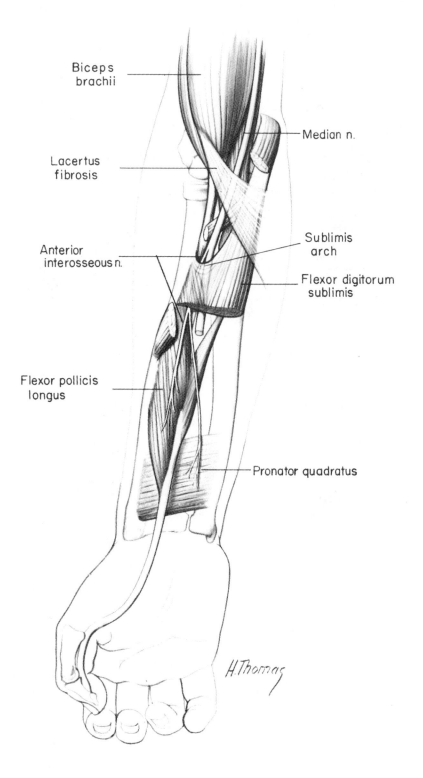

Biceps
brachii

Median n.

Lacertus
fibrosis

Sublimis
arch

Anterior
interosseous n.

Flexor digitorum
sublimis

Flexor pollicis
longus

Pronator quadratus

H.Thomas

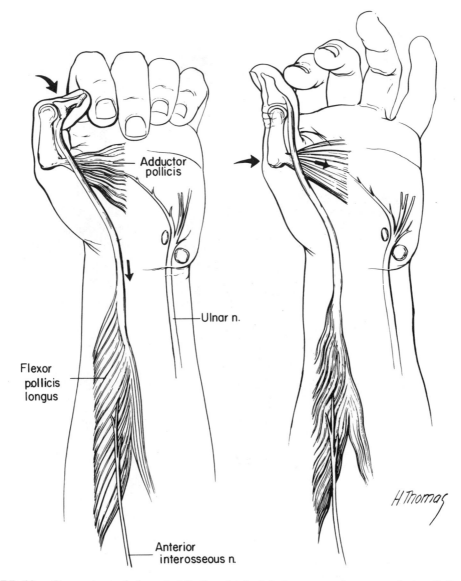

Adductor
pollicis

Ulnar n.

Flexor
pollicis
longus

Anterior
interosseous n.

H Thomas

FIGURE 59. Comparison of characteristic thumb pinch between an ulnar nerve lesion (*left*) and an anterior interosseous nerve lesion (*right*). In an ulnar nerve lesion the flexor pollicis longus substitutes for the weakened adductor pollicis, resulting in marked flexion of the IP joint during pinch (Froment's sign). In the uncommon AIN paralysis, the patient loses the ability to actively flex the IP joint and achieves pinch force by using the adductor pollicis. (From Liveson, J. A., and Spielholz, N. I.: *Peripheral Neurology*. F. A. Davis, Philadelphia, 1979, with permission.)

Muscles affected: Flexor pollicis longus, pronator quadratus, and the flexor digitorum profundus to the index and middle fingers.[65]

Muscles to monitor: This condition is so rare that it is usually not part of a routine assessment. However, evaluation of the flexor pollicis longus can help distinguish between a high (forearm) and a low (wrist) entrapment of the median nerve. Patients with a complete lesion (usually traumatic) demonstrate a characteristic two-point pinch in which the thumb IP joint and the index DIP joint are in neutral extension during prehension. This pattern may not be as easily recognized in a partial lesion.

DOUBLE CRUSH SYNDROME

Occasionally a patient with cervical spine arthritis develops nerve root compression and median nerve compression at the same time, a condition referred to as the double crush syndrome.[66] It is theorized that the cervical lesion causes primary damage to the nerve fibers, which renders them more vulnerable to a superimposed entrapment.[66] This condition can also affect the ulnar nerve.

Ulnar Nerve Entrapment

ULNAR NERVE ENTRAPMENT AT THE ELBOW

Compression of the ulnar nerve at this location (ulnar groove, posterior to medial epicondyle) is quite common in the presence of severe elbow synovitis. It occurs only occasionally in *early* rheumatoid arthritis. There is considerable variability in the depth of the ulnar groove. When a patient has a shallow groove, there is less space to accommodate any synovitis and higher risk of traumatizing or subluxing the ulnar nerve. The nerve is most vulnerable to pressure when the elbow is flexed.[63] So the patient with elbow synovitis and a flexion contracture is particularly at risk. Ulnar nerve compression can also result from improper positioning following upper extremity surgery.

Typically, conservative management includes a steroid injection to reduce synovitis and ice compresses for acute episodes. Occasionally splinting (with the elbow in extension) is helpful on a temporary basis to reduce inflammation or alleviate pressure on the nerve.

Muscles affected: flexor carpi ulnaris, flexor digitorum profundus to the ring and little fingers, all hypothenar muscles (palmaris brevis, abductor digiti quinti, opponens digiti quinti, flexor digiti quinti), lumbricals to the ring and little fingers, all interossei, flexor pollicis brevis (deep head), and the adductor pollicis.[8]

Sensation affected: palmar and *dorsal* surface of the little finger, the medial half of the ring finger, and ulnar side of the hand.[8] Sensation to the dorsum of the little finger is a key area to test to distinguish between elbow and wrist compression syndromes, because the dorsal cutaneous branch is proximal to the wrist. Thus, if the dorsal sensation is diminished, the lesion is above the wrist. If only the volar sensation is altered, the lesion is at Guyon's canal or lower.

Muscles to monitor: The first dorsal interosseous and the adductor pollicis. Patients with an ulnar nerve lesion demonstrate a characteristic pinch, in which there is marked flexion of the thumb IP joint and extension or hyperextension of the thumb MCP joint during active prehension due to substitution of the FPL for the weak adductor pollicis (see Figure 59). This prehension pattern is referred to as Froment's sign for ulnar nerve palsy. It is also important to observe for clawing of the ring and little fingers, which is characteristic of ulnar nerve compression.[8]

Symptoms: Paresthesias along both the dorsal and volar ulnar distribution and pain radiating down the forearm or occasionally upward to the arm.[8]

ULNAR NERVE ENTRAPMENT AT THE WRIST (AT GUYON'S CANAL)

Guyon's canal is between the pisiform bone and the hook of the hamate bone. It is covered by the pisohamate ligament, thus forming a fibro-osseous tunnel (Fig. 60). Compression can be in the canal or just distal to it. The most common sources of compression are carpal synovitis, trauma, deep ganglions, and occupational stress.[8,63] Motor branches arise within the canal to the hypothenar muscles. Innervation of other intrinsic muscles occurs distal to the canal; therefore, different patterns of involvement can result, depending on the specific side of the compression.

Entrapment of the ulnar nerve at the wrist is less common than at the elbow, but comprehensive hand assessments often reveal ulnar sensory loss that is apparently overshadowed by coexistent carpal tunnel syndrome. This is easy to understand when you consider that sensory skills in the ulnar fingers are not as critical as those in the median fingers, and atrophy and weakness of the intrinsic muscles may be masked by chronic rheumatoid disease and joint contractures.

Muscles affected: Palmaris brevis, abductor digiti quinti, opponens digiti quinti, flexor digiti quinti, lumbricals to the ring and little fingers, all interossei, flexor pollicis brevis (deep head), and the adductor pollicis. (The FDP and FCU are unaffected.)[8]

Sensation affected: Only the palmar surface of the little finger and medial side of the ring finger. Dorsal sensation is normal, since the dorsal cutaneous branch is proximal to the wrist.[8] If dorsal sensation is diminished the lesion is above the wrist. Compare sensation with the contralateral hand.

Muscles to monitor: Little finger abductor and adductor.

Symptoms: Decreased sensation, paresthesias along the ulnar half of the hand. There may be marked tenderness over Guyon's canal, compared with the contralateral hand.[8]

Radial Nerve Entrapment

Impingement of this nerve occurs in the elbow and forearm.

POSTERIOR INTEROSSEOUS NERVE (PIN) SYNDROME

The PIN is a motor branch of the radial nerve (Fig. 61). Elbow synovitis can impinge on this nerve as it passes through the supinator muscle in the forearm. This condition is considered uncommon in association with trauma, tumors, ganglions, or bursitis and rare in association with rheumatoid arthritis.[9]

Muscles affected: The PIN has two branches: the first is usually compressed; the second branch may be involved or spared. First branch: extensor carpi ulnaris, extensor digiti quinti, extensor communis. Second branch: extensor pollicis longus, extensor pollicis brevis, abductor pollicis longus, and extensor indicis proprius.[9]

Sensation affected: None.

Symptoms: Typically, there is a history of elbow synovitis with pain anterior to the elbow, which can radiate both proximally and distally along the radial distribution. Over a period of days, the patient develops weakness in the fingers and partial or complete inability to extend the MCP joints, and possibly the thumb. Wrist extension may be in a radial direction owing to compression of the first branch and loss of the extensor carpi ulnaris. This condition can mimic extensor tendon rupture; however, the presence of tenodesis motion can confirm tendon integrity.[9] Weakness of the finger extensors may also be confused with dislocation of

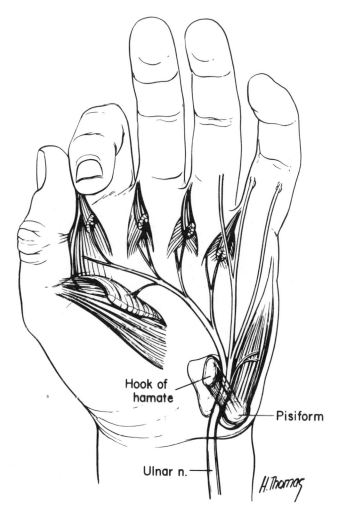

FIGURE 60. This shows the course of the ulnar nerve through Guyon's canal. Within the canal, the ulnar nerve is both motor and sensory; but beyond the hook of the hamate, the nerve divides into a separate deep motor branch and sensory fibers to the ring and little fingers. Therefore, lesions distal to the hamate may cause pure motor or sensory loss. (From Liveson, J. A., and Spielholz, N. I. *Peripheral Neurology*. F. A. Davis, Philadelphia, 1979, with permission.)

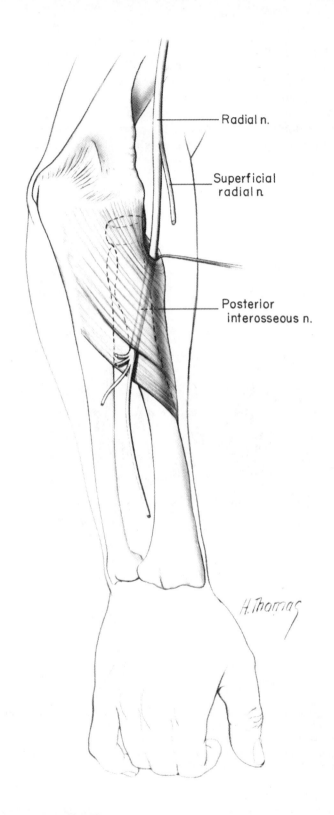

Radial n.

Superficial
radial n

Posterior
interosseous n.

H. Thomas

the EC tendons. This can be demonstrated by the ability to maintain MCP extension once positioned.

RADIAL TUNNEL SYNDROME (RTS)

The radial tunnel refers to a 5-cm area where the radial nerve crosses anterior to the radiohumeral joint and courses between the supinator and the arcade of Frohse (see Figure 61). As the nerve travels through this area, one or all of the following structures can impinge on the nerve.[67,68] The fibrous origin of the ECRB can create a flat rigid medial edge to the tunnel and may be densely adherent to the underlying fibrous origin of the supinator. The transverse fibrous bands that cross the nerve anterior to the head of the radius can become thickened. A fan of radial recurrent vessels crosses over and is often interwoven into the structure of the posterior interosseous nerve. The arcade of Frohse can become thickened and fibrous with age.

Patients with radial tunnel syndrome complain primarily of aching pain localized to the extensor muscle mass just below the elbow. The pain is initiated and intensified by repetitive motion involving forearm pronation or pronation and wrist flexion. Grip strength may be diminished secondary to pain. Generally these patients do not have any sensory or motor loss.[67,68]

Initially, these patients may appear to have tennis elbow (lateral epicondylitis), but they do not respond to conservative treatment, i.e., steroid injections, splints, or exercise, because they have a structural compression not a tendinitis. Since 1972 when this syndrome was first described, many cases of resistant tennis elbow have been identified as radial tunnel syndrome.[68]

Lister, Belsole, and Kleinert have described four diagnostic procedures for distinguishing RTS from tennis elbow.[67]

1. The point of maximum pain as indicated by history and by indirect testing is over the radial tunnel, not the lateral epicondyle.
2. The point of maximum tenderness is over the radial tunnel.
3. Resistance applied to the proximal phalanx of the middle finger, with the elbow and wrist extended, produces more pain in the radial tunnel than does resistance to the ulnar fingers or passive stretching of all the extensors. Resistance to the middle finger (occasionally the index finger) transmits the force directly to the insertion of the ECRB, which forms the lateral edge of the tunnel.[67]
4. Pain is elicited over the radial tunnel when supination is resisted, with the elbow in extension.[67] Lister, Belsole, and Kleinert also note that it is not uncommon for patients to have multiple compression syndromes and that it is possible for a patient to have both RTS and tennis elbow.[67]

Thoracic Outlet Syndrome

Entrapment of the neurovascular supply to the upper extremity as it passes through the thoracic outlet can be due to bony, fascial, or muscular impingement.[69,70] This condition is not

---

FIGURE 61. The course of the posterior interosseous branch of the radial nerve through the radial tunnel deep to the supinator muscle. (From Liveson, J. A., and Spielholz, N. I.: *Peripheral Neurology*. F. A. Davis, Philadelphia, 1979, with permission.)

specifically related to arthritis, but it is included here because its presence may first be detected during a hand assessment.

One of the first symptoms that patients often complain of is numbness only when they elevate the arm overhead. More severe symptoms include pain throughout the upper extremity and numbness and paresthesias, often perceived in the C-8–T-1 dermatome.

Compression of the subclavian artery can result in numbness, coldness, and weakness in the upper extremity.[69,70] There are several specific maneuvers that help locate the area of compression.[70] If this condition is suspected by the therapist, patients should be advised to bring the symptoms to the attention of the physician.

EVALUATION OF SENSATION FOR PERIPHERAL NERVE ENTRAPMENT

For all practical purposes in rheumatologic rehabilitation of the hand, sensation is evaluated to determine if median or ulnar nerve entrapment has affected sensory nerves. It provides a guidepost for appreciating the severity of the compression and in the early stages provides a guide for determining the effectiveness of conservative measures. Damaged sensation should return to normal if conservative measures are effective. If it does not, the patient is a candidate for surgery. For these purposes the most efficient and reliable quantitative sensory assessments are the Weber two-point discrimination (2PD) test and the moving two-point discrimination (M2PD) test. These tests are the most valuable to use because the results of these tests correlate highly with function.[72,73]

There is a wide range of other sensory assessments. Each is effective for determining a certain aspect of sensibility. No single test provides a complete assessment. The sensory nerve conduction study is considered the most sensitive means of determining the integrity of median and ulnar sensory nerves. It can be a valuable diagnostic tool, but it is expensive and must be administered by a physician. It is not indicated in all cases and is not feasible as an initial screening tool. The Weinstein-Semmes monofilament provides a precise means for mapping light touch and point localization for the documentation of injury, anomalous innervation, and nerve regeneration. However, this assessment is time consuming and thus costly. It should be reserved for cases in which the outcome of the sensory evaluation will alter or determine the treatment to be administered.[74] Testing sharp-dull discrimination provides information about protective sensibility but does not provide quantitative measures that correlate with function.[72] The Weber two-point and the moving two-point discrimination tests are efficient, inexpensive, and reliable and can be administered in all clinical settings.

Weber Two-Point Discrimination Test

The static two-point discrimination test (Fig. 62) developed by Weber in 1835 is a measure of the shortest distance at which a person perceives two distinct points touching the skin.[72] At a lesser distance the person perceives two points as one. This test has long been considered to have a direct positive correlation with hand function, that is, as the 2PD distance increases (becomes less sensitive), patients have increasing difficulty performing tasks. It is currently considered to have a strong positive correlation with the ability to perform various grips, but it does

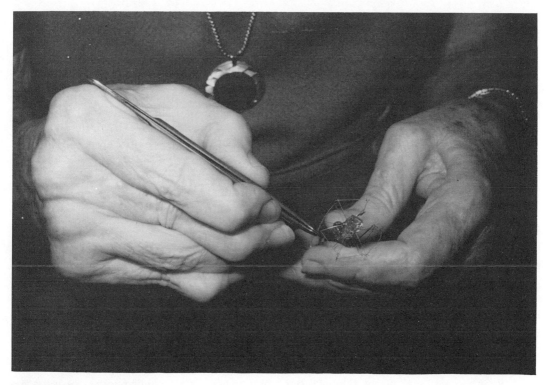

FIGURE 62. Functional assessment of the hand is a critical aspect of arthritis hand management. Rarely is it possible to predict functional skills simply from the appearance of the hand alone. This woman clearly illustrates this point. Despite severe fixed deformities, she is able to perform the dexterous skills required in her work as an electronics parts assembler.

not always correlate with tactile gnosis. Many patients have demonstrated higher tactile gnosis skills than would normally be expected considering their 2PD.[73]

From personal experience in working with hundreds of patients with rheumatic diseases, the Weber 2PD test has proven to be an excellent and reliable measure that correlates strongly with the patient's subjective report of functional skills. For example, if a patient's 2PD is 3 mm on all digit finger pads, except the median innervated fingers on the right hand which are 1 to 5 mm, the patient will report slight difficulty using those fingers for fine dexterous tasks. When 2PD reaches 7 mm patients have significant difficulty and often avoid using the affected fingers for certain tasks. For example, if the loss is in the median fingers, the patient may start gripping things with his or her ulnar fingers and palm for better control. At 10 mm of 2PD, patients have great difficulty and avoid using the fingers if possible. This test is not the most sensitive for mapping regeneration or measuring tactile gnosis, but is very effective for quantitating sensory loss owing to peripheral nerve entrapments, particularly if the patient's normal 2PD is used for a comparison with the affected area.

The measures cited in the above examples refer to the finger pad area. There are different norms for 2PD in various areas of the hand; the finger pad area is the most sensitive area. The norms in this area are 3 to 5 mm.[72] However, each person has his or her own normal distance. The majority of adults have 3 to 3.5 mm 2PD; some have 2 mm 2PD; and a few have 4 to 5 mm. Generally people with a distance of 5 mm perform heavy work and have thickened skin. When the evaluation is done, it is important that the patient's own normal 2PD be determined. This is done by comparing the ulnar and median fingers bilaterally. Gellis and Pool tested 105 normal subjects and found all subjects had less sensation in their thumb and index finger; the middle finger had the same 2PD as the ring and little fingers.[75] (This may be because the ulnar fingers are used less and are therefore more sensitive.) This finding indicates that the median nerve compression may be most clearly detected by comparing the 2PD of the middle finger with the 2PD of the little finger. They also found that sensitivity varied between age groups. Subjects 10 to 19 years of age had an average 2PD of 2 mm. Subjects 70 to 79 years of age had an average of 3 to 3.5 mm in the middle, ring, and little fingers and 4 to 5.5 mm in the index finger and thumb.

Method: First, all therapists should experience this test before they administer it to a patient.

Equipment: a 2- or 3-point anesthesiometer (available from Fred Sammons, Inc.) or a Boley gauge or dull-pointed eye calipers. The instrument used should not have sharp points that elicit a pain response. (Some professionals use a reshaped paper clip, but with this device it is difficult to keep the points even or to insure consistency among different evaluators.)

1. Explain the test and demonstrate the procedure while the patient is observing. It is often helpful to demonstrate how 2PD sensitivity increases from the palm to the fingertip.
2. Have the patient close his or her eyes or occlude vision in some manner.
3. Alternate touching the skin with one point or two points simultaneously. Ask the patient to identify if he or she feels one or two points. (The pressure from the instrument should not blanch the skin, and the two points need to touch with even pressure.) The recommendations for a correct response vary. Some surgeons recommend that 2 out of 3 correct responses are needed; others say 7 out of 10 correct answers are needed.[72,74,75] Basically you need sufficient applications to insure that the patient is perceiving the points and not guessing at the answer.
4. Generally it is easiest to start at 3 mm. If the patient can distinguish at 3 mm easily, test at 2 mm. If the patient cannot discern two points at 3 mm, gradually increase the testing 1 mm at a time, attempting at least three tries at each distance. If the person does not have 10 mm it is usually sufficient to indicate his or her sensation at greater than 10 mm and not continue testing.
5. When this test is done for evaluation of hand trauma in which the digital nerve may be damaged, the points should be applied in a longitudinal axis of the finger.[72] For nerve entrapment syndromes the placement does not alter the response.
6. Explain the results of the test to the patient.

Moving Two-Point Discrimination

This test was developed by Dellon as a means for quantitating a person's ability to discern moving touch.[73] The test is fairly new and was introduced in 1978. The test is based on the theory that the sensation of touch is mediated by two types of nerve fibers: quickly adapting fibers (which innervate Meissner's and Pacini's corpuscles) that are detectors of transient touch, that is, movement and vibration; and slowly adapting fibers that mediate the sensation of pressure by responding to increasing frequency of indentation of the skin.[73]

The test is performed in a manner similar to the Weber 2PD test, only the finger is stroked instead of touched (see method below). Dellon has reported a limited study, using the test on 39 normal hands and 63 patients with nerve injuries. Only the finger pad areas were tested, using a reshaped paper clip. Dellon found that in this population the average or normal M2PD was 2 mm in the thumb pad. Some of the normal subjects had a M2PD on 3 mm. The response was equal bilaterally, except in one person. In 25 hands ipsilateral digits were compared. In 17 of these hands, the thumb and little finger were equal; in 7 of the hands the thumb had a M2PD of 2 mm and the little finger had 3 mm. In one hand the little finger was more sensitive than the thumb. Static and moving 2PD were equal in 30 hands, and in the remaining 9 hands the M2PD was 2 mm and the static 2PD was 3 mm. (In this study Dellon found the average Weber 2PD to be 2 mm, which differs from the averages in other studies.) In the patient population studied, there was a much wider variation in the distances between 2PD and M2PD. It was also found that following nerve repair, moving 2PD returned faster than static 2PD. This variability between these two sensory functions appears to account for the discrepancy between tactile gnosis and static 2PD seen in the clinic.[73]

The moving 2PD test appears to be more sensitive than the static 2PD test for evaluating sensory regeneration and tactile gnosis. It also adds additional information regarding functional sensibility.[73] However, only one limited survey has been reported and the data conflict with previously reported larger studies on the Weber 2PD test. This may be due to different testing instruments or procedures. The moving 2PD is easier to perceive because considerably more skin is touched than with the static 2PD. This factor has not been integrated into the theory proposed by Dellon.

For purposes of evaluating sensory involvement in nerve entrapment syndromes, both the static and moving 2PD tests can be used effectively. More experience is needed in using the moving 2PD in this area. Future studies and experience may reveal that the moving 2PD is more sensitive for this function also. Therapists are encouraged to use both tests to determine the more effective test for their clinical needs.

Method: Described by Dellon

1. A paper clip is rearranged so the points are even and any sharp barbs are not touching the patient.
2. The hand to be tested is supported on a table.
3. Patient is oriented to the test. The technique is demonstrated.
4. Patient is stroked along the length of the finger pad with the points 5 to 8 mm apart and then proceeding in stages down to 2 mm apart. Vision is occluded. Stroking is parallel to the long axis of the finger at an angle to the majority of the fingerprint ridges.
5. The testing stimulus is alternated between one and two points. If the patient perceives the changes correctly, the next lower value is tested. Seven out of 10 correct responses are required before going to the next level.

Dellon does not describe the amount of pressure used, that is, whether the skin is blanched or not; nor is the exact length of the stroke described. Both of these variables could certainly affect the outcome. It is recommended that the technique used be as similar as possible to the method used for static 2PD.

ASSESSMENT OF HAND FUNCTION

Measurement of Range of Motion and Muscle Strength

Methods of assessing range of motion (ROM) and strength of the hand are discussed in detail in Evaluation of Range of Motion, Chapter 22, and Evaluation of Muscle Strength, Chapter 23.

Descriptive and Quantitative Assessment of Functional Hand Ability

The purpose of a functional hand assessment is to determine both *functional ability* of the patient, that is, how the patient can use his or her hand in spite of limitation, and *functional disability* in order to plan treatment and assess treatment effectively. The ROM and strength assessments provide some of this information, but they do not demonstrate how the patient can use muscular substitutions and adaptive methods to perform a functional task. In fact, one extensive study concluded that there is no direct correlation between hand ROM and the patient's ability to perform functional activities.[17]

There are many types of functional hand assessments currently in use, ranging from simple to complex, quantitative to nonquantitative, and standardized to nonstandardized. The type best suited to a clinic depends on the patient population and the specific reasons for assessment.

Since no single assessment method can be recommended for all clinics, this section reviews the basic functional components of the hand, the relationship to treatment for arthritis, and a description of published functional hand assessments. The assessment summary at the end of this chapter is included primarily as a reference source for therapists interested in designing their own evaluations or adopting an established test.

FUNCTIONAL COMPONENTS OF THE HAND

Essentially all hand activities involve precision or power or a combination of the two.[76] These components are applied through various prehensile and nonprehensile patterns.[77]

FINGER-THUMB PREHENSION. The holding of objects between the thumb and fingers of a single hand (Figs. 63, 64, and 65). This includes all forms of pinch: lateral, palmar, and tip. The object can be any size, that is, the fingertips do not have to be approximated.

FULL HAND PREHENSION. The holding of an object so that the palm forms one of the gripping surfaces (Figs. 66 and 67). This includes all of the typical grasps: gross (palmar), power, and cylinder.

NONPREHENSION. The following are nonprehensile uses of the hand.

1. Use of the hand as a base for the application of upper extremity strength. This includes hookgrip (when the fingers literally form a hook at the end of the forearm) and use of the extended hand to push large objects (Fig. 68).
2. Use of the fingers to apply pressure such as in patting soil around a plant (Fig. 69), smoothing cloth while ironing, tucking in a shirt at the waist, or tucking in sheets.
3. Use of the fingertip, usually the index or middle finger, for precision sorting motions such as sorting coins on a counter (Fig. 70), dialing a telephone, or pushing buttons.
4. Use of the heel of the hand or the ulnar edge of the palm to apply pressure.

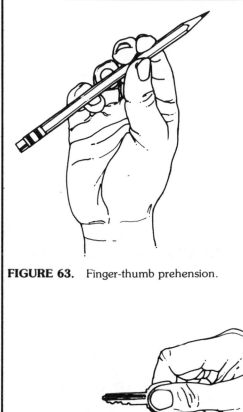
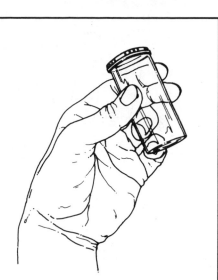

FIGURE 63. Finger-thumb prehension.   **FIGURE 64.** Finger-thumb prehension.

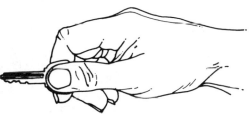

FIGURE 65. Finger-thumb prehension.

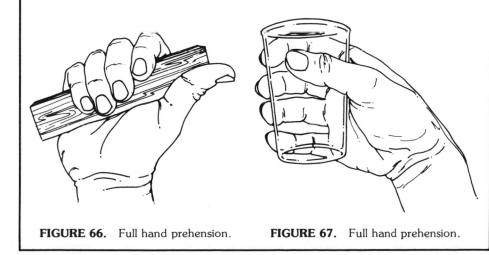

FIGURE 66. Full hand prehension.   **FIGURE 67.** Full hand prehension.

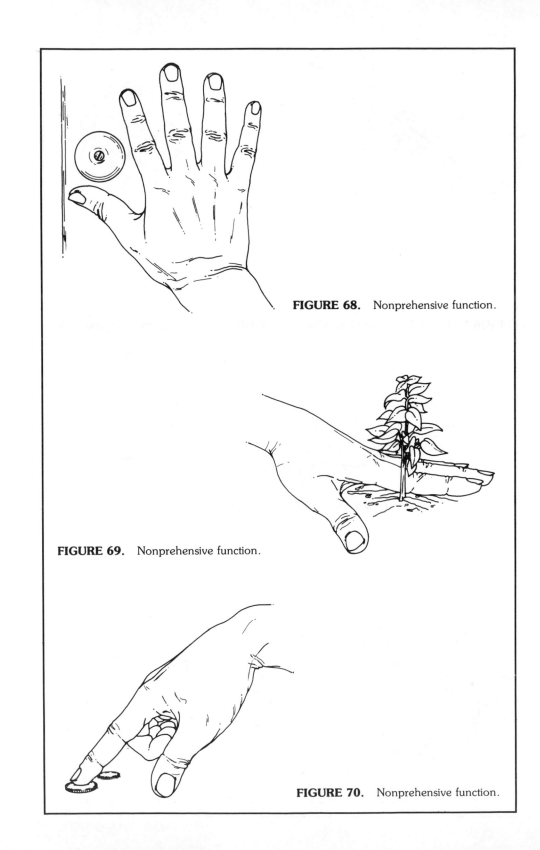

FIGURE 68.   Nonprehensive function.

FIGURE 69.   Nonprehensive function.

FIGURE 70.   Nonprehensive function.

BILATERAL PREHENSION. This is the holding of objects between the palmar surfaces of both hands as in unilateral nonprehension. The hand functions as a static extension of the upper extremity. Prehension is performed because both hands are used. It is essentially used to hold objects too large or too heavy to hold with a single hand.

RELATIONSHIP OF PREHENSION TO TREATMENT OF ARTHRITIS. The prehension patterns represent function unique to the hand. It is difficult to substitute for them if the hand is damaged; therefore, they constitute an area of prime concern in surgical hand reconstruction.

The nonprehension and bilateral prehension skills are not basic to hand function: most of them could be performed even if the fingers were amputated. However, they play an important role in activities of daily living and in rehabilitation for arthritis. Patients with various hand problems, such as metacarpophalangeal synovitis, wrist involvement, ruptured extensor tendons, metacarpophalangeal subluxation, and boutonniere deformities, frequently report difficulty or inability in performing nonprehension tasks.

One of the major goals in preventive treatment for the arthritic hand is to substitute nonstressful hand use for that which is stress-producing. For the rheumatoid hand with active synovitis all of the prehensile patterns carry a potential for deformity when used with significant pressure. However, the nonprehension and bilateral prehension patterns do not present the same potential for deformity. Additional instruction in compensatory adaptive methods or assistive equipment is indicated for patients with difficulty in performing nonprehension tasks. (See Assistive Equipment, Chapter 27.)

DOCUMENTATION OF HAND INVOLVEMENT

Purpose of Documentation

The primary purpose of documenting hand involvement is communication. It assists in the following:

1. Documentation is effective if another therapist or physician, in re-evaluating the patient's condition several months later, can determine the alterations from the documentation. Phrasing or recording should be directed toward facilitating the re-evaluator's assessment.
2. The written description is an effective method for learning and teaching how to do hand assessments simply because it requires a full qualitative evaluation.

Methods of Documentation

There are two principal ways of documenting hand involvement:

1. Photograph the hands and add a written description of aspects that cannot be pictorially displayed such as instability, triggering, or ankylosis. This is the most efficient method, but it is time consuming and requires photographic skills.
2. Write a systematic description of involvement, itemized by joints or anatomic areas in paragraph form, or create a form to document measurements and a summary of the assessment.

The hand evaluation form at the end of this chapter was developed by the Occupational Therapy staff at the Robert B. Brigham Hospital to provide an organized method for recording and documenting hand status. The form allows for flexibility in recording methods and was designed to meet the therapists documentation needs. A brief summary of the patient's hand status accompanied the form in the medical chart to facilitate physician and team communication. The use of this form was designated for patients with active complex hand involvement who could benefit from a systematic review and documentation process. It was not indicated for patients with minimal involvement, for example, carpal tunnel syndrome or monoarticular arthritis, or patients with severe burned out, end-stage deformity who were not candidates for hand therapy.

Documentation Procedures

PHOTOGRAPHIC DOCUMENTATION

Procedure

When using photographic documentation of hand involvement it is helpful to have a standard protocol for positioning the hands. *All members of the team involved with the photography must be aware of the positioning procedure.*

For some deformities, positioning is crucial in order to obtain a reliable interpretation of the photograph. For example, it is impossible to evaluate the degree of MCP ulnar drift present in a photograph unless it is known whether the fingers are in active or passive extension. (See Evaluation of Range of Motion, Chapter 22, for discussion on how to assess ulnar drift.) Medical photographers commonly use the same positioning procedures used in radiology for taking x-ray pictures. This method involves placing the hands on a table which means passive pressure from the table can distort the degree of ulnar deviation and the degree of finger flexion deformities. This method does not allow for accurate assessment of ulnar drift. *The fingers should be off the table and in active extension to assess MCP involvement.*

Photographic Views

The six standard photographic views are

> posteroanterior (PA), dorsal (Fig. 71 left)
> anteroposterior (AP), ventral (Fig. 71 right)
> ulnar, medial (Fig. 72 left)
> radial, lateral (Fig. 72 right)
> ulnar oblique (Fig. 73 left)
> radial oblique (Fig. 73 right)

Note the proper positioning of the camera for each view. The view recommended depends on the type of problem demonstrated and the number of photographs to be taken. Doctor Adrian Flatt describes the 16 standardized views that he uses for surgical documentation in his book, *Care of the Rheumatoid Hand.*[17]

Joint structures are more readily visible from the dorsum of the hand; therefore, the dorsal (PA) approach is usually the view used for most common joint deformities such as bouton-

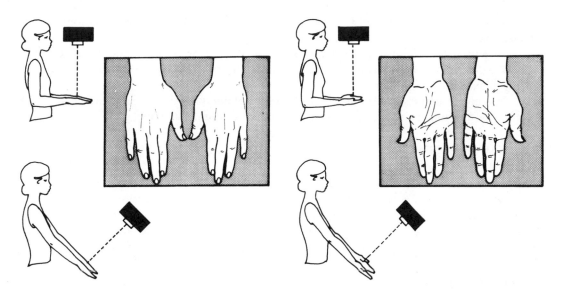

FIGURE 71. Photographic fields. *Left,* Posteroanterior (PA) view; *Right,* Anteroposterior (AP) view.

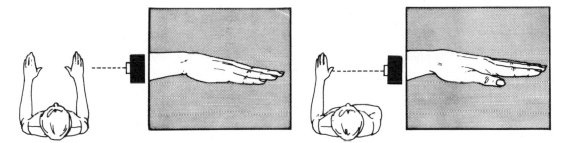

FIGURE 72. Photographic fields. *Left,* Ulnar (lateral) view; *Right,* Radial (medial) view.

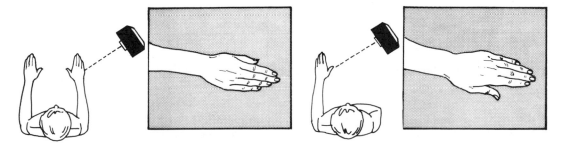

FIGURE 73. Photographic fields. *Left,* Ulnar (oblique) view; *Right,* Radial (oblique) view.

niere, swan neck, ulnar drift, wrist deviation, and synovitis or when only one photograph is to be taken to document multiple joint problems.

A radial, ulnar, or oblique view may be more effective for documenting decreased finger extension resulting from triggering, Dupuytren's contracture, ruptured extensor tendons, and MCP subluxation.

In addition to the standard views, photographs of the hand during functional use such as in pinch or grip may be a helpful adjunct for certain treatment situations.

Patient Consent Form

Every hospital has a patient release or consent form that should be signed by any patient even if only the hands are photographed. Make sure it includes patient permission to use the photos in professional publications. Many publishers will not use a photo unless there is a written consent form. Sometimes a publisher will use the photo without consent but will block out the eyes.

Background

Background color is an important consideration in photography and can significantly influence the appearance of the skin color. Red tones tend to reflect off the hand and increase any redness present. Very pale colors and white tend to reflect light; this results in diminished skin tone. Warm tones such as brown and gold usually do not provide sufficient contrast.

Moderate intensity shades of blue or green (e.g., surgery green, sky blue) or *flat black* (for light skin) provide the overall best results. A black background provides optimal contrast for black and white photographs for publication. When doing re-evaluations of the same hand it is helpful to use the same background color with each documentation.

Lighting

Usually regular clinic lighting with flashbulbs or a strobe light is sufficient; if extra lighting is used, it should be kept consistent in re-evaluations. For close-up hand photography a weak flash light is needed. If the strobe or bulb is too bright it will reflect off the hand, leaving a light or washed-out area in the center of the hand. The strobe light can be muted by putting white paper tape directly on the strobe light or covering it with any thin white opaque material, e.g., tissue paper.

Film

The selection of film depends on the type of camera used. Top quality film should be used for color slides and prints.

Kodachrome (ASA 64) is often recommended for close up photography because it offers the highest resolution. Ectachrome can also be used. It offers the advantage of a faster speed but has less resolution. If you need the slides in a hurry, keep in mind that Kodachrome may take up to a week to be developed because it has to be sent to an authorized center for processing. Only high-speed films can be processed in one day at most photo centers.

There are two excellent publications available for therapists interested in pursuing clinical photography: Clinical Photography, No. N-3, 1972, 117 pages, cost approximately $2.95; and Planning and Producing Slide Programs, 1975, 68 pages, cost $4.00. Both books are available from Eastman Kodak Co., Department 454, Rochester, N.Y. 14650.

REFERENCES

1. Polley, H. F., and Hunder, G. G.: *Rheumatological Interviewing and Physical Examination of the Joints*, ed. 2. W. B. Saunders, Philadelphia, 1978.
2. D'Ambrosia, R. D.: *Musculoskeletal Disorders: Regional Examination and Differential Diagnosis.* J. B. Lippincott, Philadelphia, 1977.
3. Hoppenfeld, S.: *Physical Examination of the Spine and Extremities.* Appleton-Century-Crofts, New York, 1976.
4. Kapandji, I. A.: *The Physiology of the Joints.* Vol. 1. *Upper Limb.* Churchill-Livingstone, Edinburgh, 1968.
5. Jackson, R.: *The Cervical Syndrome*, ed. 4. Charles C Thomas, Springfield, Ill., 1978.
6. Cailliet, R.: *Neck and Arm Pain.* F. A. Davis, Philadelphia, 1964.
7. Kozin, F.: *Painful shoulder and the reflex sympathetic dystrophy syndrome.* In McCarty, D. J. (ed.): *Arthritis and Allied Conditions.* Lea and Febiger, Philadelphia, 1978, pp. 1091-1120.
8. Nakano, K. K.: *Entrapment neuropathies.* In Kelley, W. M., et al. (eds.): *Textbook of Rheumatology.* W. B. Saunders, Philadelphia, 1981.
9. Millender, L. H., Nalebuff, E. A., and Holdsworth, D. E.: *Posterior interosseous nerve syndrome secondary to rheumatoid synovitis.* J. Bone Joint Surg. 55A(4):753, 1973.
10. Coonrad, R. W., and Hooper, W. R.: *Tennis elbow: Its course, natural history, conservative and surgical management.* J. Bone Joint Surg. 55A:1177, 1973.
11. Lehman, J. L., and Kushner, S.: *Tennis elbow.* Physiotherapy (Can) 31(5):251, 1979.
12. deAndrade, et al.: *Joint distension and reflex muscle inhibition in the knee.* J. Bone Joint Surg. 47A:313, 1965.
13. Vasey, J. R., and Crozier, L. W.: A neuromuscular approach to knee joint problems. Physiotherapy 66(6):193, 1980.
14. Huskisson, E. C.: *Measurement of pain.* Lancet 2(7889):1127, 1974.
15. DeCeulaer, K., and Dick, W. C.: *The clinical evaluation of antirheumatic drugs.* In Kelley, W. M. et al. (eds.): *Textbook of Rheumatology.* W. B. Saunders, Philadelphia, 1981.
16. McCarty, D. J., and Gatter A.: *A dolorimeter for quantification of articular tenderness.* Arthritis Rheum. 8:551, 1965.
17. Flatt, A. E.: *Care of the Rheumatoid Hand.* C. V. Mosby, St. Louis, 1974.
18. Lampe, E.: *Surgical Anatomy of the Hand.* CIBA Pharmaceutical Co., Summit, New Jersey, 1969. (Still available in 1981).
19. Hunter, J. M., and Mackin, E. J.: *Edema and bandaging* In Hunter, J M, Schneider, L. H., Mackin, E. J., and Bell, J. A.: *Rehabilitation of the Hand.* C. V. Mosby, St. Louis, 1978.
20. Wright, V.: *Psoriatic arthritis.* In Kelley, W. M., et al. (eds.): *Textbook of Rheumatology.* W. B. Saunders, Philadelphia, 1981.
21. Harris, E.: *Rheumatoid arthritis: The clinical spectrum.* In Kelley, W. M. et al. (eds.): *Textbook of Rheumatology.* W. B. Saunders, Philadelphia, 1981, p. 951.
22. Ginsberg, M. H., Genant, H. K., Yu, T. F., and McCarty, D. J.: *Rheumatoid nodulosis: An unusual variant of rheumatoid disease.* Arthritis Rheum. 18:49, 1975.
23. Angelides, A. C., and Wallace, P. F.: *The dorsal ganglion of the wrist—Its pathogenesis, gross and microscopic anatomy and surgical treatment.* J. Hand Surg. 1(3):228, 1976.
24. Calabro, J: *Rheumatoid arthritis.* Clinical Symposia, CIBA, Vol. 23, No. 1, 1971.
25. Brandt, K. D.: *Pathogenesis of osteoarthritis.* In Kelley, W. M., et al. (eds.): *Textbook of Rheumatology.* W. B. Saunders, Philadelphia, 1981, p. 1463.
26. Swanson, A. B., Goran-Hagert, C., and Swanson, G. dG.: *Evaluation of impairment of hand*

function. In Hunter, J. M., Schneider, L. H., Mackin, E. J., and Bell, J. A. (eds.): *Rehabilitation of the Hand*. C. V. Mosby, St. Louis, 1978.

27. Dell, P. C., Brushart, M. D., and Smith, R. J.: *Treatment of trapeziometacarpal arthritis: Results of resection arthroplasty*. J. Hand Surg. 3(3):243, 1978.
28. Lockie, L. M.: *Examination of the arthritic patient*. In Hollender and McCarty (eds.): *Arthritis and Allied Conditions*. Lea and Febiger, Philadelphia, 1972, p. 87.
29. Rosenthal, E. A.: *The extensor tendons*. In Hunter, J. M., Schneider, L. H., Mackin, E. J., and Bell, J. A. (eds.): *Rehabilitation of the Hand*. C. V. Mosby, St. Louis, 1978, pp. 206-210.
30. Kleinert, H. E., and Frykman, G.: *The wrist and thumb in rheumatoid arthritis*. Orthop. Clin. North Am. 4:1085, 1973.
31. Boyes, J. H.: *Bunnell's Surgery of the Hand*, ed. 5. J. B. Lippincott, Philadelphia, 1970.
32. Eaton, R. G.: *Joint Injuries of the Hand*. Charles C Thomas, Springfield, Ill., 1971.
33. Fess, E. E., Gettle, K. S., and Strickland, J. W.: *Hand Splinting—Principles and Methods*. C. V. Mosby, St. Louis, 1981.
34. Palmer, A. K., and Louis, D. S.: *Assessing ulnar instability of the MCP joint of the thumb*. J. Hand Surg. 3(6):542, 1978.
35. Wilson R. L., and Carter, M. S.: *Joint injuries in the hand: Preservation of proximal interphalangeal joint function*. In Hunter, J. M., Schneider, L. H., Mackin, E. J., and Bell, J. A. (eds.): *Rehabilitation of the Hand*. C. V. Mosby, St. Louis, 1978, p. 172.
36. Nalebuff, E. A. and Garrett, J.: *Opera-glass hand in rheumatoid arthritis*. J. Hand Surg. 1(3):210, 1976.
37. Forrester, D., Brown, J. C., and Nesson, A.: *The Radiology of Joint Disease*. W. B. Saunders, Philadelphia, 1979.
38. Adamson, J. D.: *Treatment of the stiff hand*. Orthop. Clin. North Am. 1:467, 1970.
39. Entin, M. A., and Wilkinson, R. D.: *Scleroderma hand: A reappraisal*. Orthop. Clin. North Am. 4:1031, 1973.
40. Pahle, J. A., and Raunio, P.: *The influence of wrist position on finger deviation in the rheumatoid hand*. J. Bone Joint Surg. 51B:664, 1969.
41. Taleisnik, J.: *Rheumatoid synovitis of the volar compartment of the wrist joint: Its radiological signs and its contribution to wrist and hand deformity*. J. Hand Surg. 4(6):526, 1979.
42. Chaplin, D., Pulkki, T., Saarimaa, A., and Vainio, K.: *Wrist and finger deformities in juvenile rheumatoid arthritis*. Acta Rheum. Scand. 15:206, 1969.
43. Backhouse, K. M.: *The mechanics of normal digital control in the hand and an analysis of the ulnar drift of rheumatoid arthritis*. Ann. R. Coll. Surg. Engl. 43:154, 1968.
44. Hakstian, R., and Tubiana, R.: *Ulnar deviation of the fingers: The role of joint structure and function*. J. Bone Joint Surg. 49A:299, 1967.
45. Smith, E. M., Juvinall, R. C., Bender, L. F., and Pearson, J. R.: *Flexor forces and rheumatoid metacarpophalangeal deformity*. J.A.M.A., 198:130, 1966.
46. Laine, V. A. I., Sairanen, E., and Vainio, K.: *Finger deformities caused by rheumatoid arthritis*. J. Bone Joint Surg. 39A(3):527, 1957.
47. Swezey, R. L., and Fiegenberg, D.S.: *Inappropriate intrinsic muscle action in the rheumatoid hand*. Ann. Rheum. Dis. 30(6): 619, 1971.
48. Smith, R. J., and Kaplan, E. B.: *Rheumatoid deformities at the MCP joints*. J. Bone Joint Surg. 49A:31, 1967.
49. Swanson, A. B.: *Flexible Implant Resection Arthroplasty in the Hand and Extremities*. C. V. Mosby, St. Louis, 1973, p. 109.
50. Nalebuff, E. A., and Millender, L. H.: *Surgical treatment of swan neck deformities in rheumatoid arthritis*. Orthop. Clin. North Am. 733, 1975.
51. Souter, W. A.: *The problem of the boutonniere deformity*. Clin. Orthop. 104:116, 1974.

52. Nalebuff, E. A.: *Diagnosis, classification and management of rheumatoid thumb deformities.* Bull. Hosp. Joint Dis. 24:119, 1968.

53. Phalen, G. S.: *The carpal tunnel syndrome: Seventeen years experience in diagnosis and treatment of 654 hands.* J. Bone Joint Surg. 48A:211, 1966.

54. *Guide for Muscle Testing of the Upper Extremity.* Occupational Therapy Department, Rancho Los Amigos Hospital. Published by the Professional Staff Assoc. of RCAH. Downey, California, 1976.

55. Kendall, H.O., Kendall, F. P., and Wadsworth, G. E.: *Muscles — Testing and Function*, ed. 2. Williams and Wilkins, Baltimore, 1971.

56. Daniels, L., and Worthingham, C.: *Muscle testing: Techniques of Manual Examination.* W. B. Saunders, Philadelphia, 1972.

57. Millender, L. H., and Nalebuff, E. A.: *Preventive surgery — Tenosynovectomy and synovectomy.* Orthop. Clin. North Am. 6(3):765, 1975.

58. Medl, W. T.: *Tendinitis, tenosynovitis, "trigger finger," and Quervain's disease.* Orthop. Clin. North Am. 1:375, 1970.

59. Nalebuff, E. A.: *The recognition and treatment of tendon ruptures in the rheumatoid hand.* In American Academy of Orthopedic Surgeons, *Symposium on Tendon Surgery in the Hand.* C. V. Mosby, St. Louis, 1975.

60. Gray, R. G., Kiem, I. M., and Gottlieb, N. L.: *Intratendon sheath corticosteroid treatment of RA, associated and idiopathic hand flexor tenosynovitis.* Arthritis Rheum. 21(1):92, 1978.

61. Soter, N. A.: *Cutaneous manifestations of rheumatic disorders.* In Kelley, W. M., et al. (eds.): *Textbook of Rheumatology.* W. B. Saunders, Philadelphia, 1981.

62. Leroy, E. C.: *Scleroderma (systemic sclerosis).* In Kelley, W. M., et al. (eds.): *Textbook of Rheumatology.* W. B. Saunders, Philadelphia, 1981, p. 1217.

63. Spinner, M.: *Injuries to the Major Branches of Peripheral Nerves of the Forearm.* W. B. Saunders, Philadelphia, 1972.

64. Johnson, R. K., Spinner, M., and Shrewsbury, M. M.: *Median nerve entrapment syndrome in the proximal forearm.* J. Hand Surg. 4(1): 48, 1979.

65. Nakano, K. K., Lundergan, C., and Okihiro, M. M.: *Anterior interosseous nerve syndrome. Diagnostic methods and alternative therapies.* Arch. Neurol. 34:477, 1977.

66. Upton, A. R. M., and McComas, A. J.: *The double crush in nerve entrapment.* Lancet 2:359, 1973.

67. Lister, G. D., Belsole, R. B., and Kleinert, H. E.: *The radial tunnel syndrome.* J. Hand Surg. 4(1):52, 1979.

68. Roles, N. C., and Maudsley, R. H.: *Radial tunnel syndrome — Resistant tennis elbow as a nerve entrapment.* J. Bone Joint Surg. 54:499, 1972.

69. Urschell, H. C., and Razzuk, M. A.: *Management of the thoracic outlet syndrome.* N. Engl. J. Med. 286:1140, 1972.

70. CIBA Symposia: *Thoracic Outlet Syndrome.* CIBA Pharmaceutical Co, Summit, New Jersey, 1970.

71. Britt, L. P.: *Nonoperative treatment of the thoracic outlet syndrome symptoms.* Clin. Orthop. 51:45, Mar-Apr, 1967.

72. Omer, G. E., Jr., and Spinner, M: *Peripheral nerve testing and suture techniques.* American Academy of Orthopedic Surgeons Instructional Course Lectures, Vol. XXIV, C. V. Mosby, St. Louis, 1975.

73. Dellon, A. L.: *The moving two-point discrimination test: Clinical evaluation of the quickly adapting fiber/receptor system.* J. Hand Surg. 3(5):474, 1978.

74. Bell, J. A.: *Sensibility evaluation.* In Hunter, J. M., Schnieder, L. H., Mackin, E. J., and Bell, J. A. (eds.): *Rehabilitation of the Hand.* C. V. Mosby, St. Louis, 1978.

75. Gellis, M., and Pool, R.: *Two-point discrimination distances in the normal hand and forearm.* Plast. Reconstr. Surg. 59:57, 1977.

76. Landsmeer, J. M.: *Power grip and precision handling.* Ann. Rheum. Dis. 21:164, 1962.

77. Napier, J. R.: *The prehensile movements of the human hand.* J. Bone Joint Surg. 38B:902, 1956.

ADDITIONAL SOURCES

Doyle, J. R.: *Anatomy of the flexor tendon sheath and pulleys of the thumb.* J. Hand Surg. 2(2):149, 1977.

Kaplan, E. B.: *Functional and Surgical Anatomy of the Hand,* ed. 2. J. B. Lippincott, Philadelphia, 1965.

Linscheid, R. L., and Dobyns, J. H.: *Rheumatoid arthritis of the wrist.* Orthop. Clin. North Am. 2:649, 1971.

Napier, J. R.: *The form and function of the CMC joint of the thumb.* J. Anat. 89:362, 1955.

Neviaser, J. S.: *Musculoskeletal disorders of the shoulder region causing cervicobrachial pain: Differential diagnosis and treatment.* Surg. Clin. North Am. 43:1703, 1963.

Makuc, D., Utginger, P. D., Yount, W. J. Slosser, D., and Moskowitz, N.: *Hand structure and function in an industrial setting.* Arthritis Rheum. 21(2):210, 1978.

Smith, R. L.: *Intrinsic muscles of the fingers: Function, dysfunction, and surgical reconstruction.* American Academy of Orthopedic Surgeons, Instructional Course Lectures, XXIV, St. Louis, C. V. Mosby, 1975.

Taleisnik, J.: *The ligaments of the wrist.* J. Hand Surg. 1:110, 1976.

Wyke, B.: *The neurology of joints: A review of general principles.* Clinics of Rheumatic Diseases, Vol. 7, No. 1. W. B. Saunders, Philadelphia, April, 1981. (Excellent description of joint pain mechanisms.)

Understanding or Developing Functional Hand Assessments

Lansbury, J.: *Methods for evaluating rheumatoid arthritis.* In Hollander, J. L. (ed.): *Arthritis and Allied Conditions,* ed. 7. Lea and Febiger, Philadelphia, 1966, pp. 269–291. (Also in ed. 6., 1960. The same chapter in ed. 8, is abbreviated. Contains a review of evaluations of joint status.)

Landsmeer, J. M.: *Power grip and precision handling.* Ann. Rheum. Dis. 21:164, 1962

Napier, J. R.: *The prehensile movements of the human hand.* J. Bone Joint Surg. [Br] 38:902, 1956.

Robinson, H. S., et al.: *Functional results of excisional arthroplasty for the rheumatoid hand.* Can. Med. Assoc. J. 108:1495, 1973. (Application of C.A.R.S. hand function assessment to document surgical treatment contains normative data on grip strength using a sphygmomanometer.)

Sherik, S., Weiss, A. E., and Flatt, A. E.: *Functional evaluation of the congenitally anomalous hand.* Part I. Am. J. Occup. Ther. 25:98, 1971.

Swanson, A. B.: *Flexible implant resection arthroplasty in the hand and extremities.* C. V. Mosby, St. Louis, 1973.

Taylor, N., Sand, P. L., and Jebson, R.: *Evaluation of hand function in children.* Arch. Phys. Med. 54:129, 1973.

Weiss, A. E., and Flatt, A. E.: *Functional evaluation of the congenitally anomalous hand.* Part II. Am. J Occup. Ther. 25:139, 1971.

Summary of Published Functional Hand Evaluations

See table 4 on pages 273 to 277.

TABLE 4 Summary of published functional hand evaluations (listed in chronological order)

Author	Title	Where published	Test items	Grading system	Method standardized*	Normative data
Carroll, D.	A Quantitative Test of Upper Extremity Function	J. Chronic Dis. 18:479–491, 1965	*Timed Functional Tasks:* 1. Moving a series of items from a table to a shelf 14" higher than the table. Items include: graduated wooden blocks, metal pipe, spheres, a slate of wood, a washer, an iron 2. Pouring water: pitcher to glass, glass to glass, using pronation and then supination. 3. Placing hand: behind head, top of head, and at mouth. 4. Writing name	Thirty-three sub-tests, each item rated on a scale of 0–3; grade equals total score.	Yes	Yes
Carthum, C. J., Clawson, D. K., and Decker, J. L.	Functional Assessment of the Rheumatoid Hand	Am. J. Occup. Ther. 23:122–125, 1969	*Hand Strength:* 1. Grip (sphygmomanometer). 2. Pinch (adapted sphygmomanometer). 3. Cylindrical (adapted dowel and weights). 4. Finger flexion (special measurement device). *Disease status:* Presence of: pain, heat, tenderness and crepitation indicated by color coded chart. *ROM:* using a goniometer. *Timed Functional Tasks:* 1. One-handed activities: opening and closing a safety pin, unbuttoning and buttoning button boards, cutting out a square and straight line with scissors. 2. Two-handed activities: cutting plasti-cized clay with knife and fork, unlac-ing relacing, and tying a shoelace.	Based on percen-tage of norma-tive time.	Yes	Yes

Table 4   Summary of published functional hand evaluations (listed in chronological order) (Continued)

Author	Title	Where published	Test items	Grading system	Method standardized*	Normative data
Jebsen, R. H.	An Objective and Standardized Test of Hand Function	Arch. Phys. Med. Rehabil. 50: 311–319, 1969	*Timed Functional Tasks:* 1. Writing a short sentence. 2. Turning over 3 × 5 inch cards. 3. Picking up small objects and placing them in a container. 4. Stacking checkers. 5. Simulated eating. 6. Moving empty large cans on a table. 7. Moving weighted large cans.	Timed individual subtest scores	Yes	Yes (Extensive N = 360)

MacBain, K. P. (Assessment used at C.A.R.S.— British Columbia)	Assessment of Function in the Rheumatoid Hand	Can. Occup. Ther. J. 37:95–102, 1970	*Hand Strength:*
			1. Grip (sphygmomanometer).
			2. Pinch (sphygmomanometer).
			3. Hook grasp (weight-pulley system).
			
			ROM:
			1. Fingertip inches to crease.
			2. Hand tracing
			
			Timed or weighted functional tasks:
			1. For applied strength:
			  a. Cutting playdough with a knife and fork.
			  b. Pouring a full kettle of water into a bowl.
			  c. Pouring from a large measuring cup into a teacup.
			2. For precision:
			  a. Buttoning and unbuttoning a Montessori board.
			  b. Pinning and unpinning a safety pin into cloth.
			  c. Threading and tying a shoelace.
			  d. Opening, closing, and locking a model door.
			  e. Picking up and retaining 3 coins.
				Based on percentage of normative time	Yes	Yes

Author	Title	Reference	Description	Scores		
Kellor, M., et al.	Technical Manual Hand Strength and Dexterity Norms	1. Sister Kenny Institute Pub. #721 2. Am. J. Occup. Ther. 25:77-83, 1971	*Hand Strength:* 1. Grip (dynamometer). 2. Pinch: palmar, lateral, 3-point (pinch meter). *Dexterity:* Placing and removing 9 pegs in a board.	Individual subtest scores.	Yes	Yes (Extensive for: age, sex, hand dominance)
Treuhaft, P. S., Lewis, M. R., and McCarthy, D. J.	A Rapid Method for Evaluating the Structure and Function*† of the Rheumatoid Hand	Arthritis Rheum. 14:75-86, 1971	*RCM:* 1. Active ROM is measured on all joints. 2. Grades of range are assigned a numerical score. *Structure:* Common hand pathologies, e.g., ulnar deviation and instability, are assigned a numerical rating. *Scores:* Written on a hand outline (functional activities not included).	Sum of subtest ratings.	Yes	Yes
Potvin, A. R., et al.	Simulated Activities of Daily Living Examination	Arch. Phys. Med. Rehab. 53:476-486, 1972	*Timed functional tasks:* There are 7 subtests that involve walking, standing, or dressing. *Additional hand function subtests include:* 1. Unbuttoning and buttoning buttons on a cloth board. 2. Opening and closing a zipper on a cloth board. 3. Putting on garden gloves. 4. Tying a bow in shoelaces. 5. Opening and closing a safety pin. 6. Unwrapping a Bandaid. 7. Squeezing toothpaste. 8. Threading a needle. 9. Picking up coins. 10. Dialing a telephone. 11. Cutting soft plastic substance with a knife. 12. Using a fork.	Timed individual subtest scores.		Yes

Table 4 Summary of published functional hand evaluations (listed in chronological order) (Continued)

Author	Title	Where published	Test items	Grading system	Method standardized*	Normative data
Smith, H.	Smith Hand Function Evaluation	Am. J. Occup. Ther. 27:244-251, 1973	*Timed Functional Tasks:* 1. Unilateral Grasp-Release Tasks: 　a. Placing and replacing 3 graduated blocks to a prescribed position on the table. 　b. Placing 4 graduated nails in a glass. 　c. Placing 4 coins in a glass. 　d. Placing 16 pegs in a board (8 small, 8 large). 2. Activities of Daily Living: 　a. Opening and closing a safety pin. 　b. Unbuckling and buckling a belt on a cloth board. 　c. Unbuttoning and buttoning three buttons on a cloth board. 　d. Opening and closing a zipper on a board. 　e. Tying a double knot in shoelaces on a board. 　f. Tying a bow with shoelaces on a board. 　g. Simulated shoelacing on a cloth board. 3. Writing Sample: 　Write name, trace rectangle and a curved line. *Hand Strength:* 　Grip (dynamometer).	Separate timed scores for each subtest.	Yes	Yes

Bell, E., Jurek, K. and Wilson, T. Physical Capacities Evaluation of Hand Function (PCE) Am. J. Occup. Ther. 30(2): 80-6, 1976

(Article titled: Hand Skill Measurement.)

Timed subtest scores.

Averaged total.

Yes

Yes (N = 50)

Unilateral Tasks:
1. Picking up straight pins
2. Peg, washer, sleeve assembly
3. Nut, bolt assembly
4. Card Sorting
5. Turning blocks over

Bilateral Tasks:
1. Erector set assembly
2. Removing coins from purse
3. Peg washer assembly
4. Nut, bolt assembly
5. Card sorting
6. Bennet Hand Tool Dexterity Test
7. Turning blocks over

Strength:
Dynamometer

*Method is described in adequate detail for reproduction.
†In this study, function is defined as active ROM.

OCCUPATIONAL THERAPY
ARTHRITIS HAND EVALUATION

☐ INPATIENT   ☐ OUTPATIENT

Dx:_____ Onset: _____ Age: _____ Date:_____ Time:_____

Referral:_____ Occupation: _____

Medications/Surgeries: _____

Prior OT/PT _____ ARA Class __

JOINT INVOLVEMENT   Right   Left

	Right	Left
Neck		
Shoulders		
Elbows		
Forearms		
Wrists		

RIGHT HAND

		Thumb		Index	Middle	Ring	Little
	CMC		MCP				
	MCP		PIP				
	IP		DIP				

Type _____ Fingertip to Palm Crease: T_____ I_____ M____ R _____ L _____ cm
Comments:

LEFT HAND

		Thumb		Index	Middle	Ring	Little
	CMC		MCP				
	MCP		PIP				
	IP		DIP				

Type _____ Fingertip to Palm Crease: T_____ I_____ M____ R _____ L _____cm
Comments:

Circle Dominance

Note the following conditions in above section.

Pain	Crepitation (Crep)	Synovial Hyper. (Syn Hyp)	Synovitis (Syn)
Swelling	Osteophytes	Dislocation (Disloc)	Ankylosis (Anky)
Nodules	Boutonniere (Bout)	Bone Resorption (Resorp)	Mallet
Lag	Subluxation (Sublux)	Ulnar Drift (Ul-Dr)	Swan Neck (S-N)

MUSCLE INVOLVEMENT   RIGHT   LEFT

Intrinsic Muscle atrophy		
Intrinsic Muscle strength		
Abd. Pollicis Brevis Strength		
Intrinsic Tightness		

TENDON INVOLVEMENT

Flexor Tenosynovitis Wrist and Digits		
Trigger Finger		
Flexor Tendon Excursion		
Extensor Tenosynovitis		
DeQuervain's (APL, EPB) Finklestein Test		
Tendon Ruptures EDQ, EDC, EIP, EPL, FPL, FDP		

SKIN/NEUROVASCULAR INVOLVEMENT

Skin Integrity/ulcers		
Raynaud's Phenomenon		
Sensation med./ul. nerve		

PREHENSION

	RIGHT		LEFT		Comments
	able	unable	able	unable	
Full Grip					
Palmar Grip					
Lateral Pinch					
2 Pt. Pinch					

Morning Stiffness _____

ADL STATUS _____

_____

_____

MAIN FUNCTIONAL HAND LIMITIATIONS: _____

_____

TREATMENT RECOMMENDATIONS/PLAN: _____

_____

_____

Therapist: _____

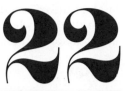

EVALUATION OF
RANGE OF MOTION

The Range of Motion (ROM) evaluation not only provides information on the degrees of motion present but also affords the therapist an opportunity to assess joint status in general, pain tolerance, and, in part, functional ability. A system of recording joints that (1) are painful with motion, (2) are painful without motion, and (3) manifest crepitation during the ROM evaluation is recommended as a simple means of charting disease activity as well as providing an easy reference for treatment planning. In addition, *the time of the assessment and the amount and type of anti-inflammatory or analgesic medication taken prior to the assessment should be noted, since these medications can significantly affect objective assessments.*

METHOD OF MEASUREMENT

The method for measuring joint range of motion in this chapter is based on procedures for measuring and recording adopted by the American Academy of Orthopedic Surgery (AAOS) in 1965. This method assumes the extended "anatomical position" of extremity joints as zero degrees rather than 180 degrees. All motions of a joint are measured from a starting position defined as zero degrees; the degrees of motion of a joint are added in the direction the joint moves from the zero starting position.

The AAOS manual published by the American Academy of Orthopedic Surgeons entitled "Joint Motion—Method of Measuring and Recording"[1] defines the direction, range, and axis of all joint motions. Although it *does not* show the actual positioning of the goniometer, lines depicting the axis of the joint suggest its appropriate placement. In addition to the procedures outlined in the manual for measuring normal joints, special considerations are needed to insure consistent and accurate measurement of the arthritic joint.

The procedures and rationales in this chapter supplement the content of the AAOS manual. However, only joint motions that need special consideration are included here.

JOINT MEASUREMENT USING A GONIOMETER

Shoulder

The patient may not be able to perform pure abduction or flexion because of pain or joint changes. Frequently this patient will substitute flexion on an oblique plane. Therefore motion in other than a standard plane should be noted. It is important to have the patient externally rotate the arm when performing abduction so there will be no interference from the greater tuberosity of the humerus jamming against the acromion process.

Elbow

When the elbow is in full extension, the radius and ulna do not extend in a straight line from the humerus but are at an angle. This is often referred to as the carrying angle or cubitus valgus[2] (Fig. 74). The angle is usually greater for females than for males. This angle can easily be confused with flexion or extension range, especially if forearm rotation is limited.

The standard procedure of measuring elbow range is with the forearm supinated (anatomic position), but frequently this is not possible with patients who have arthritis. When elbow range is being measured precisely for surgical or splinting treatment, accuracy can be enhanced by also noting the degree (or position) of forearm rotation.

Forearm

When evaluating forearm supination or pronation, it is essential that the elbow be at a 90-degree angle and next to the side of the body to prevent substitution of shoulder rotation.

Wrist

FLEXION AND EXTENSION

Placement of the goniometer for evaluation of the wrist varies from clinic to clinic. The AAOS manual diagrams indicate placement for flexion over the dorsum of the wrist joint, but common arthritic wrist deformities (e.g., synovial hypertrophy or subluxation) often prohibit accurate measurement with this method. The following method is recommended for consistent measurement of both flexion and extension on patients with or without wrist involvement.

Alignment of the axis of the goniometer with the axis of the radiocarpal joint. The stable bar of the goniometer is placed along the shaft of the radius and the movable bar is placed along the shaft of the second metacarpal bone (Fig. 75). Alignment with the second metacarpal is preferred over the fifth metacarpal because (1) wrist motion takes place principally at the radiocarpal joint, and (2) rotational forces on the fifth metacarpal distort the measurement of wrist motion.

Although wrist flexion and extension ranges are determined by measuring the angle between the shaft of the second metacarpal and the shaft of the radius, orthopedic surgeons may refer to wrist flexion and extension as the angle between the scaphoid (or carpal navicular) and the shaft of the radius rather than the second metacarpal. There is a difference of about 10 to 15 degrees between these two reference points. This is a minor point, but it will facilitate communication if the therapist is aware that the physician *may* have a different frame of reference in discussing joint range. An example of this is the surgeon may state that he fused the wrist at 15 degrees of flexion to facilitate perineal care but the therapist's measurement may read neutral or zero degrees.

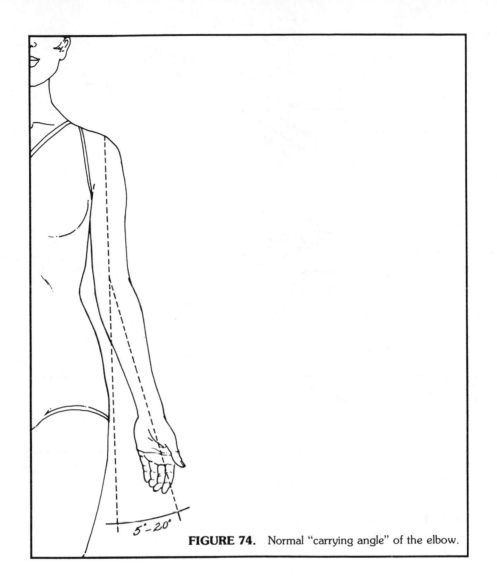

5°-20°

FIGURE 74. Normal "carrying angle" of the elbow.

ULNAR AND RADIAL DEVIATION

Align the stable bar along the median of the forearm and the movable bar with the shaft of the third metacarpal. The end of the bar should be directly over the third metacarpal joint (Fig. 76).

Fingers

When evaluating fingers, remember that *the goal is to measure the angle between the shafts of the bones.* Thus, when subluxation is present, the true axis of the joint is lost and only approx-

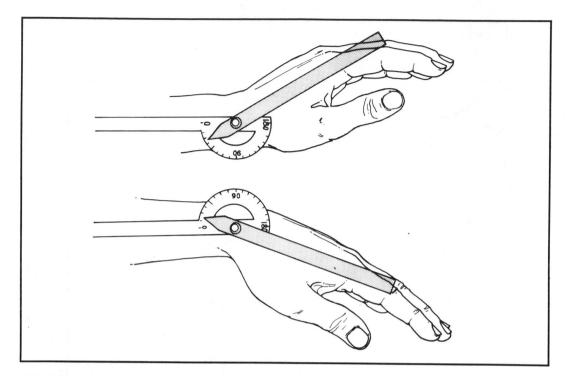

FIGURE 75. Measurement of wrist flexion and extension.

imate, not accurate, measurements can be obtained with a goniometer. It is recommended that a cut off 180 degrees goniometer (with the goniometer arms measuring about two and a half inches from the axis) be used for the fingers.

FLEXION AND EXTENSION

Flexion of all joints is most accurately measured by placing the goniometer over the dorsum of the joint; however, if deformities, swelling, or nodules make placement difficult, move the goniometer *slightly* lateral to the protuberance and align the arms of the goniometer with the shafts of the bones being measured.

Metacarpophalangeal Joints

(MCP joints are commonly termed proximal finger joints by surgeons.)

The directive, "make a fist," often is effective to elicit full PIP flexion but *not effective* for eliciting full MCP flexion, because full power grip ("fist") limits MCP flexion of the index and middle fingers. To measure MCP flexion have the patient bend his knuckles as far as possible (with the PIP joints relaxed).

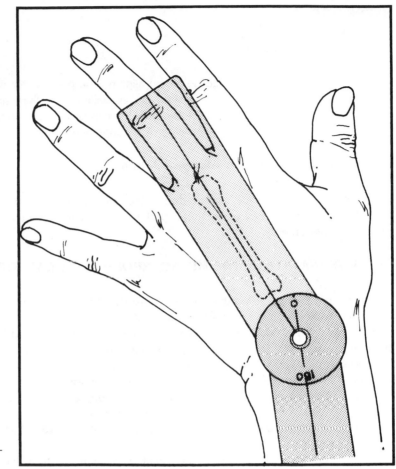

FIGURE 76. Measurement of wrist deviation.

Proximal Interphalangeal Joints (Middle Finger Joints)

Caution: The AAOS manual indicates that measurement of the DIP and PIP joints should be done with the MP joints in extension. This method will give an inaccurate measurement if the patient has intrinsic muscle tightness. (See Chapter 21 for information on intrinsic tightness.)

Measurement of the PIP joint should be done with the hand in a comfortable position with MCP joints flexed (in about midrange).

Distal Interphalangeal Joints (Distal Finger Joints)

The DIP joints should be measured in the position that allows maximal DIP flexion.

HYPEREXTENSION

Metacarpophalangeal Joints

Measure the index and little finger joints by aligning the goniometer with the metacarpal and proximal phalangeal bones and estimating or "eyeballing" the third and fourth MCP ranges. Measurement over the volar aspect of the MCP joints is less accurate because of poor landmark identification, especially if there is swelling or derangement.

Proximal and Distal Interphalangeal Joints

Place the goniometer on the *lateral* edge of the joint aligning the axis of the goniometer with the axis of the joint. Lateral placement is preferred over volar because volar fat pads can distort goniometer placement.

ULNAR DEVIATION OF THE METACARPOPHALANGEAL JOINTS

The technique for measuring this motion is probably the most controversial of all the joints. A variety of methods can be found throughout the country. Some therapists measure the MCP joint in active extension; others measure the MCP joint with the hand lying on a table; and still others measure it with the hand in a resting position.

Measuring the joint in active extension appears to be the most accurate and consistent method. It offers several advantages over the other methods.
1. Measurement in this position reflects the degree of deviation present during functional extension activities, for example, reaching for a glass.
2. The goniometer can be placed directly on the bones. This is not possible with the hand in a resting position.
3. There is usually greater ulnar deviation present during active extension than there is when the hand is resting flat on the table. It also eliminates the problem of determining how much passive distortion occurs when the hand is resting on a surface.
4. In the normal hand the MCP joints abduct towards neutral or zero deviation during active extension, thus, theoretically, active extension represents a zero starting position.

Method of measurement using active extension: Have the patient hold his or her hand in pronation, in midair and raise his or her fingers toward the ceiling without trying to correct the drift. For some patients it may be necessary to stabilize the palm. The axis of the goniometer is placed over the dorsum of the MCP joint and the arms of the goniometer are aligned with the proximal phalanx and metacarpal bone (Fig. 77). Care should be taken *not* to align the goniometer with the extensor tendons. When measuring the MCP joints it is also important to keep in mind that the index finger normally has about 20 degrees of ulnar deviation.[3] Thus, if a patient had 10 degrees of drift in the middle, ring, and little fingers and 30 degrees of drift in the index finger, only 10 degrees of the index measurement would be pathologic, and it would be appropriate to report that the patient has 10 degrees of MCP ulnar drift. Most clinics record the 30 degrees because it is the goniometric reading.

Degrees of range are recorded as a single measurement and not as a range, e.g., 40-degree ulnar deviation and not 0 to 40 degrees.

Additional information regarding the integrity of the joint and muscles can be obtained by measuring the degree of active drift correction. Have the patient actively extend his or her fingers, place the palm of the hand on the table, relax the fingers; then have the patient radially deviate each finger to neutral. Measure at the point of maximal correction.

A two-axis goniometer has been developed by Hasselkus and associates for measuring MCP joint subluxation.[5] The need for this amount of precision should be carefully considered.

Thumb

Metacarpophalangeal and Interphalangeal Joints.

Flexion, extension, and hyperextension are measured in the same manner as the finger PIP joints.

Carpometacarpal joints

Two measurements of the CMC joint are commonly taken: palmar abduction, with the thumb at a right angle to the plane of palm (this position is actually abduction and opposition of the CMC joint); and abduction in extension, with the thumb in the same plane as the palm. The first one, abduction-opposition, is more important for functional use, since this motion is necessary for grasping objects. The second one, abduction-extension, provides information about the integrity of the joint. RA or DJD of the CMC joint frequently limits full extension. Measurement of this motion is referred to as an abduction measurement because of the bony landmarks used. We do not have a defined method for measuring pure CMC joint extension (considered here as the opposite of flexion).

Precise measurement of CMC joint extension is necessary in therapy following CMC joint arthroplasty, because the prescribed postoperative immobilization creates an adduction contracture and the specific therapy is to regain CMC extension. In search of a method for documenting CMC joint extension I have used a palm print on a Harris mat with success. A Harris mat is a thin rubber grid sheet used to determine pressure areas on the sole of the foot. (It is available from podiatric supply distributors.) The grid is inked with a roller and covered with a sheet of typing paper; with the grid on the table, the patient presses his other palm on the paper, creating a grid imprint on the reverse side of the paper. If the person has a CMC joint adduction contracture, there is great pressure over the CMC joint and less surface contact with the remaining palmar surface. As the contracture is reduced, greater surface contact is demonstrated on the print. The Harris mat is only one method of taking a palm print. Other methods using finger paints, carbon sheets, and a photocopying machine need experimentation in this context.[4] The most difficult aspect of this technique is adjusting the height of the table to the patient's height and setting standards for the amount of force that the patient applies while making the print.

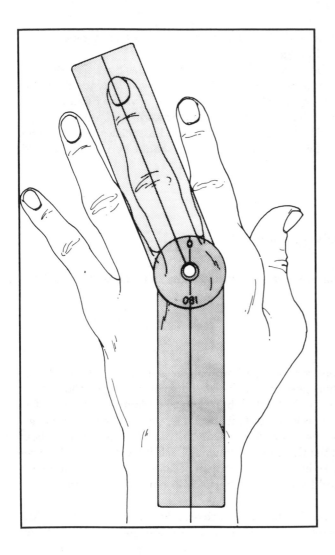

FIGURE 77. Measurement of metacarpophalangeal deviation during active extension.

ALTERNATE METHODS OF ASSESSING ROM

Functional ROM

This type of assessment involves having the patient touch various body landmarks to determine if there is sufficient ROM to accomplish self-care tasks in each body region (Table 5). Consequently this method provides information about multiple joint range rather than a single specific joint.

This method can be useful as a rapid clinical screening procedure. It provides information concerning mobility for all self-care activities, except perineal care. This needs to be considered separately.

TABLE 5.   Landmarks for assessing functional range of motion

Common body landmarks	Range of Motion for:
Top of head	Hair care, face hygiene, shoulder abduction, and flexion.
Back of neck	Neck hygiene, managing clothes, shoulder abduction, and external rotation.
Mouth	Feeding and dental hygiene.
Back of waist	Managing clothes and shoulder internal rotation.
Toe of shoe (while sitting)	Lower extremity dressing (assess back, hip, and knee flexion and elbow extension).

Composite Flexion ROM of the Fingers

1. Measurement of distance between fingertip and the distal palmar (midpalmar) crease.
   a. Equipment:
      1. Ruler with a zero starting edge[1]
      2. Digit-o-meter[1]
   b. Procedure: Have the patient flex his fingers and measure the distance between either the tip of the fingers (not the pad) or the fingernail edge and the distal palmar crease (Fig. 78). For greater accuracy the distance of the tips proximal or distal to the crease should be noted, e.g., 1 inch from crease *proximal* + $1/2$ inch off of palm indicates greater MCP flexion, whereas 1 inch from crease *distal* + $1/2$ inch off of palm indicates very little MCP flexion. The landmark (tip or fingernail) selected for measurement is arbitrary but should be used consistently throughout the clinic. Personally, I have found the fingernail edge less accurate, as many patients do not have fingernails that extend to the end of the finger.

2. Measurement of distance between fingertips and distal wrist crease. This method is recommended only for hands with severely limited finger flexion.

Finger Abduction and Web Space Excursion

1. Measurement of finger abduction span from tip of the little finger to tip of the index finger[1] and from tip of the little finger to the tip of the thumb.
   a. Procedure: Have the patient abduct fingers on a piece of paper. Place a dot above the tip of the little finger and above the tip of the index or thumb. Remove the hand and measure the distance between the dots. *Note:* MCP ulnar drift may influence the accuracy of this form of measurement.

   This method is particularly valuable for documenting abduction mobility for people with scleroderma. A copy of their hand outline and documented finger span can be given to them to use at home as a guide for maintaining mobility.

2. Measurement of web space for patient with ulnar drift or thumb IP hyperextension: Measure from the center of the thumb IP crease to the end of the thenar crease on the radial edge of the palm.[7]

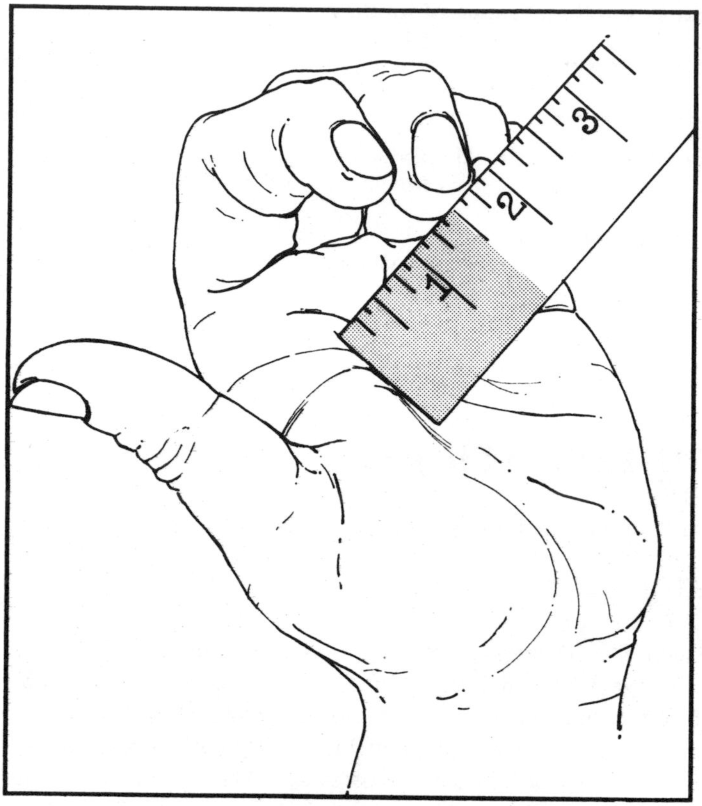

FIGURE 78. Measurement of composite finger flexion.

Wrist or Finger Deviation

A record can be kept of the degree of deviation by tracing an outline of the hand and forearm. With one color of ink, trace the position of greatest deviation, and with another color, trace the position of active correction.

REFERENCES

1. *Joint Motion—Method of Measuring and Recording.* American Academy of Orthopaedic Surgeons, Chicago, 1966.
2. Smith, F. M.: *Surgery of the Elbow,* ed. 2. W. B. Saunders Co., Philadelphia, 1972, pp. 19–20.
3. Flatt, A.: *Care of the Rheumatoid Hand,* ed. 3. C. V. Mosby, St. Louis, 1974, p. 250.
4. Brown, M. E.: *Rheumatoid arthritic hands. Tactual-visual evaluation approaches.* Am. J. Occup. Ther. 20(1): 17, 1966.
5. Hasselkus, B. R., Kshepakaran, K. K., Houge, J. C., and Plautz, K. A.: *Rheumatoid arthritis: A two-axis goniometer to measure metacarpophalangeal laxity.* Arch. Phys. Med. Rehab. 1980.
6. Brayman, S.: *Measuring device for joint motion of the hand.* Am. J. Occup. Ther. 25:173, 1971.
7. Personal communication from K. P. MacBain, Canadian Arthritis and Rheumatism Society (C.A.R.S.), Vancouver, British Columbia.

23

EVALUATION OF MUSCLE STRENGTH

Assessment of muscle strength in patients with rheumatic diseases commonly involves three forms of testing:

1. Manual group muscle test
2. Manual individual muscle test
3. Objective grip and pinch strength test

For most clinical needs, a group muscle test is sufficient. Testing of individual muscles is indicated when assessing specific neurologic impairment, e.g., ulnar nerve entrapment, or in documenting progression of postoperative strengthening.

Because a manual test can determine only gross differences in muscle strength and is inadequate for determining increments of normal (Grade 5) strength (e.g., both a 30-pound grip and a 70-pound grip would test as normal on a manual test), objective measures are employed for hand strength assessment.

This chapter discusses the specific considerations needed when performing measurements of manual or objective strength on patients with joint disease. Individual muscle testing for patients with arthritis is the same as muscle testing for neurology patients.[1,2]

MANUAL MUSCLE TEST FOR PATIENTS WITH ARTHRITIS

Method

Basic information on specific positioning and grading procedures for both group and individual tests can be found in the major texts on muscle testing.[1,2] However, the procedures in these books are designed for patients with normal joints and therefore need to be adapted for evaluation of the patient with arthritis.

The important difference in assessing strength of patients with arthritis versus other disability groups is that *resistance should be applied within the patient's pain-free range and not at the end of his or her active range.* (Standard muscle testing procedure involves application of resistance at the end of complete range.)

Patients with arthritic joints frequently have pain at the end of active range or have marked discomfort the last 30 to 40 degrees of active motion. Resistance should be applied when the joint is positioned within the pain-free range because this avoids pain-inhibition of muscle strength and is the range of the patient's functional strength.

For example, Mr. S. has shoulder flexion range 0 to 120 degrees passively and 0 to 90 degrees actively (with pain at the end of range). If the shoulder flexor muscles are tested at the end of active range, they may be scored as a Grade 3 (Fair—unable to take resistance against gravity) due to pain inhibition, but if tested at 45 degrees of flexion (within the pain-free range) they may be scored as a Grade 4 (Good—able to take moderate resistance). The amount of resistance this patient can take within the pain-free range will be indicative of the kinds of functional tasks he can perform. For instance, Mr. S. could probably lift or transport moderate weight items or lift pans when cooking. Reporting a Grade 3 for this patient would not accurately portray his actual muscle strength.

Grading Terminology

The most common system of grading utilizes descriptive terms such as Good or Fair to convey degrees of muscle strength. The inherent problem with this terminology is that the connotations of the terms are in conflict with the precise definition ascribed them. For example, a grade of Good indicates a muscle is able to move the joint through complete range of motion against gravity and hold against some resistance.[3] But, a Good muscle is not *good*; it is a damaged or weakened muscle. The term Fair implies okay; but a Fair muscle is not *okay*; it is severely damaged. Likewise muscle strength with a grade of Normal may not be *normal* for that particular individual. This descriptive terminology can be misleading and hinder communication with health professionals, especially with physicians or nurses who are not familiar with the precise clinical definitions ascribed by therapists.

A solution to this semantic conflict is to substitute a numerical scale for the descriptive terms. The system which follows was first published in 1946 by the National Foundation for Infantile Paralysis.[3]

5 = Normal (able to take full resistance against gravity)
4 = Good (able to take moderate or some resistance against gravity)
3 = Fair (not able to take resistance against gravity)
2 = Poor (able to move part through complete ROM with gravity eliminated)
1 = Trace (muscle contraction can be palpated)
0 = Zero (no palpable contraction)

When using a numerical system it is helpful to report the baseline score. This indicates the points achieved compared with the total possible, e.g., Elbow flexors: 4/5 (4 out of 5 points). Muscle strength that is between two scores can also be represented numerically instead of by a plus-minus system, e.g., a score of 3.5 can be used instead of Fair plus (F +) to indicate a muscle that can take *slight* resistance against gravity.

Recording

Either a special form should be used or a notation should be made on a general recording form, noting that the grades represent the degree of resistance the muscles could sustain within a (relatively) pain-free range.

A special notation is required *when painful joints prohibit application of full or moderate resistance.* If this occurs, an accurate evaluation is not possible, although it is usually possible to determine if the muscles can take at least slight resistance.

It is valuable to determine if the muscles can take at least slight resistance (Grade 3.5) as this is the minimal amount of strength required to counteract opposing muscle groups (important in preventing contractures). Sample notation: "Accurate evaluation not possible because of pain; elbow and shoulder muscles can take at least slight resistance."

The form should also note the time of day and amount of anti-inflammatory or analgesic medication taken (prior to assessment) since these medications can significantly affect objective assessments.

OBJECTIVE ASSESSMENTS OF HAND STRENGTH

Grip Strength

EQUIPMENT

For patients with hand or wrist involvement, it is recommended that an adapted sphygmomanometer be used to measure grip strength. It is comfortable to hold and is a sensitive measuring device for weak hands.

The standard dynamometer is *not recommended* because its inflexibility and hardness can produce pain, which causes muscle inhibition, and it is difficult for patients with moderate or severe deformity to grasp adequately.

A standard mercury sphygmomanometer can be used with all patients who have less than 300 mm Hg grip strength. It is necessary to use a dynamometer in patients with about 70 lb grip or greater.

METHODS FOR ADAPTING

The sphygmomanometer is adapted by rolling up the cuff and securing it so that when inflated to a specific point the cuff attains a constant circumference. The point of inflation and the size of the circumference are arbitrary. The most common circumference sizes are 6, 7, and 8 inches with starting points of 20, 30, and 40 mm Hg respectively. However, the only normative data gathered to date have been on a cuff with an 8-inch circumference and starting point of 40 mm Hg.[1]

NOTE: When ordering a sphygmomanometer for this purpose, request a cloth arm cuff. The newer models come with a nylon cuff that is difficult to roll and to stabilize.

PROCEDURE

The following are two methods for adapting a sphygmomanometer for grip strength (Fig. 79). An aneroid sphygmomanometer may be used; however, it is easier to maintain the starting point with a mercury sphygmomanometer.

Method I (Fig. 79).

1. Make a bag to hold the cuff using a nonslippery, nonstretch, washable preshrunk material.
2. The size of the bag should allow the cuff to expand to the desired circumference when inflated to the initial starting point, e.g., a 3½-inch wide bag will allow for a 7-inch circumference.

Method II (Fig. 79).

1. Roll up the cuff starting with the bladder end until it is about 6 inches in circumference when deflated. Tape with masking tape.
2. Inflate the cuff to the selected starting point, either 20, 30, or 40 mm Hg. Adjust the cuff until it has the desired circumference of 6, 7, or 8 inches.
3. Remove tape and pin and whip stitch the edges, being careful not to puncture the rubber.

Have the patient seated for the procedure. Inflate the sphygmomanometer to the designated starting point, e.g., 30 mm Hg. (Be sure there is no pressure on the cuff when this is done.) Have the patient grip the cuff as hard as possible. Test each hand three times, alternating hands to minimize the fatigue factor. The forearm or hand *should not* rest on the table or lap and should be in midrotation to start with. After each recording, make sure the mercury returns to the designated starting point.

Every method possible for recording results has been reported in the literature; however, the following method is recommended.

1. Record three readings and report an average of the three; this can significantly reduce the error factor. (In a study on grip strength in Scotland, investigators found

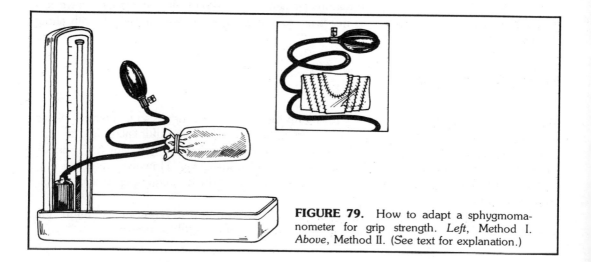

FIGURE 79. How to adapt a sphygmomanometer for grip strength. *Left*, Method I. *Above*, Method II. (See text for explanation.)

the first reading had a significantly higher range of error over the second and third readings.)[5]

2. Record the highest sustained pressure with each test. This can be difficult. If the patient grips slowly there is no problem. But, if he or she grips hard or fast, the mercury will show a high initial spurt because of the momentum of the mercury (not muscle strength). Do not record spurts that appear as a result of momentum but record the sustained high point.

CAUTION: If the purpose of the test is to determine the patient's functional strength, the mercury column *should not* be in view of the patient nor should the therapist offer verbal encouragement. However, if the purpose is to determine absolute muscle function, e.g., in a drug study, encouragement or visual feedback may be desired. *Whatever is done must be consistent with each patient and each retest.*

Pinch Strength

EQUIPMENT

Since the surface contact between the measuring device and the fingers is minimal the design of the equipment is not as crucial as it is for measuring grip strength. Most standard pinch gauges are sensitive enough for low measurements.

Kellor and associates have collected normative data on pinch strength, using a sample of approximately 500 people. The testing procedures for lateral and 3-point palmar pinch, as well as normative data for handedness, age, and sex, are available from the Sister Kenny Institute, Publication no. 721, 1800 Chicago Avenue, Minneapolis, Minnesota 55404.

REFERENCES

1. Daniels, L., and Worthingham, C.: *Muscle Testing: Techniques of Manual Examination.* W. B. Saunders Co., Philadelphia, 1972.
2. Kendall, H. O., Kendall, F. P., and Wadsworth, G. E.: *Muscles: Testing and Function,* ed. 2. Williams and Wilkins, Baltimore, 1971.
3. Daniels, L.: Muscle Testing, p. 3.
4. Robinson, H. S., et al.: *Functional results of excisional arthroplasty for the rheumatoid hand.* Can. Med. J. 108: 1495, 1973.
5. Lee, P., et al.: *An assessment of grip strength measurement in rheumatoid arthritis.* Scand. J. Rheum. 3:17, 1974.
6. Kellor, M., et al.: *Hand strength and dexterity: Norms for clinical usage: Age and sex comparisons.* Am. J. Occup. Ther. 25:77, 1971.

ADDITIONAL SOURCES

Measurement of Grip Strength for Both Sphygmomanometer and Dynamometer

Anderson, W. F., and Cowan, N. R.: *Hand grip pressure in older people.* Br. J. Prev. Soc. Med. 20: 141, 1966.

Bechtol, C. O.: *The use of a dynamometer with adjustable handle spacings.* J. Bone Joint Surg. 36:4, 1954.

Caleb, B.: *Fluid squeeze dynamometer.* Physiotherapy 48:3, 1968.

Carthum, C., Clawson, D., and Decker, J.: *Functional assessment of the rheumatoid hand.* Am. J. Occup. Ther. 23:122–125, 1969.

Cousins, G. F.: *Efffects of trained and untrained testers upon the administration of grip strength tests.* Research Quarterly 26:273, 1955.

Fisher, M. B., and Birren, J. B.: *Standardization of a test of hand strength.* J. Appl. Psychol., 1946, pp. 380–387.

Kai-nan, A., Chao, E. Y. S., and Askew, L. J.: *Hand strength measurements* (*using special designed strain-gauge instruments*). Arch. Phys. Med. Rehab. 61:366, 1980.

Kellor, M., et al.: *Hand strength and dexterity: Norms for clinical usage: Age and sex comparison.* Am. J. Occup. Ther. 25:2, 1971.

Lee, P., et al.: *An assessment of grip strength measurement in rheumatoid arthritis.* Scand. J. Rheumatol. 3:17, 1974. (Using a sphygmomanometer.)

MacBain, K. P.: *Assessment of function in the rheumatoid hand.* Can. J. Occup. Ther. 37:95, 1970. (Describes use of a sphygmomanometer.)

Myers, D. B., Grennan, D. M., and Palmer, D. G.: *Hand grip function in patients with rheumatoid arthritis* (*using an electronic dynamometer*). Arch. Phys. Med. Rehab. 61:369, 1980.

Rose, G. A., et al.: *A sphygomomanometer for epidemiologists.* Lancet 1:296, 1964.

Schmidt, R. T., and Toews, J. V.: *Grip strength as measured by the Jamar dynamometer.* Arch. Phys. Med. Rehab. 5:321, 1970.

Scott, J. T.: *Morning stiffness in rheumatoid arthritis.* Ann. Rheum. Dis. 19:361, 1960. (Describes use of an adapted sphygmomanometer that records up to 600 mm Hg.)

Wainerdi, H. R.: *Simple ergometers for measuring strength of hand grip.* J.A.M.A. 144:8, 1950.

Wright, V.: *Some observations on diurnal variation of grip.* Clin. Sci. 18:17, 1959.

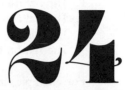

EVALUATION OF ACTIVITIES OF DAILY LIVING

Procedures for evaluation of Activities of Daily Living (ADL) are the same for rheumatic disease patients as they are for any other physical disabilities group. However, the purpose is different and some additional factors in regard to morning stiffness, fatigue, positioning during rest, and taking medication need special consideration.

Purpose of the Evaluation

The primary goal of the evaluation is to provide a data base necessary for effective treatment planning that will (1) reduce pain from needless stress, (2) increase functional independence, and (3) prevent unnecessary deformity (through patient education). Secondarily the assessment can serve as a measure of change following treatment. The ADL assessment should answer the following questions:

1. Is the patient performing any daily tasks that are causing needless or potentially deforming stresses to his or her involved joints?

and

Are there adaptive methods or equipment that could minimize or eliminate the joint stress in these activities?

2. Is the patient limited in performing daily tasks as a result of a physical limitation?

and

Are there adaptive methods or equipment that could increase the patient's independence or ability in these tasks?

Method of Assessment

The evaluation procedure can take several forms: interview, observation of patient performance (timed or untimed), or patient self-report. Usually a full evaluation is a combination of all three. The choice depends on:

1. The nature of the patient's disability.
2. The patient's reliability in reporting.
3. The clinical setting in which the evaluation is taking place.
4. The reason for the assessment.

For example, interview and patient self-report may be sufficient for an ADL assessment on an employed man with chronic degenerative joint disease of the knees in an outpatient clinic; however, interview, self-report, and demonstration of tub/shower transfer ability may be indicated for a severely disabled inpatient. *Interview and self-report are not sufficient and patient demonstration is essential for accurate assessment of functional ability in patients with (1) severe multiple joint involvement, (2) recent onset of disease or an increase in debility (when they may not be aware of their limitations), or (3) psychological overlay.*

Special Factors to Consider

Factors that are typical to rheumatic disease patients and that need special consideration in the ADL evaluation are

1. Morning stiffness (duration, location, severity).
2. Percent of good days versus bad days.
3. Fatigue (time of onset, duration) and endurance.
4. Medication (amount, type, when taken, if taken).

These factors are discussed in detail in Chapter 20, Evaluation of Medical History and Symptoms. In addition to these medical conditions, six activity areas need special attention.

1. Positioning at night and during leisure activities such as watching television or reading.
2. Use and height of seats for lower extremity problems (bed, chairs, toilet) in the home or at work.
3. Amount of stair climbing for patients with lower extremity involvement.
4. Use and height of work surfaces and materials for neck and back involvement.
5. Ability of the patient to use private or public transportation.
6. Taking medication (ability to open bottles, swallowing, or problems with remembering).

When the Evaluation Should Be Done

The time of the day that the evaluation is done is an important factor. This is especially true for the patient with morning stiffness or poor endurance. An ADL evaluation (with demonstration) done on a patient with rheumatoid arthritis at 2:00 p.m. only provides information about how the patient performs in the afternoon and this can be quite different from the person's performance in the morning when stiffness is at a maximum.

In assessing outpatients it is important to determine their early morning functional status as well as their ability during the clinic evaluation. In assessing inpatients, an early morning (before breakfast) evaluation has the advantage of providing information about the patient's most dysfunctional state, but this may not be representative of their average level throughout the day. A more representative assessment is possible for both inpatients and outpatients, when it precedes hydrotherapy.

The time of day of the assessment also needs to be taken into account when doing re-evaluations and longitudinal comparisons.

Emotional Factors to Consider During the Assessment

Regardless of whether an interview or demonstration is done the ADL evaluation is a very personal procedure. It is as personal as going into the doctor's office and undressing for an examination. Not only is the patient going through a literal or figurative undressing, but also, as the procedure takes place, the patient has to discuss his or her worst attributes, that is, list inabilities.

No matter how empathetic the therapist is, there is no way of completing an ADL assessment by stressing only the positive aspects. One avenue open for positive counteraction is in giving the patient feedback about the positive things that can be done to increase his or her independence. But, in order for the therapist to be able to give this kind of feedback, the therapist needs to know the patient's physical status before starting the ADL evaluation.

Literature on ADL Assessments

Most of the research and development of ADL assessments in occupational therapy has been done on an individual clinic basis. Each clinic has either adapted an established assessment or developed its own evaluation forms and procedures.

Most assessments involve an ADL analysis checklist with or without a scoring procedure. Two reports which utilize a standardized ADL assessment procedure with rheumatic disease patients have been published and are mentioned here for therapists who wish to develop or incorporate a quantitative ADL assessment procedure in their program. Dr. Edward Lowman used an itemized ADL assessment (106 items) scored on the basis of "percentage of functional deficiency" (percentage of items the patient was not capable of performing).[1] Dr. H. Robinson and Ms. D. Bashall, OT Reg., at the Canadian Arthritis and Rheumatism Society (C.A.R.S.) in British Columbia developed a timed "Self-Care Assessment" which quantitates the patient's performance as a percentage of normal time range for all basic dressing tasks, for example, putting on a blouse: normal time 15 to 25 seconds.[2]

K. P. MacBain, O. T. Reg., has published the only functional assessment specially related to children with arthritis. I. L. Coley, O.T.R., has published a text addressing evaluation of self-care skills in children. (See end of chapter for complete reference.)

Home Assessment

The ideal method for a home assessment is an on-site home visit. It affords a unique opportunity to

1. Assess architectural barriers in the home that limit the patient's functional independence.
2. Give the patient specific instructions on how to adapt his or her furniture or home to minimize joint stress and improve function.

3. Assess the quality of home life in terms of family attitudes, interpersonal relationships, cooperation, and stress factors that significantly influence patient compliance.
4. Assess the ease or difficulty of maintaining the house and yard. (Homes that are cluttered or have poorly divided work areas require more energy to maintain than homes with adequate space.)

The procedure for the home assessment depends primarily on the client's ambulation status. When ambulation aids or wheelchairs are involved the assessment is essentially the same as for patients with ambulation aids in nonarthritic disorders. There are a few exceptions. The height of chairs or seats is an important consideration for joint protection of the knees for people using crutches, canes, or walkers. The type and height of chairs can also influence neck positioning during reading or leisure activities.

The type of handrim is a special consideration for people using wheelchairs. Regular wheelchair handrims increase ulnar drift deformity. For clients with beginning ulnar drift (or the potential for it), handrims with projections are preferred since they can be used in a nondeforming manner. However, these projections increase the width of the wheelchair and may limit accessibility through inside passageways and doorways.

In general the home assessment should include the following:

1. Evaluation of the safety and accessibility of entrances and passageways.
2. Types of floor coverings, especially if ambulation aides or a wheelchair is used.
3. Patient's ability to open, close, and lock windows and doors. (If a person is severely disabled, methods of escape in event of fire should be explored.)
4. Accessibility of light switches, outlets, and heat controls.
5. Height of counters, tables, tub, bed, and chairs.
6. Consideration of work areas in regard to work simplification and energy conservation measures.

The slide/tape program developed by Tillman and Haviland is an excellent resource for reviewing these criteria. (See resource list at the end of the chapter.)

SAMPLE ADL AND HOME ASSESSMENT FORMS

Two ADL and home assessment forms are included here as samples to stimulate thinking and to provide a starting point for therapists to develop their own forms. Each occupational therapy clinic serves a unique population and each therapist has a different assessment bias or technique. Forms developed in a clinic should reflect these differences.

The first sample form is a screening form developed at the Los Angeles County-University of Southern California (LAC-USC) Medical Center for use in the Arthritis Medical Clinic by an occupational therapist. This screening interview takes approximately 10 to 15 minutes and was designed as a case-finding tool—to determine if patients could benefit from a complete evaluation and treatment. A copy of the form was kept in the patient's clinic chart for a medical record and to orient resident physicians as to some of the activities of daily living that need consideration. Notations on status were spelled out for physicians not familiar with jargon.

The second form is a complete ADL assessment developed for patients with rheumatic diseases. Parts 1 and 3 were designed at the LAC-USC Medical Center. Part 2 was developed by the Canadian Arthritis and Rheumatism Society (C.A.R.S.) of British Columbia. The sequence of the C.A.R.S. form has been reordered and items on female hygiene, child care, endurance, and housework assistance added. Part 3, Occupational Therapy Recommendations, has proven extremely valuable for emphasizing or summarizing the many joint protection or safety suggestions made to patients during the ADL assessment or treatment sessions. For example, a therapist may consider a recommendation to put safety strips or a safety mat in the tub to be a casual, common sense suggestion. Formally writing it out as a professional recommendation often makes the patient appreciate the structure and purpose of the ADL assessment.

FUNCTIONAL ASSESSMENTS VERSUS ADL ASSESSMENTS

A major area of concern in the treatment of chronic disease is the determination of patient progress or outcome as a result of medical, surgical, or rehabilitative intervention. A wide range of instruments described as functional assessments has been developed for this purpose. These functional assessments differ from ADL assessments in that they tend to be more general and are designed to be administered by physicians or research assistants with the overall objective of measuring change in the patient. ADL assessments are primarily designed for treatment planning and therefore are very detailed in format. For example, most functional assessments do not include specific questions about the patient's ability to write or to open food packages.

REFERENCES

1. Lowman, E. W.: *Rehabilitation of the rheumatoid cripple: A five year study.* Arthritis Rheum. 1:38, 1958.
2. Robinson, H., and Bashall, D.: *Functional assessment in rheumatoid arthritis.* Can. J. Occup. Ther. 29: 123-138, 1962. (Reprinted in: Ehrlich, G. (ed): *Total Management of the Arthritic Patient.* J. B. Lippincott Co., Philadelphia, 1973.)

ADDITIONAL SOURCES

Home Assessment

Buchwald, E.: *ADL for Physical Rehabilitation.* McGraw-Hill Book Co., New York, 1963. (Primary transfer training, functional assessment carried out by physical therapy.)

Loomis, B.: *The home visit: An integral part of OT for patients with rheumatic diseases.* Am. J. Occup. Ther. 19:264, 1965 (Only source on home visits for people with arthritis.)

National Society for Crippled Children and Adults: *Making Buildings and Facilities Accessible to and Usable by the Physically Handicapped.* American Standards Association, 1961.

Peszczynski, M., and Fowles, B.: *Home Evaluations.* Highland View Cuyahoga County Hospital, Highland View, Indiana, 1957.

Rusk, H. A., et al.: *A Manual for Training the Disabled Homemaker.* Rehabilitation Monograph VIII, ed. 2. Institute of Physical Medicine and Rehabilitation, Bellevue Medical Center, 400 E. 34th Street, New York, New York, 11216, 1961. (Excellent resource.)

Tillman, F., and Haviland, N: *603 Elm Street: Overcoming Barriers to Independence.* This is an excellent slide/tape program designed for health professionals. Includes evaluation of home safety factors. #P116. University of Michigan Media Library, G1302 Towsley Center, University of Michigan Medical Center, Ann Arbor, Michigan, 48109.

ADL Assessment for Children

Coley, I. L.: *Pediatric Self Care Evaluation*. C. V. Mosby, St. Louis, 1978.

MacBain, K. P., and Hill, R. H.: *A functional assessment for juvenile rheumatoid arthritis*. Am. J. Occup. 27(6):326, 1973.

General Functional Evaluation

Convery, F. R., Minteer, M. A., Amiel, D., and Connett, K. L.: *Polyarticular disability: A functional assessment*. Arch. Phys. Med. Rehab. 58:494, Nov., 1977.

Conaty, J. P., and Nickel, V. L.: *Functional incapacitation in rheumatoid arthritis: Rehabilitation challenge*. J. Bone Joint Surg. 58:624, 1971. (A correlative study of function before and after hospital treatment)

Chamberlain, M. A., Buchanan, J. M., and Hands, H.: *The arthritic in an urban environment*. Ann. Rheum. Dis. 38:51, 1979.

Rosenthal, D., Boblitz, M. H., and Rao, V. R.: *Bus use by disabled arthritics: Functional requirements*. Arch. Phys. Med. Rehab. 58:220, May, 1977.

Boblitz, M. H.: *Transportation evaluation, counseling, and training*. In Ehrlich, G. E. (ed.): *Rehabilitation Management of Rheumatic Conditions*. Williams & Wilkins, Baltimore, 1980.

Sample #1

ACTIVITIES OF DAILY LIVING (ADL)

SCREENING

Name: *Jane Doe* ___ Age: *40* Hosp. #: *123456*

DX *R. A.* ___ Dominance *R* ___

A.D.L.		Date *9/4/81*	Date	Date
Dressing:	UE & torso	*indep.*		
	LE & torso	*indep*		
	fasteners	*assist needed with sm. buttons*		
Grooming		*indep.*		
Hygiene:	toilet	*indep*		
	bath	*unable to wash back*		
Transfer:	chair	*low seat causes pain*		
	bed	*indep.*		
	toilet	*causes knee pain*		
	tub	*needs a bench*		
	car	*needs assist.*		
	public trans.	*unable*		
Kitchen work		*husband helps*		
Housework		*husband helps*		
Marketing		*husband*		
Yard work		*husband*		
Vocational skills		*NA*		
Hand skills (keys, writing, jars, etc.)		*indep. except for strength tasks*		
Assistive Equipment				
splints		*none*		
ambulation aids		*cane*		
adaptive devices		*none*		
Endurance		*fair*		
ROM		*mod. limitations*		

COMMENTS: *9/4/81 patient needs a full ADL assessment*

Sample #2

ADL ASSESSMENT (PART 1)

Name_____ File No.: _____
Address _____ Age: _____
_____ ARA Functional Class:* _____
Phone _____

Diagnosis: (*onset joint involved*)†
_____
Ambulation Status: (*household, community, etc. + gait*)_____
Posture: _____
Handedness: Dominant Hand_____   Preferred Hand_____
Morning Stiffness: From_____ to about_____;   Average_____ hours.
Percent of good days vs. bad days: _____
Energy Pattern:
    Hours of sleep/night? _____hrs. from _____   to   _____ .
    Rest breaks during day? _____
    Rest time of day? _____
    Amount of fatigue? (*onset, duration*)_____
Medications: (*type + quantity*)_____

Home Assessment

Home and Family Situation: (*type of home; people in home, their age & health*)_____
_____

Entrances: (*steps, rails, inclines?*)_____
Inside Passageways: (*width, loose rugs, electrical cords?*)_____
Types of Floor Covering: Kitchen_____
    Living Room _____   Hall_____
    Bedrooms _____   Bathroom _____
Door & Windows: (*ability to open, close, lock*)_____
Height of:
    Tub: Inside:_____ outside_____   Toilet bowl (excluding seat)_____
    Bed_____   Sofa_____
    Dining room chair_____   Living room chair_____
    Kitchen counter_____
Wheelchair Measurements
    Height of seat_____   Width_____
    Type_____   Type of handrim (*regular or with projections?*)_____

Transportation: (*method, transfer ability?*)_____

Vocation Assessment

Type of Work Setting: _____
Physical Layout‡ (*problems or hindrances*)_____
Use of Entrances _____
Use of Lavatories_____
Amount of:
    Lifting _____
    Bending _____
    Walking _____
    Sitting _____
Height of work surface _____
Height and type of chair used: _____

SPECIAL OR ADAPTIVE EQUIPMENT (currently used by patient at home or work):_____
_____

*This is discussed in Medical History, Chapter 20.
†Notations in parentheses are not included on the original form but are included here to indicate some of the factors considered in each section.
‡When indicated have patient draw a house plan or work layout and furniture arrangement on back of paper.

ADL ASSESSMENT (PART 2*): ACTIVITY ANALYSIS

Name: _____

Date: _____

The purpose of this questionnaire is to discover any difficulties you might have in the stated area which the therapist may be able to help you with.

Please complete the following questionnaire putting a check in the appropriate column or drawing a line through the question if it is not applicable.

I. SELF CARE SECTION

BEDROOM: Can you ... ?	Easily	With diff.	Not at all	Solution
move from place to place in bed				
roll to right and then to left side				
turn and lie on abdomen				
sit up in bed				
get into bed				
get out of bed				

DRESSING: Are you able to put on and take off the following articles?	Easily	With diff.	Not at all	Solution
Women				
brassicrc				
girdle				
garter belt				
panties				
slip				
stockings				
socks				
shoes				
dress with front opening				
dress with side opening				
dress with back opening				
blouse				
skirt				
sweater				
coat				
hat				
gloves				
slacks				

*Adapted from material from the Canadian Arthritis and Rheumatism Society (C.A.R.S.), British Columbia.

	Easily	With diff.	Not at all	Solution
Men				
vest or undershirt				
shorts				
trousers				
shirt				
sweater				
socks				
shoes				
suit jacket				
tie				
coat				
hat				
gloves				
Men and women: Can you manage. . . ?				
zippers				
buttons: large				
small				
hooks and eyes				
snap dome fasteners				
buckles				
safety pins				
belts				
putting hand in: back pocket				
side pocket				
brushing clothes				
hanging up or putting away clothes				
putting on working or resting splints				
TOILET: Can you manage . . . ?				
getting on and off toilet				
adjusting clothing for toilet needs				
using toilet paper				
flushing toilet				
maneuvering bedpan				
getting to toilet at night				
BATH: Can you manage . . . ?				
getting into a bath				
out of a bath				
into a shower				
out of a shower				
turning taps (tub & sink)				

	Easily	With diff.	Not at all	Solution
BATHING: Can you manage ... ?				
washing: feet				
hands				
back				
chest				
neck				
face				
hair				
drying self				
drying between toes				
PERSONAL CARE: Can you manage ... ?				
Men and Women				
brushing teeth				
using dental floss				
using electric razor				
safety razor				
cutting: fingernails				
toenails				
brushing and combing hair				
Women				
applying makeup				
setting hair				
shaving legs				
shaving underarms				
using sanitary napkins or tampons				
douching				
grooming eyebrows				
application of contraceptives				
AMBULATION: Can you ... ?				
walk unaided or with cane				
with crutches				
walk: up steps (if applicable)				
down steps				
up a slope				
down a slope				
turn around				
walk on rough ground				
get up and down a curb				
cross a street in 30 seconds on green light				
get down to the floor and up again				

	Easily	With diff.	Not at all	Solution
stand for more than half hour while working				
get on and off living room chair				
get on and off kitchen chair				
EATING: Can you ... ?				
use a fork				
use a spoon				
cut meat				
butter bread				
drink from a cup				
from a glass				
stir coffee, tea, etc.				
open a bottle				
pour from a bottle				
pour a cup of tea or coffee				

II. HOUSEHOLD ACTIVITY SECTION

FOOD PREPARATION: Can you ... ?

	Easily	With diff.	Not at all	Solution
do grocery shopping				
open: tin cans				
jars				
packaged goods				
reach shelves: above countertop				
below countertop				
prepare vegetables: peel				
slice				
bake a cake or cookies:				
measure dry ingredients				
measure liquids				
break an egg				
use an eggbeater				
stir batter				
knead dough				
pour batter into pan				
open oven door				
place pan in oven				
roll dough				
use a saucepan				
fill a saucepan				
carry pan to stove				
remove hot dish from oven				
drain vegetables				
pour hot water from kettle				
pour tea and/or coffee into cups				

	Easily	With diff.	Not at all	Solution
DINING: Can you ... ?				
set table				
carry to table: full glass				
full cup & saucer				
full plate				
hot casserole				
(other)				
CLEAN UP: Can you ... ?				
scrape and stack dishes				
wash dishes				
scrub pots and pans				
pick up object from floor				
wipe up spills on floor				
sweep floor				
use dustpan				
mop floor				
shake mop				
wash floor				
clean refrigerator				
clean oven				
dispose of garbage				
(other)				
OTHER HOUSEHOLD ACTIVITIES: Can you manage ... ?				
laundry: handwashing				
wringing				
machine washing				
machine drying (open dryer door?)				
hanging on line				
ironing blouse or shirt				
folding sheets				
hanging dress on hanger				
dusting/cleaning—high and low surfaces				
vacuuming/carpet sweeper				
making beds				
changing beds				
cleaning bathtub				
picking up a pin				
threading a needle and sewing				
using scissors				
handling coins				

	Easily	With diff.	Not at all	Solution
feeding pets				
(other)				
TRANSPORTATION: Can you ... ?				
get onto a bus				
stand on bus holding overhead bar				
descend from bus				
get into a car (open car door)				
out of a car				
drive a car				
MISCELLANEOUS: Can you ... ?				
manage medicine bottles				
take own medicine				
use a telephone				
open an envelope				
write for 15 minutes				
hold a book				
turn the pages				
shuffle and hold a hand of cards				
strike a match (use cigarette lighter)				
smoke a cigarette or pipe				
wind a clock				
a watch				
type				
care for garden				
mow lawn				
sweep porch				
open and close: a door				
window				
drawer				
reach shelves at head level				
open milk cartons				
turn taps on and off				
use pull-chain light				
use light switches				
manage wall-plugs				
push buzzer, doorbell				
use spray cans				
open doors with knobs				
with keys				
pour milk from bottle to glass				
operate stove burners and oven				
operate sink taps				

	Easily	With diff.	Not at all	Solution
open and close refrigerator				
use wall plug				
(other):				

CHILD CARE OR GRANDCHILD CARE: Can you ... ?

	Easily	With diff.	Not at all	
lift a small child (e.g. under age two)				
bathe a child				
fix child's hair				
dress small child				
change diapers				
do personal hygiene for small children				

ENDURANCE:

Does an average day's housework make you:				
extremely tired				
quite tired				
only slightly tired				

What activity during the week is the most strenuous for you?

_____

ASSISTANCE:

Who will do heavy cleaning duties, e.g. waxing floor, washing windows?

_____

How often is he/she available?

_____

DAILY ROUTINE:

    Briefly describe your average daily routine or schedule:

_____
_____
_____
_____
_____

RECREATIONAL OR LEISURE INTERESTS: Difficulties with these activities due to the arthritis? Please list:

_____
_____
_____
_____
_____

OCCUPATIONAL THERAPY (PART 3)

RECOMMENDATIONS BASED ON ACTIVITY OF DAILY LIVING ASSESSMENT*

For: _____ File No.: _____

Rest/Sleep:

Morning Stiffness:

Ambulation:

Entrances, steps:

Inside Passageways:

Floor Coverings:

Doors and Windows:

Seating Heights:

Wheelchair:

Bedroom:

Toilet:

Bathing:

Washing:

Personal Care:

Dressing:

Eating:

Meal Preparation:

HOUSEHOLD ACTIVITIES

Best height for:
      toilet
      dining chair
      kitchen stool
      living room chairs or sofa
      bed

EQUIPMENT RECOMMENDATIONS:

_____ O.T.R.

_____ Date

*Complete this form in duplicate, one copy for patient.

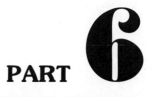

OCCUPATIONAL THERAPY MODALITIES

25

SPLINTING FOR ARTHRITIS OF THE HAND

This chapter describes the key issues in splinting for arthritis of the hand. The various processes involved with the use of splinting as a treatment modality for patients with arthritis that will be discussed are

Indications and Rationale
Patient Evaluation
Design and Fabrication
Splint Evaluation (Index)
Patient Education

The functional properties of the splinting materials are reviewed, and seven basic splint types are discussed in terms of specific treatment application.

INDICATIONS AND RATIONALE

Therapeutic Splinting

Joint motion appears to aggravate inflammation and increase pain and secondary muscle spasm. Splinting or immobilization supports the joint, reduces stress to the capsule, allows muscles to relax, and eliminates pain with motion; and through these processes, a decrease in inflammation results.[1,2,3]

Splinting is also used therapeutically in selected situations to correct or minimize joint contractures through application of gentle passive stretch. Serial casting is an example of this concept.[4]

The symptoms of median nerve compression (carpal tunnel syndrome) are alleviated in some patients with a splint that eliminates wrist flexion.[5]

Preventive Splinting

Splints are excellent for positioning the hand, and it is clear that deformity resulting from chronic improper positioning can be *prevented* with the use of splints. Splints cannot eliminate or prevent fibrosis, but they can prevent contractures from developing in a nonfunctional position. The two most common contractures of the hand that can be prevented are wrist flexion and thumb adduction.

An issue of major concern is the role of splinting for prevention of deformities caused by musculotendon imbalance and dynamic forces. Can these deformities be prevented or their progress slowed? Or is their course inevitable? It appears there are several points at which preventive intervention is possible and can affect the final outcome. But the key to success is truly in prevention, for there is almost no recourse in corrective intervention, except for surgery.[6]

ULNAR DRIFT

There is no evidence that absolute prevention of MCP ulnar drift is possible, but there is clinical and research evidence that hand-wrist dynamics have an effect on this deformity.[7,8]

Three causal factors of ulnar drift lend themselves to preventive intervention. They are:

Position of the Wrist. People with radiocarpal subluxation and radial deviation of the wrist and coexistent MCP synovitis have a greater tendency toward ulnar drift (zig-zag phenomenon) than those with ulnar subluxation and ulnar deviation of the hand.[7,8] Consequently, splinting to maintain ulnar deviation of the wrist can reduce or eliminate radial deviation as a contributing factor to ulnar drift. (See Chapter 21, Hand Pathodynamics and Assessment, for detailed discussion.)

Chronic Synovitis of the MCP joints. Deformity and laxity of the MCP ligaments and capsule take place during periods of synovitis; therefore, reduction of inflammation and protection of the supporting joint structures during exacerbations are key elements for prolonging joint integrity.[9]

Role of the Flexor Tendons. The manner in which the flexor tendons pull across the MCP joint during grasp and pinch is a major contributing factor to overstretching of vulnerable joint ligaments.[10] (See Figure 32.) Splinting to alter the line of pull during functional activities can be another method of therapeutic intervention in selected patients.[10]

WRIST SUBLUXATION

Volar subluxation of the carpus with radial deviation of the hand on the forearm is the typical wrist deformity of adult rheumatoid arthritis (RA) and, as noted previously, a contributing factor to MCP drift. A major causal factor of this deformity is the laterovolar displacement of the extensor carpi ulnaris tendon. Once displaced it can no longer counterbalance the strong radioflexor muscles.[8] Ulnar styloid synovitis is often one of the initial sites of RA. Early splinting to protect the extensor carpi tendon and maintain ulnar deviation of the wrist may be a viable intervention. Flexible gauntlet splints (e.g., Futuro splints) reduce stress to wrist structures by restricting circumduction motion during daily activities.

SWAN NECK DEFORMITIES

There are four etiologic factors in swan neck deformities. (See pathodynamics of swan neck deformity in Chapter 21, Hand Pathodynamics and Assessment, and in Chapter 13, Hand,

Wrist, and Forearm Surgery.) The most common etiologic factor in rheumatoid arthritis is tightness of the finger intrinsic muscles secondary to MCP inflammation, a condition that creates a pull on the lateral bands. Splinting and exercise to stretch the intrinsic muscles and encourage proximal interphalangeal (PIP) flexion with the MCP joints in extension can be effective in eliminating intrinsic muscle tightness as a deforming force.

INTRINSIC PLUS DEFORMITY

Some patients develop a deformity of MCP joint flexion and PIP joint extension (without swan neck deformities). In some instances it appears that spasm of the intrinsic muscles and continual intrinsic plus positioning during functional activities are causal factors for this condition. In other cases it appears that the intrinsic muscles become shortened secondary to MCP volar subluxation. If detected early, night splinting of the MCP joints in extension can stretch the intrinsic muscles and reduce the possibility of deformity and limited dexterity.

Functional Improvement

Wrist pain is a common limitation to hand function. Muscle inhibition secondary to pain can cause the wrists to give way during grasp or severely diminish functional grip strength.[11] Stabilization splints for the wrist minimize or alleviate wrist pain during grasp and thus can increase functional grasp strength.[11,12]

This process can often be clearly seen in patients with traumatic wrist injury and normal fingers. It is more difficult to discern in patients who also have painful MCP, PIP, and CMC joints.

Postoperative Splinting

Splinting following surgical restoration is designed to maintain surgically achieved mobility and alignment; to assist postoperative strengthening; and to prevent or minimize postsurgical adhesions. In certain implant arthroplasties, dynamic splinting provides a means for shaping the capsular scarring (encapsulation) process to allow the desired alignment and mobility.

PATIENT EVALUATION (Figs. 80, 81, 82, and 83)

A thorough physical and functional hand assessment is essential both before and after splinting. The initial assessment is necessary to determine the type of splint to use and the post-assessment is necessary to determine if the splint is of value. (Methods of physical and functional hand assessments are described in detail in Hand Assessment, Chapter 21.)

After each assessment the therapist should be able to answer the following questions:

1. What hand functions can the client perform? (Lateral pinch, hook grasp, power grasp, opposition, manipulation, ADL, strength)
2. What is the quality of performance? Are the functions done easily, with effort, slowly, or with or without pain? (This is an important assessment because frequently clients

can do the same number and kinds of tasks with a splint as without it; however, if pain is relieved, its use is justified.)

3. When there is functional limitation, what is the cause? (Pain, muscle tightness, fibrosis, triggering, weakness, instability, limited ROM, malalignment?)

When ready to recommend splinting to the physician, the therapist should be able to specify the client's need for the splint and the splinting objectives.

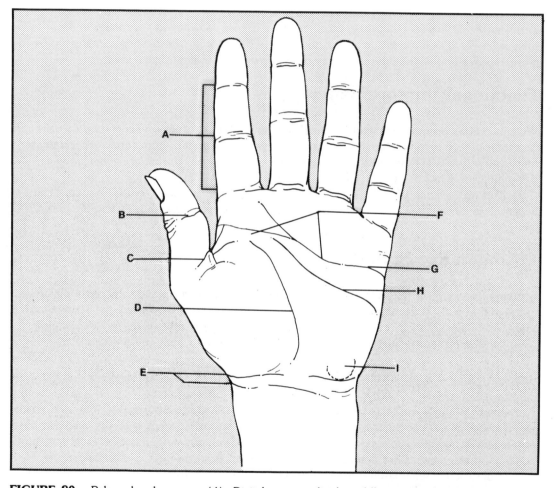

FIGURE 80. Palmar hand creases: (*A*), Digital creases; distal, middle, proximal; (*B*), Distal thumb crease; (*C*), Proximal thumb creases; (*D*), Thenar crease; (*E*), Wrist creases; (*F*), Composite (midpalmar crease); (*G*), Distal palmar crease; (*H*), Proximal palmar crease; (*I*), Pisiform bone.

The palmar hand creases are important because they delineate where joint motion takes place. The thenar crease (*D*) defines the area of thumb motion. The composite or midpalmar crease (*F*) delineates MCP joint flexion. The proximal palmar crease (*H*) indicates motion of the carpal-metacarpal joints of the fourth and fifth digits. The proximal palmar crease is frequently absent.[14]

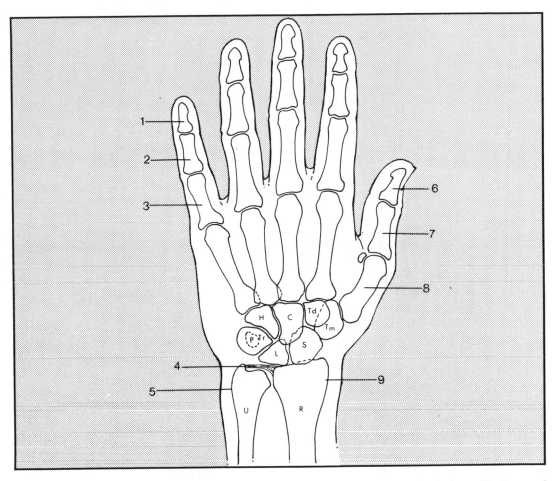

FIGURE 81. Bones of the hand and wrist: (*1*), Distal phalanx; (*2*) Middle phalanx; (*3*) Proximal phalanx; (*4*), Triangular fibrocartilage; (*5*), Ulnar styloid; (*6*), Distal phalanx; (*7*), Proximal phalanx; (*8*), Metacarpal; (*9*), Radial styloid; H, Hamate; C, Capitate; Td, Trapezoid; TM, Trapezium; S, Scaphoid (navicular); L, Lunate; Tr, Triquetrum; P, Pisiform; U, Ulna; R, Radius.

DESIGN AND FABRICATION

DESIGN

Since each splint is designed to accomplish a particular function, the design and materials used can vary considerably as long as the desired function is achieved and the splint is well tolerated and cosmetically acceptable. Specific design requirements for each type of splint commonly used for arthritic hand problems are reviewed later in this chapter. Specific splinting procedures, patterns, and use of materials are not covered in this chapter because there are two excellent updated resources compiled by Maude Malick, O.T.R., which cover the topic thoroughly: *Manual on Static Hand Splinting* (1973)[13] and the *Manual on Dynamic Hand Splinting with Thermoplastic Materials* (1974).[14] Polyethylene is the only material commonly used with arthritis patients that is not covered in these manuals; for this reason procedures and resources for polyethylene are given in Appendix 3 of this book.

FABRICATION

Special precautions and considerations needed when constructing splints for arthritic joints are:

1. *Fitting the splint.* There may be discomfort to the client during fitting of the splint because of temperature, compression over synovitis, or sudden passive movements by the therapist.
2. *The orthosis may affect the other joints of the same extremity.* For example:
   a. Immobilization of a joint may cause increased compensatory stress to adjacent joints.
   b. A heavy wrist splint can aggravate an involved elbow or shoulder joint.
3. *The client's ability to put on and remove the splint.* This factor is especially important when bilateral splinting is involved.
4. *The weight of the splint.* Plaster is often the ideal material used for certain short term splints but frequently is too heavy for clients with arthritis. A plaster splint requires careful construction to be lightweight. (Table 6)
5. *The degree and fluctuation of joint and periarticular swelling.* This is an important consideration for circumferential splints. Splints fabricated during the day need to allow room for nocturnal swelling, and splints made for severely swollen joints will have to be adjusted as the swelling or inflammation decreases.
6. *Compatibility of the splint material with the client's activities of daily living.* For example, thin low temperature plastics can change shape during dishwashing. (Table 6)

OPTIMAL SPLINT FIT

Suggestions for achieving optimal fit of the splint are the following:

1. *Ulnar Styloid:* For clients with rheumatoid arthritis and wrist involvement, pressure over the ulnar styloid can be prevented by padding the styloid area on the positive mold or on the client *before* shaping the splint.
2. *Swelling:* Some clients have a swelling pattern. For example, they may swell consistently during the night. A night splint fitted for these clients during the middle of the day needs to be designed in a manner to accommodate night swelling.
3. *Perspiration:* Some splinting materials have a high sweating factor; the use of talcum powder or cotton stockinette liners can increase wearing comfort and reduce skin irritation at night. Moleskin is *not recommended* since it cannot be cleaned. It is helpful to show patients how to make their own stockinette liners, so they can keep them clean and not have to contact the therapist to obtain new ones.

SPLINT EVALUATION INDEX

The purpose of this section is the evaluation of a hand splint on a particular patient. The hand splints are described on pages 326 and 348.

TABLE 6. Splinting materials

Materials	Advantages	Disadvantages
Orthoplast	Easy to work with, contours readily, requires hot water or heat gun for shaping, and can be formed on the patient. Can be reshaped and is easily adjustable Has self-adhering properties when heated and is available in perforated form. Recommended for short-term splints.	Cannot be used in household tasks involving heat, e.g., washing dishes, cooking. Difficult to keep clean; scratches easily. Can overstretch with repeated use (especially slip-on splints).
Aquaplast (1/16″ thick)	High cosmetic acceptance, high contour property. The lightest, thinnest splint material available. Excellent for children and adolescents. Can be stretched for specific needs.	With constant use, wearing time may be limited to 1 year. High contour ability and rigidity requires precision finishing techniques. May discolor with age and use.
(3/8″ thick)	Moderate-high contour and shaping properties. Cosmetic appearance and cleans easily.	Rigidity and high contour properties may be a disadvantage for adult arthritis wrist splints.
Polyform and Kay Splint	Moderate-high contour property. High flexibility, can be easily stretched for specific splint requirement. Can be easily formed to adapt to assistive devices.	Rigidity can be a disadvantage for patients with arthritis. Contour shaping may not accommodate joint swelling and changes over time.
Plastazote	Soft, comfortable, lightweight, and has high skin tolerance. Porous and therefore causes less sweating.	Poor wearing properties (wearing ability about 3 months). Recommended only for splints involving low stress. Requires plastic reinforcement to provide stability or correction. Bulky.
Leather	High cosmetic and skin tolerance; greater male acceptance. Available in a variety of colors and thicknesses. Flexibility and nonslip surface helpful for some vocational demands.	Poor hygienic properties. Requires metal, elastic, or plastic reinforcement to provide stability. Circumferential splints create warmth and swelling.
Polyethylene (low density) (See Appendix)	Long wearing, cleans easily, maintains shape, and has cosmetic appearance.	Requires oven heating and positive mold. May shrink with heating.
Polypropylene	Inexpensive. Can be worn in hot water tasks. Thickness determines rigidity.	Slippery palmar surface may hinder gripping.

TABLE 6.   Splinting materials (*continued*)

Materials	Advantages	Disadvantages
Plaster of Paris bandage	Fast curing, easy to use, requires no heat. Optimal contour property. Inexpensive. Recommended for short-term splints on patients who can tolerate weight or as an immediate temporary splint. It can be lightweight, attractive and comfortable if skillfully constructed.	Breaks down with stress and exposure to water. Cannot be cleaned or remolded. It is heavy, bulky, and unattractive if constructed using a standard cast technique.
Lightcast	Lightweight, fast curing, and water proof. Easily applied in the operating room as a postoperative splint. Fabric-like material becomes rigid with curing.	Requires a special curing light. Bulky and has rough edges. Curing odor may bother some people. Not recommended for hand splints.
Fiberglas	Long wearing, cleans easily. Rigid; available in brown tones. Intermediate contouring ability. Fabric-like material becomes rigid with curing.	Difficult to work with and to adjust. Requires oven heating and a positive mold. Rigidity is not well suited to functional splints.

DESIGN INDEX

If the splint is well designed and of optimal value to the client, the following questions *should be answered yes.*

1. Does the splint conform to and maintain the normal transverse and longitudinal arches of the hand and wrist?[14]
2. Does the splint position the wrist in 5 to 10 degrees ulnar deviation?[15] (This only applies if the client can tolerate this position.)
3. When the splint is worn for a half hour and used in functional tasks, is the client's hand free of persistent redness caused by splint or strap pressure?
4. If MCP flexion is desired, does the palmar end extend *only to* the distal or mid-palmar crease?[14] If fourth and fifth metacarpal rotation is desired for power grasp, the splint should extend one-half inch proximal to the distal palmar crease or to the proximal palmar crease.[14]
5. If MCP joint protection is desired, does the palmar end extend to the middle of the proximal phalanx?[10]
6. When thumb motion is desired, does the thenar clearance allow for full opposition?
7. Is the splint sturdy enough to provide the desired stability for the wrist when the client is using his hands?

8. Does the fit of the splint allow for distribution of pressure over the widest area possible?
9. When fitted, is the client free of any pain caused by the splint? (It should not push the wrist into too much dorsiflexion or cause pressure over the ulnar styloid.)
10. Can the client put on and take off the splint without causing stress to the opposite hand?
11. If the patient has carpal tunnel syndrome or wrist flexor tenosynovitis, is his or her wrist splinted in 10 degrees of extension? (The angle that maximizes the carpal tunnel space.)

FUNCTIONAL INDEX

When the splint is designed to increase hand function, an objective assessment of hand function should be made with and without the splint to determine if the splint is effective. Determining grip and pinch strength with and without the splint provides a rapid and objective means of assessing a wide range of functional factors. However, the more subtle motions of hand function are often hampered by a splint; therefore, manipulation tasks are equally important. Many of the subtests in standard functional hand evaluations can be adapted to provide effective assessments for specific splints. (A review of some of the published assessments is printed at the end of Hand Pathodynamics and Assessment, Chapter 21.)

PATIENT EDUCATION

A splint is of value only if it is worn correctly. Because of the problems that may occur secondary to incorrect use of a splint, effective education regarding splint instruction is essential. To

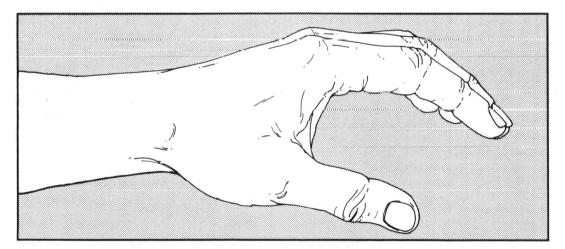

FIGURE 82. Functional position of the hand, lateral view: 20 to 30 degrees wrist extension, thumb in opposition, finger joints slightly flexed. (MCP joints in 30 to 45 degrees of flexion.)

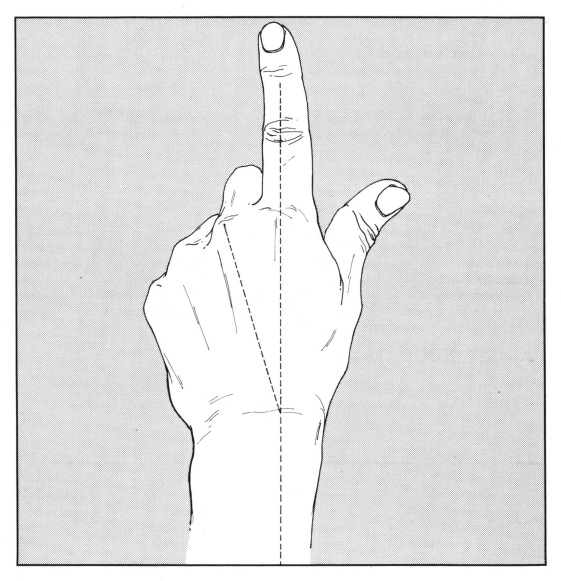

FIGURE 83. Functional position of the hand, dorsal view. Second metacarpal is in a straight line with the radius; wrist is in 5 to 10 degrees of ulnar deviation.

facilitate assessment of patient instruction and learning, information regarding splint usage has been delineated into behavioral objectives.

THERAPIST'S INSTRUCTIONAL OBJECTIVE

The objective is to teach the patient the following information in such a manner that the patient can achieve his or her objectives:

1. The purpose of the splint, including the advantages and disadvantages.
2. When and for how long the splint should be worn.
3. What exercises to do in conjunction with the splint.
4. How to take the splint on and off.
5. How to determine if the splint is positioned correctly.
6. How to care for and clean the splint.
7. How to check the skin for pressure areas.
8. Who to call or see, if problems with the splint should arise.

PATIENT OBJECTIVES

Before the splint is issued or the patient is discharged, the patient should be able to

1. Tell the therapist the purpose of the splint and when it should be worn.
2. Demonstrate prescribed exercises.
3. Put the splint on and take it off independently, without any verbal or nonverbal cues from the therapist.
4. Identify the landmarks to look for in order to determine if the splint is positioned correctly.
5. Explain to the therapist what has to be done to the splint to care for it properly.
6. Describe what to look for when checking the skin for pressure areas.

SPLINTS COMMON TO ARTHRITIC HAND TREATMENT

WRIST-HAND RESTING SPLINT

The wrist-hand resting splint is a static splint that immobilizes the wrist, thumb, and fingers.

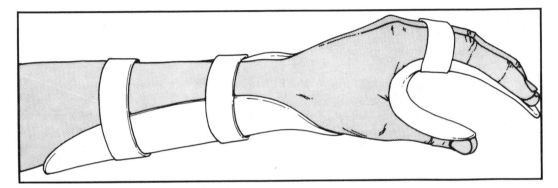

FIGURE 84. Full hand resting splint with C bar. In this figure, the wrist is in 30 degrees of extension. Patients with RA, wrist flexor tenosynovitis, or carpal tunnel syndrome should be splinted in 10 degrees of extension to maximize the carpal space. Thirty degrees of extension is appropriate for patients who are losing extension and appear to be developing wrist drop or wrist flexion contractures. The MCP joint should be in 35 to 45 degrees of flexion.

DESIGN

It is a volar splint that extends from the tip of the fingers to the proximal half of the forearm and maintains the hand in the functional position. There is a three-point dorsal strap closure and an optional thumb strap. It usually is constructed of thermoplastic or plaster or Paris. The C bar is also optional.

TREATMENT CONSIDERATION

The splint should be kept as small and light as possible. It *should extend just distal to the involved finger joints;* for example, if the wrist and MCP joints are involved, the splint should extend to the middle of the proximal phalanges.[10] The C bar (thumb abduction section) should be removed as soon as it is no longer needed so patients can manage bedclothes more easily and maintain thenar muscle tone.

Positioning

Wrist. Five to 10 degrees ulnar deviation (the normal functional alignment of the wrist) and in *maximal pain-free* extension up to 30 degrees (i.e., if there is pain beyond 20 degrees extension, the wrist should be splinted in 20 degrees extension and not in 30 degrees).

TABLE 7. Indications and goals for the wrist-hand resting splint

Indications	Goals
Acute synovitis of the wrist, fingers, and thumb.	To provide localized rest to the involved joints, thereby decreasing inflammation and pain.
Wrist and finger extensor and/or thumb abductor muscles are less than Grade 3.5 (not able to take slight resistance against gravity due to weakness).	To maintain optimal range until extensors are strong enough to counterbalance flexors (splint should be used in conjunction with a strengthening program).
Beginning multiple joint contractures.	To insure proper positioning and maintain optimal range of motion during sleep.
Patients with arthritis, severe disability, or peripheral nerve damage, who are not actively using their hands.	To obtain proper position and maintain optimal joint range and web space.

Patients with carpal tunnel syndrome and wrist flexor tenosynovitis should be splinted in 10 degrees of extension to maximize the carpal space. Since carpal tunnel syndrome is so common in RA, it is recommended that all patients with RA be splinted in 10 degrees of extension, unless they appear to be developing a wrist flexion contracture.

Thumb. Abduction and opposition (volar to the second metacarpal, not lateral).

Fingers. Third MCP joint in zero deviation with second, fourth, and fifth approximated to the third, but not crowded.

Spacers between the fingers may be needed to maintain optimal position, or an ulnar ridge may be indicated to keep the fifth in alignment.

(*Note:* From a dorsal view of the normal hand in the functional position, the index MCP joint should appear in slight ulnar deviation and the fourth and fifth MCP joints should appear in slight radial deviation.[17])

The MCP joint should be in 35 to 45 degrees of flexion—the greater the extension the more likely the possibility that the collateral ligaments can become tight in a shortened position. The PIP joints should also be in about 45 degrees of flexion and the DIP joint in slight flexion.

PRECAUTIONS

1. Pressure against skin over bony prominences should be avoided.
2. Proper positioning is stressed.
3. Guard against aggravation of elbow or shoulder involvement due to a heavy plaster splint.
4. Daily ROM should be done to prevent contractures.

PATIENT INSTRUCTION

These instructions are in addition to general instructions given earlier in this chapter.

1. If splint is to be worn at night only, patient may remove it to accomplish self-care tasks.

2. If the patient has bilateral splints, the straps on the dominant hand should be such that they can be opened independently (e.g., with teeth) in order to get out of bed in a hurry or in an emergency.

3. If the patient needs bilateral splints and cannot manage both splints at the same time, it is sometimes effective to have the patient wear the splints on alternate nights.

FUNCTIONAL WRIST STABILIZATION SPLINT

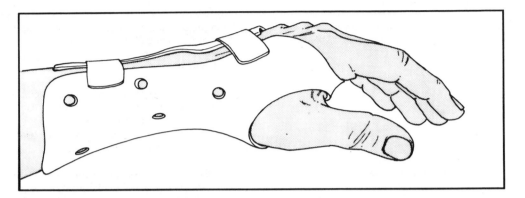

FIGURE 85. Polyethylene gauntlet splint.

The functional wrist stabilization splint is an orthosis that partially or completely immobilizes the wrist but allows for full MCP joint and thumb mobility.

DESIGN

It can be a slip-on gauntlet style or a modified gauntlet. The amount of dorsal coverage may vary considerably as long as the desired goal is achieved.

The volar aspect extends from the proximal palmar crease (see Figure 80) to the proximal third of the forearm with a cutout for the thenar eminence. When a patient does not have a proximal palmar crease or when it is too proximal to insure an adequate splint surface, extend the splint to one-half inch proximal to the distal crease.

Custom-made splints use thermoplastic materials, whereas commercial splints are usually made of leather, vinyl, or vinyl and elastic.

TREATMENT CONSIDERATIONS

In some clients with active wrist and MCP joint synovitis this splint can create or accentuate stress on the MCP joints and exacerbate the synovitis in these joints. The more severe or acute the MCP joint involvement is, the more vulnerable the MCP joints seem to be to any additional stress.

Two factors seem to contribute to this process. First, immobilization of the wrist and carpal bones requires that all motion take place in the finger and elbow joints. The importance of this particular factor seems to depend on the type of work or hand skills a person does with the splint on. The heavier the work is, the more stress is involved. (I refer to this as compensatory stress.) Second, in a plastic splint the palmar piece prevents sensation in that area. The only palmar area with sensation is over the MCP joints. This *may* require a person to apply more pressure to insure a tight grip when picking up an object.

TABLE 8. Indications and goals for the functional wrist stabilization splint

Indications	Goals
Hand function limited by wrist pain (patient may report dropping things or wrist giving way).	To improve hand function and grip strength (immobilization of the wrist relieves pain with motion and consequently muscle inhibition secondary to pain[11]).
Severe chronic wrist pain or inflammation	To provide localized rest to the joint, decrease inflammation and pain, and protect extensor tendons from attrition and rupture.[5] (See discussion on extensor tendon rupture in Chapters 13 and 21.)
Some cases of persistent carpal tunnel syndrome.[5]	To relieve pressure on the median nerve. *Note:* splints that involve high cost or extensive construction time are not recommended for short-term use (less than 8 weeks); wrist cock-up splints that maintain the wrist in 10 degrees of extension are suggested instead.

Those factors are described in conditional terms because the theory about this process is based on personal observation. Studies are needed on how wrist splints affect digital joints. The hand is a complex mechanism. Immobilization of a major component is bound to have some effect on the adjacent structures. A review of the literature has not revealed any research on this topic.

In my clinical experience I have seen two patients develop severe MCP subluxation in an inordinately short period of time (4 to 6 weeks), following daytime use of a plastic wrist gauntlet splint. Also, several other patients have complained of increased pain and swelling in the MCP joints while using these splints. Therefore, I am very cautious about daytime use of these splints. I have found the program for splinting outlined below to be the most effective one for managing wrist synovitis in patients with coexistent MCP synovitis. There are several kinds of splints that can be used, depending on the severity of the wrist involvement. The primary guideline is: the more active or acute the MCP joint involvement, the less restrictive is the wrist splint used during the day. (This is in conjunction with a thermoplastic wrist splint at night.)

1. Severe, acute wrist synovitis and minimal MCP joint involvement. The patient with this condition may benefit the most from a thermoplastic splint with instruction to monitor the MCP joints carefully. If the splint appears to be making the MCP joints worse, a change to a more flexible splint is advised.
2. Moderate wrist synovitis and moderate MCP synovitis. The optimal splint is a flexible elastic-vinyl gauntlet (commercial) splint with the metal reinforcement included. These splints allow approximately 50 degrees of wrist flexion-extension but prevent circumduction; so they reduce considerable rotation forces to the wrist but do not alter flexion and extension dynamics as much as a rigid splint. However, for most patients to use these splints comfortably during the day, the splints need to be cut back

at the thenar and distal edges, and this often requires a commercial sewing machine, which is not available in all clinics.

3. Moderate wrist synovitis and acute MCP synovitis. If the PIP joints are not involved, a thermoplastic wrist-MCP stabilization splint may be ideal. If the PIP joints are inflamed this type of splint may cause compensatory stress to the PIP joints. For these patients it may be necessary to use a flexible commercial splint with the metal bar removed.

These examples of splinting apply to patients with early active disease. For patients with damaged unstable wrist joints and essentially inactive MCP joint disease, thermoplastic wrist gauntlet splints are often ideal for daytime use.

PRECAUTIONS

1. Splint may increase deforming stresses to the MCP joints.
2. Distal end of the splint should not extend past the distal palmar crease.
3. Full thumb opposition should be possible.
4. Thumb web space section can irritate or cut the skin. (Edges should be smoothed, rolled, or padded.) It is usually most comfortable if it does not impinge against the index MCP joint.
5. There should not be any pressure over the ulnar styloid.

PATIENT INSTRUCTION

These instructions are in addition to the general instructions given earlier in this chapter.

1. If the purpose of the splint is to decrease pain and increase hand function, the splint should be worn during hand activities and be removed when the patient is at rest.

2. If the splint is prescribed for positioning or to help reduce wrist pain at night, it can be worn day and night. For some patients it may be necessary to have a separate (clean) splint for night use.

3. The patient should remove the splint several times during the day or when needed; the wrist should be ranged and the skin should be checked for pressure areas.

4. When this splint is prescribed to increase hand function and is to be worn during activities, it is important that the patient has realistic expectations of the splint. The splint may relieve wrist pain, but the palmar piece reduces dexterity and many activities may seem more difficult. Unrealistic expectations can lead to disappointment and discarding of the splint.

PROTECTIVE MCP SPLINT

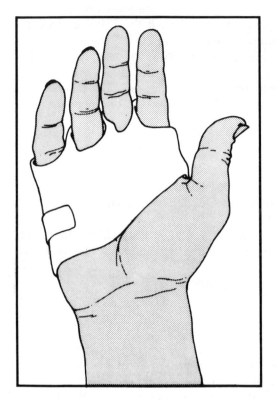

FIGURE 86. Palmar metacarpophalangeal stabilization splint (Johnson-Johnson pattern).

The protective MCP splint maintains the MCP joints in normal alignment with a 0- to 25-degree MCP flexion to protect the joints from ulnar deviating or volar subluxating forces created by the flexor tendons during pinch and grasp activities. (See Figure 32 in Chapter 21, Hand Pathodynamics and Assessment.)

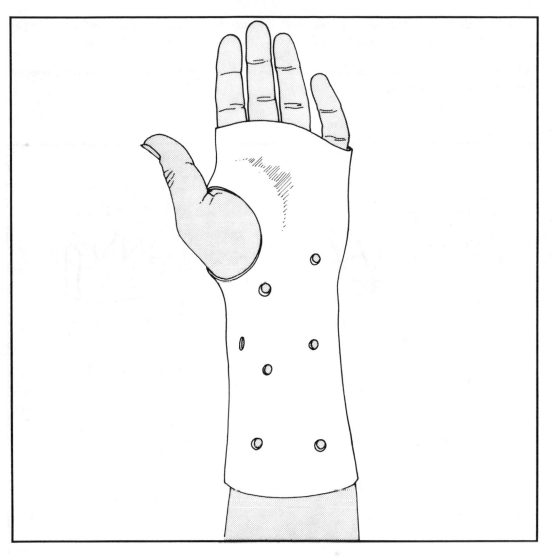

FIGURE 87. Polyethylene gauntlet splint (distal and extended to stabilize the metacarpophalangeal joints).

DESIGN

Variable basic designs include:
1. Static short splint that fits entirely on the hand with a palmar piece over the MC heads and individual finger separators (Fig. 86).
2. Static wrist stabilization splint that extends to the middle of the proximal phalanges. This is used when there is both wrist and MCP joint involvement[10] (Fig. 87).

3. A static volar wrist cock-up splint with an extended palmar piece and individual finger separators. It may have an optional thumb post and ulnar ridge (Fig. 88).

These splints are custom-fitted and commonly made from thermoplastic. Type and number of closures vary with the design.

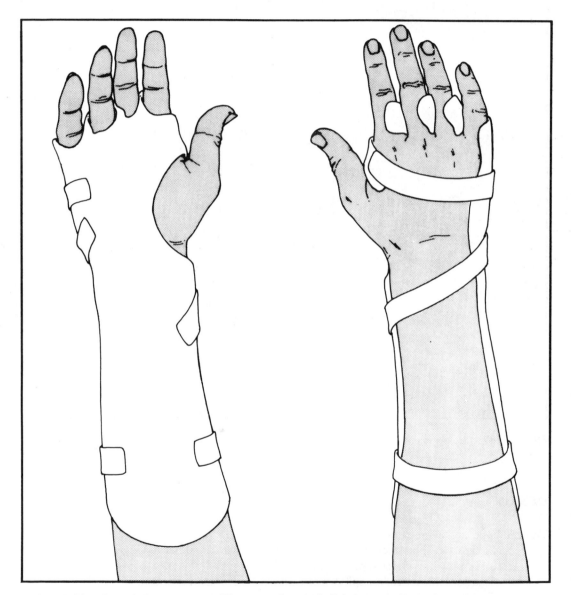

FIGURE 88. Extended static wrist stabilization splint: *Left,* Palmar view; *Right,* Dorsal view.

TABLE 9. Indications and goals for the protective MCP splint

Indications	Goals
MCP synovitis with zero to moderate ulnar drift.	To prevent overstretching of the capsule during phases of inflammation and swelling. The capsular and articular ligaments are distended by joint effusions and are extremely vulnerable to overstretching during these phases. These splints minimize the two most damaging forces: 1. pull of the flexor tendons in strong grasp and pinch. [10] 2. passive pressure toward ulnar deviation. They also help minimize the effect of reflex intrinsic spasm.
Beginning MCP volar subluxation, beginning swan neck deformities, or intrinsic tightness.	To counteract the influence of tight intrinsics by keeping the MCP joints in extension and allowing PIP flexion, [18] thereby producing gentle repetitive stretch to the instrinsic muscles.

TREATMENT CONSIDERATIONS

Restriction of motion at one joint may increase stress to adjacent joints. If the patient has PIP involvement, it is important to determine the effect of the splint on these joints.

The MCP joints should be positioned in full extension (neutral) or as close to that position as possible to stretch the intrinsic muscles.

If there is active MCP synovitis, the primary goal is to protect the joints rather than stretch the intrinsics.

Counterpressure with a soft, padded strap over the dorsum of the MCP heads may be facilitative if there is an additional goal to help reduce MCP volar subluxation. [19]

Either the splint should be made of a high temperature plastic if it is to be used during activities involving heat, such as dishwashing or bathing, or strong rubber gloves should be used to protect low temperature plastics.

Patients must be told that this splint (like all hand splints) does *decrease* hand dexterity, thus making some hand skills awkward.

PRECAUTIONS

1. Careful frequent skin inspection must be carried out for splints with finger separators. Patients with dry, atrophied, tissue paper skin resulting from long-term steroid use may be prone to breakdown with these splints.

2. Maximal allowance for the thenar eminence is necessary for hand function.

3. *Splinting of the MCP joints in extension can cause shortening of the collateral*

ligaments in diagnoses other than MCP synovitis. In the presence of chronic MCP synovitis the radial collateral ligaments become overstretched. It is possible that splinting in extension may cause a desirable shortening of these ligaments, but further experimentation is needed in this area.

PATIENT INSTRUCTION

These instructions are in addition to the general instructions given earlier in the chapter.

1. For MCP protection, the splint is preferably worn both day and night with removal for ROM exercises and brief periods throughout the day when the patient is at leisure. If the patient cannot tolerate day and night wear, then the daytime hours, when hand function is greatest, are recommended for splint use. Jim Hammond, OTR, Mount Sinai Hospital, Florida, started a program of using protective MCP splints at night and has reported a reduction of ulnar drift in patients in this program.[20]

2. If the splint is used for protection, its purpose is to counteract the ulnar deviating and subluxating forces that are created by the long finger flexors on the MCP joint capsule during grasp and pinch activities. (See Hand Pathodynamics and Assessment, Chapter 21, for pathodynamics of ulnar drift.) This is a difficult concept for patients to understand, but they need to have an awareness of the process in order to know how to protect their joints. They also must receive instruction in how to manage tasks in a protective manner when they are not wearing the splint, e.g., during bathing and while handling sheets and blankets in bed. (See Joint Protection and Energy Conservation Instruction, Chapter 26.)

3. Treatment of intrinsic tightness is still experimental. It may be necessary to wear the splint as little as one hour twice a day or as much as all day long, or even during the night, depending upon severity of the tightness and the treatment objective.

ULNAR DRIFT POSITIONING SPLINT

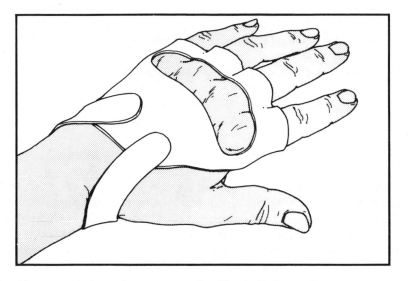

FIGURE 89. Metacarpophalangeal positioning splint (Quest-Cordery splint).

The ulnar drift positioning splint encourages optimal alignment of the MCP joints to facilitate dexterity during functional activities.

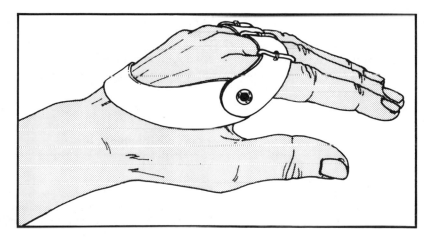

FIGURE 90. Metacarpal ulnar drift (MUD) splint.

DESIGN

The basic designs are:

    1. Short splint that fits entirely on the hand with individual spaces for each finger[11] (Fig. 89).
    2. Short splint with a dorsal bar to position the fingers[22] (Fig. 90).

These splints are custom fitted using a thermoplastic material. The type and number of closures vary considerably with design. Table 10 lists indications and goals for its use.

TREATMENT CONSIDERATIONS

These splints often are difficult to fit, and not all patients with severe ulnar drift are candidates for this splint. Ulnar drift may make hand skills more awkward, but it does not necessarily limit total functional ability particularly if the patient has good flexion and extension. This splint may not increase total ability but may make overall function easier and less awkward particularly when instability is severe. (Note: Initially anti-ulnar deviation splints were designed to correct (cure) established deformity. To date there has been no documentation of splinting actually reversing established ligamentous deformity.)[6]

The splint checkout should include a functional task performance, e.g., making a bed, making a sandwich, or buttoning to determine if the splint slips or binds or is effective. The Jebsen Hand Function test provides a fast standardized test for evaluating splint effectiveness. (See Table 4, Chapter 21.)

PRECAUTIONS

    1. Proper effective fit is crucial.
    2. Pressure over the dorsum of MCP joints should be avoided.
    3. Make sure there is no pressure of the fifth finger against the ring finger.

TABLE 10. **Indications and goals for the ulnar drift positioning splint**

Indications	Goals
Severe ulnar drift of the MCP joints that interferes with function.	To block ulnar drift during pinch and grasp activities. To reduce pain and improve function. (Splints are worn during activities and generally not at rest.)
Ulnar subluxation of the fifth MCP joint that interferes with function.	To reposition the finger in optimal alignment. (This is particularly important if the fifth finger is traumatized frequently because of its deviated and subluxed position.)

PATIENT INSTRUCTION

These instructions are in addition to the general instructions given earlier in this chapter.

1. The patient needs to be an active participant in the evaluation of the splint.
2. Since this is an elective splint, the patient's subjective appraisal of its effectiveness is the most important criterion. Therefore, no matter how favorable the objective evaluations are, if the patient does not feel that the splint is helping, there is no reason to issue it.

POSTSURGICAL SPLINT

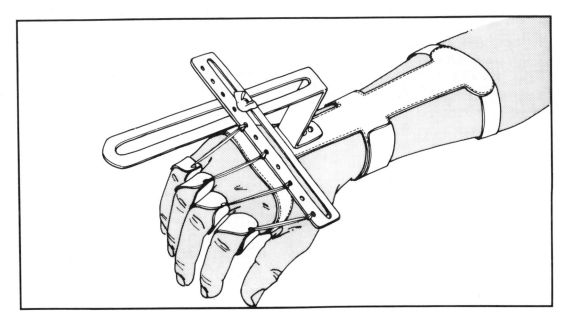

FIGURE 91. Swanson metacarpophalangeal postsurgical splint with extensor assist. An elbow strap (not shown) is often used to reduce forward sliding of the splint.

The postsurgical splint positions and supports the wrist, dynamically controls position and alignment of the fingers, and assists MCP flexion or extension as indicated. When used in the management of an MCP arthroplasty the splint allows application of tension to individual fingers to encourage desired encapsulation (Fig. 91). (See Surgical Rehabilitation, Chapter 13, for specific surgical procedures and timing of splint application.)

DESIGN

The postsurgical splint is a volar or dorsal static wrist splint. There are attachments for both finger flexion assists (flexion cuff, slings, or fingernail hooks) and extension assists (outrigger with individual finger slings). The initial basic splint may be made of plaster of Paris bandage. Later splints usually are prefabricated from wire[23] or metal[24] and custom-contoured for fit or custom-made from thermoplastic.[25] The specific design of the splint does not matter as long as the desired goals are achieved. It is recommended that the splint have a transverse outrigger that allows individual alignment of the fingers. Table 11 lists indications and goals for its use.

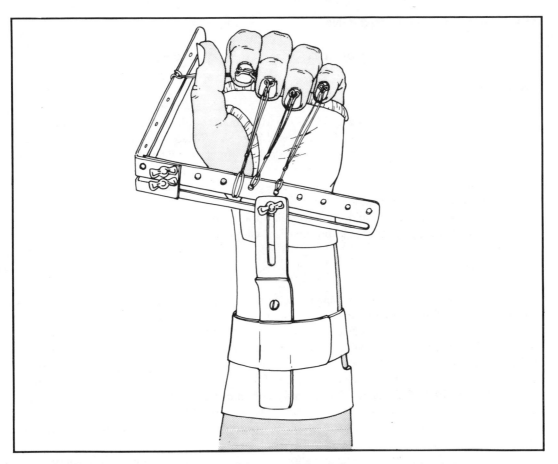

FIGURE 92. Volar thermoplastic wrist stabilization splint with flexion assist and index supination assist attached by fingernail hooks.

TABLE 11. Indications and goals for the postsurgical splint

Indications	Goals
Post-MCP synovectomy and extensor tendon relocation with or without prosthetic implant.	To optimally position the wrist. To position the fingers in optimal dorsovolar, radioulnar, and rotational alignment (at rest and in motion) to facilitate optimal encapsulation. To minimize ulnar deviating forces. To reduce extensor lag, thereby increasing the mechanical advantages and functional strength of the extensor communis. To increase MCP flexion range. To prevent or minimize postsurgical adhesion.

TREATMENT CONSIDERATIONS

Effective positioning and tension of the flexor and extensor assists are crucial.

Static Splint Base

1. The wrist should be positioned in 5 to 10 degrees of ulnar deviation (if tolerated) and in neutral or 10 degrees of extension if possible. (More than 10 degrees of wrist extension places the long extensors on slack and makes it difficult to maintain MCP joint extension.)
2. The palmar piece should not extend beyond to the proximal palmar crease in order to allow full MCP flexion.
3. Thenar clearance should allow for full opposition.
4. Length of the splint should not interfere with elbow flexion or supination.

Flexion Assists

Individual finger assists (slings or fingernail hooks) accommodate different finger ranges. Fingernail hooks (Fig. 92) allow for control of circumduction and are especially helpful when the PIP joints are stiff. Flexion cuffs do not allow for individual finger control. However, if there is active PIP synovitis and the PIP joints are unstable, finger slings may cause less stress to the PIP joint than fingernail hooks. *The pull of the rubber bands or cuff strap should be toward the scaphoid* (navicular) and not toward the center of the wrist.[26]

    FINGERNAIL HOOKS. * Temporarily bonding a hook fastener to the dorsum of a fingernail provides a stable point from which a tension-producing material can project to a given point. Depending on the location of the end point the finger can be rotated or flexed into the desired position.

    In the rheumatoid hand, indications for use of fingernail hooks are the following:

1. To assist flexion of the MCP joints, the PIP joints, and the DIP joints postsurgically for implant arthroplasty.
2. To passively flex the PIP joints while the MCP joints are stabilized volarly in extension in order to stretch out early intrinsic tightness.
   (In both of these instances, a volar outrigger that allows for correct radial-ulnar alignment is the end point.)
3. To rotate (supinate) the index finger following an MCP implant arthroplasty which involves partial transfer of the volar plate to the radial aspect of the proximal phalanx.

Postoperatively the finger tends to rotate as in pronation. By placing the hook across the nail with the hook opening on the ulnar side of the nail the tension material hooks on and passes beneath the finger to a radial outrigger attached to the splint or an independent outrigger projecting from the radial side of the hand.

---

* Developed by Dena M. Shapiro, O.T.R., Los Angeles, California.

Materials needed for fingernail hook placement are

#2 hooks (³/₈ in. long)
2 pairs needle-nosed pliers
screwdriver
cyanoacrylate adhesive (Loctite Super Bonder, Loctite Corporation, Newington, CT 06111) or epoxy resins
emery board

(*Precaution:* The above bonding agents can bond skin-to-skin surfaces rapidly. The solvent is acetone.)

The following procedure is used:

1. Shape the hook. Using needle-nosed pliers, open and spread the base of the hook, making them curved to fit the nail surface. Pry the hook open slightly with the screwdriver to facilitate application of the rubber band or other tension-producing material.
2. Prepare the nailbed. File the top of the nail to provide a rough surface for easier bonding.
3. Apply one drop of the adhesive to the nail. *Carefully* place the hook and allow to dry one to two minutes. A second drop on top of the base of the hook may be necessary. (Some therapists report gluing Velcro hooks to the nail and using Velcro pilo straps to apply tension.)

Extensor Assists

The following points must be considered in attaching the extensor assists:

1. The outrigger should be distal to the MCP joints so that the line of the pull is perpendicular to the proximal phalanx, thereby preventing jamming of the joint and facilitating extension. This also prevents the slings from pulling or cutting into the web space. However, this may not be advisable if there is a threat of dorsal displacement of the distal stem, as in severe osteoporosis.
2. The proximal phalanx should be assisted only to neutral.
3. The appropriate tension is the minimal amount that will bring the phalanges to neutral (or maximal extension if less than neutral). Care must be taken not to apply too much tension to the ring and little fingers because maximal flexion of these joints is needed for grasp.
4. The assists should pull the fingers *just beyond normal* deviation (not neutral or zero degress deviation) for the fingers in neutral, which is zero degrees for the middle finger; 5 to 20 degrees of ulnar deviation for the index finger; and slight radial deviation for the ring and little fingers. [17] (To achieve this positioning, radial positioning of the bands on the outrigger may be necessary to allow for tightening of the radial interossei.)
5. If the fingers abnormally circumduct (pronate), additional lateral assists may be necessary to correct rotation. [24]

PRECAUTIONS

1. If finger slings are too tight or of a hard nonporous material such as plastic, skin breakdown or irritation may occur.
2. Finger slings should be narrow enough to allow full PIP flexion.
3. Too much extensor band tension may cause undue joint stress; therefore, adjust to patient's tolerance.
4. Flexion assists that pull the fingers toward the center of the wrist rather than to the scaphoid may cause rotational stress to the MCP joints.
5. If swelling occurs distal to the splint or distal to the assist slings, the splint is too tight and needs adjusting. (A volar design may remedy the problem.)
6. In an attempt to gain MCP extension, the hand may inadvertently lift from the palmar piece and lose volar support. If this occurs a dorsal strap should be considererd.

PATIENT INSTRUCTION

These instructions are in addition to the general instructions given earlier in this chapter.

1. The patient should be given written instructions explaining when to wear the splint and how to position it and the assist bands. It is helpful to identify visual landmarks which he or she can use to spot check to see if the splint is positioned correctly. Usually the patient should be able to change from flexion to extension assists independently.
2. The patient should have a clear understanding of the postoperative goals and treatment procedures and the importance of positioning the splint correctly.

POSTOPERATIVE PROCEDURE

There are several excellent programs for dynamic splinting described in the literature.[24,27,28,29,30,31]

THUMB CARPOMETACARPAL (CMC) STABILIZATION SPLINT

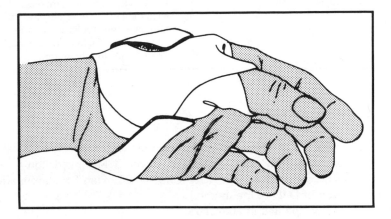

FIGURE 93. Polyethylene carpometacarpal stabilization splint.

The thumb CMC stabilization splint restricts motion of the thumb CMC and MCP joints but allows function of the IP joint and wrist.

DESIGN

It is a short, static splint that slips over the first metacarpal with a C bar. It may slip on to the hand or a strap may be used for closure. The most common splints are of leather with metal reinforcement (Fig. 93) or low and high temperature thermoplastics (Fig. 94). Indications and goals are listed in Table 12.

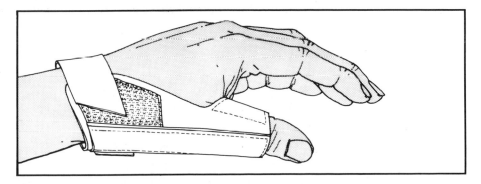

FIGURE 94. Leather metacarpophalangeal stabilization splint with metal reinforcement on the extensor surface. This allows some carpometacarpal mobility, because there is no C bar.

TABLE 12. Indications and goals for the thumb carpometacarpal stabilization splint

Indications	Goals
Thumb CMC pain with motion.	To relieve pain and increase hand function. This splint is most effective for isolated joint involvement typically seen in DJD. It is usually too restrictive for people with multiple hand joint involvement.

TREATMENT CONSIDERATIONS

Because of the structure of the thumb it is almost impossible to completely immobilize the CMC joint and simultaneously allow MP joint motion; however, CMC restriction to a 10-degree range is usually sufficient to decrease pain. (See Chapter 21, Hand Pathodynamics and Assessment, for a discussion of DJD of the thumb.)

The thumb should be splinted in abduction.

Orthoplast splints, designed to slip on, frequently overstretch with repetitive use and may require a strap closure.

Aquaplast (1/16″ thick) has proven to be an excellent material for this type of splint. Its thinness and high contour ability allow for intricate strapping around the thenar eminence and web space.

PRECAUTIONS

A careful functional performance checkout is necessary to determine such problems as slippage and binding.

PATIENT INSTRUCTION

These instructions are in addition to the general instructions given earlier in this chapter.

Usually this splint is prescribed during activities, but it also can be worn at night if it helps relieve pain.

TRI-POINT FINGER SPLINT

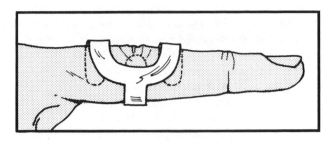

FIGURE 95. Tri-point ring finger splint (originally Bennett double ring finger metal splint).

The tri-point finger splint (1) limits PIP or thumb IP hyperextension and allows full flexion or (2) limits PIP flexion and allows full extension. Certain splint designs can be rotated to achieve either effect.

DESIGN

It is a small lightweight splint that applies pressure at three points: proximal and distal to the dorsal (or volar) surface of the joint and centrally to the opposing surface (Fig. 95). These splints are most frequently made from thermoplastic material. Aquaplast ($^1/_{16}$") can be quickly shaped to a highly cosmetic, lightweight slip-on splint. The original splints were made from metal.[26,27] Indications and goals are listed in Table 13.

TABLE 13.   Indications and goals for the tri-point finger splint

Indications	Goals
Swan neck deformities.	To maintain PIP flexion range. To improve hand function and relieve stress to the volar aspect of the PIP joint (resulting from severe hyperextension) To improve cosmesis (occasionally).
Postsurgical swan neck repair (Littler procedure).	To prevent overstretching of ligaments and expansion of fibers during postoperative healing phase.[36]
Thumb hyperextension.	To improve function, especially pinch prehension.
Boutonniere deformity.	To decrease or prevent PIP contractures usually requiring the Bunnell safety pin splint.[29,30]

TREATMENT CONSIDERATIONS

Aquaplast and ring splints appear to have the highest patient acceptance.

This method of splinting is suitable for one to three fingers in swan neck deformities, but it is not practical for all of the digits except postsurgically. (See Hand Pathodynamics and Assessment, Chapter 21, for dynamics of swan neck deformities.)

Splints for the thumb usually need to be custom contoured because they are the most difficult to fit. They can also be used to reduce lateral forces to the thumb as a protective or preventive measure during functional activities such as needlework.

The PIP joint following swan neck surgery should not extend beyond 10 degrees of flexion in order to encourage shortening of the volar structures and, it is hoped, to inhibit reoccurrence.[36]

PRECAUTIONS

In swan neck deformities the skin over the volar surface of the PIP joint may be especially tender or vulnerable as a result of the constant stretch from PIP subluxation (hyperextension).

PATIENT INSTRUCTION

See page 323 for instructions pertaining to patient education.

REFERENCES

1. Partridge, R. E. H., and Duthie, J. J. R.: *Controlled trial of the effect of complete immobilization of the joints in rheumatoid arthritis.* Ann. Rheum. Dis. 22:91, 1963.
2. Gault, S. S., and Spyker, J. M.: *Beneficial effect of immobilization of joints in rheumatoid arthritis and related arthritides: A splint study using sequential analysis.* Arthritis Rheum. 12:34, 1969.
3. Ehrlich, G. E. (ed.): *Total Management of the Arthritic Patient.* J. B. Lippincott, Philadelphia, 1973.
4. Bell, J. A.: *Plaster cylinder casting for contractures of the interphalangeal joints.* In Hunter, J. M., Schneider, L. H., Mackin, E. J., and Bell, J. A. (eds.): *Rehabilitation of the Hand.* C. V. Mosby, St. Louis, 1978.
5. Ehrlich. G. E.: *Total Management of the Arthritic Patient,* p. 48.
6. Convery, F. R., Conaty, J. P., and Nickel, V. L.: *Dynamic splinting of the rheumatoid hand.* Ortho. Prosth. March, 1968, p. 41.
7. Pahle, J. A., and Raunio, P.: *The influence of wrist position on finger deviation in the rheumatoid hand.* J. Bone Joint Surg. (Br.) 51:665, 1969.
8. Flatt, A. E.: *Care of the Rheumatoid Hand.* C. V. Mosby, St. Louis, 1974, p. 76.
9. Ehrlich, G. E.: *Total Management of the Arthritic Patient,* pp. 47–48.
10. Smith, E. M., et al.: *Flexor forces and rheumatoid metacarpophalangeal deformity.* J.A.M.A. 198:130, 1966.
11. Millender, L. H., and Nalebuff, E. A.: *Reconstructive surgery in the rheumatoid hand.* Orthop. Clin. North Am. 6:712, 1975.
12. Ehrlich, G. E.: *Total Management of the Arthritic Patient,* p. 52.
13. Malick, M. H.: *Manual on Static Hand Splinting.* Harmarville Rehabilitation Center, Pittsburgh, Pa., 1973.
14. Malick, M. H.: *Manual on Dynamic Hand Splinting with Thermoplastic Materials.* Harmarville Rehabilitation Center, Pittsburgh, Pa. 1974, p. 16.

15. Boyes, J.: *Bunnell's Surgery of the Hand*, ed. 5. J. B. Lippincott, Philadelphia, 1970, pp. 10–11.
16. Treanor, W. S.: *Motions of the hand and foot.* In Licht, S. (ed.): *Therapeutic Exercise.* Elizabeth Licht Publishers, New Haven, Ct., 1965, pp. 102–103.
17. Flatt, A. E.: *Care of the Rheumatoid Hand,* p. 250.
18. Boyes, J.: *Bunnell's Surgery,* pp. 173–174.
19. Personal communication from MacBain, K. P., Canadian Arthritis and Rheumatism Society (C.A.R.S.), British Columbia Division, Vancouver.
20. Hammond, J.: *Prevention and correction of ulnar drift and pain in patients with rheumatoid arthritis.* Presented at the annual meeting of the Allied Health Professions Section Meeting of the Arthritis Foundation, 1974.
21. Quest, D., and Cordery, J.: *A functional ulnar deviation cuff for the rheumatoid deformity.* Am. J. Occup. Ther. 25:32, 1971.
22. Houchin, R., and Cheshire, L.: *Splintage for ulnar deviation.* Engl. Occup. Ther. J. 34:9, 1971.
23. Wire-foam hand splints. L.M.B. Hand Rehabilitation Products, San Luis Obisbo, Ca.
24. Swanson, A. B.: *Flexible Implant Resection Arthroplasty in the Hand and Extremities.* C. V. Mosby, St. Louis, 1973, pp. 171–183.
25. Malick, M. H.: *Dynamic Hand Splinting,* pp. 177–183.
26. Malick, M. H.: *Dynamic Hand Splinting,* p. 7.
27. Brand, P. W.: *The forces of dynamic splinting: Ten questions before applying a dynamic splint to the hand.* In Hunter, J. M., Schneider, L. H., Mackin, E. J., and Bell, J. A. (eds.): *Rehabilitation of the Hand.* C. V. Mosby, St. Louis, 1978.
28. Carter, M. S., and Wilson, R. L.: *Postsurgical management in rheumatoid arthritis.* In Hunter, Schneider, Mackin, and Bell, J. A. (eds.): *Rehabilitation of the Hand,* C. V. Mosby, St. Louis, 1978.
29. Madden, J. W., DeVore, G., and Arem, A. J.: *A rational postoperative management program for metacarpophalangeal joint implant arthroplasty.* J. Hand Surg. 2:358, 1977.
30. Pearson, S. O.: *Dynamic splinting.* In Hunter, J. M., Schneider, L. H., Mackin, E. J., and Bell, J. A.: *Rehabilitation of the Hand.* C. V. Mosby, St. Louis, 1978.
31. Fess, E. E., Gettle, K. S., and Strickland, J. W.: *Hand Splinting: Principles and Methods.* C. V. Mosby, St. Louis, 1981.
32. Swanson, A. B., Swanson, G. G., and Leonard, J.: *Postoperative rehabilitation program for inflexible implant arthroplasty of the digits.* In Hunter, J. M., Schneider, L. H., Mackin, E. J., and Bell, J. A.: *Rehabilitation of the Hand.* C. V. Mosby, St. Louis, 1978.
33. Barr, R. N.: *The Hand: Principles and Techniques of Simple Splint Making and Rehabilitation.* Butterworth & Co., Boston, 1975. (Excellent resource. Describes method for making wire outriggers and polyethylene thumb splint.)
34. Bennett, R. L.: *Wrist and hand slip-on splints.* In Licht, E. (ed.): *Arthritis and Physical Medicine.* Elizabeth Licht Publishers, New Haven, Ct., 1969, pp. 484–485.
35. Boyes, J.: *Bunnell's Surgery,* pp. 174–175.
36. Nalebuff, E. A., and Millender, L. H.: *Surgical treatment of the swan neck deformity in rheumatoid arthritis.* Orthop. Clin. North Am. 6:733, 1975.
37. Souter, W. A: *The problem of the boutonniere deformity.* Clin. Orthop. 104:116, 1974.
38. Nalebuff, E. A., and Millender, L. H.: *Surgical treatment of the boutonniere deformity in rheumatoid arthritis.* Orthop. Clin. North Am. 6:753, 1975.

ADDITIONAL SOURCES

Splinting for Arthritis

Bennett, R. L.: *Orthotic devices to prevent deformities of the hand in rheumatoid arthritis.* Arthritis Rheum. 8:1006, 1965.
Besser, M. I.: *The conservative treatment of the swan neck deformity in the rheumatoid hand.* Hand 10(1):91, 1978.

Carr, K.: *Hand splints for rheumatoid arthritis.* Can. J. Occup. Ther. 35:17, 1978.

Convery, R. F., and Minteer, M. A.: *The use of orthoses in the management of rheumatoid arthritis.* Clin. Orthop. 102:118, 1974.

Elliott, R. A., Jr.: *Splints for mallet and boutonniere deformities.* Plast. Reconstr. Surg. 52:282, 1973.

Feinberg, J., and Brandt, K. D.: *Use of resting splints by patients with rheumatoid arthritis.* Am. J. Occup. Ther. 35(3):173, 1981.

Johnson, B. M., Flynn, M. J. G., and Beckenbaugh, R. D.: *A dynamic splint for use after total wrist arthroplasty.* (For a Meuli prothesis.) Am. J. Occup. Ther. 35(3):179, 1981.

Mikic, Z., and Helal, B.: *The treatment of the mallet finger by the Oakley splint.* Hand 6:76, 1974.

Moon, M: *Compliancy in splint wearing behavior of patients with rheumatoid arthritis.* N. Z. Med. J. 83(564):360, 1976.

Nicolle, F. V., and Presswell, D.: *A valuable splint for the rheumatoid hand.* Hand 7:67, 1975.

Redford, J. B. (ed.): *Orthotics Etcetera*, ed. 2. Williams & Wilkins, Baltimore, 1980.

Souter, W. A.: *Splintage in the rheumatoid hand.* Hand 3:144, 1971.

Williams, J. G.: *Splints for the rheumatoid hand.* Br. Med. J. 1:106, 1970.

26

JOINT PROTECTION AND ENERGY CONSERVATION INSTRUCTION

Joint protection is a *process* in which the therapist evaluates the patient's total living pattern, his or her psychological response to the arthritis, family or personal support systems, and the patient's willingness to influence his or her arthritis by modifying behavior or adapting his or her environment.

The goal or purpose of joint protection is to *reduce stress and pain* in the involved joints and consequently *to reduce inflammation* and *preserve the integrity of the joint structures.* The incorporation of energy conservation training helps the patient conserve physical resources and improve functional endurance.

When joint protection was first introduced, it was hoped that diligent application of these principles could prevent deformity.[1] But widespread clinical application demonstrated the difficulty of effecting steadfast patient compliance over long periods of time. This difficulty in achieving long-term compliance has limited our ability to demonstrate the preventive potential of joint protection methods.

The primary value of joint protection lies in its effectiveness for reducing pain, stress to the joint, and inflammation. Although studies on joint protection have not been published, the effectiveness of joint protection techniques can be easily demonstrated in the clinic. If certain techniques are recommended to reduce pain and joint stress, the effectiveness of the technique is generally immediate. This can be demonstrated by having the patient perform a task, such as picking up a saucepan, in a routine fashion and then having the patient repeat the task using joint protection techniques. When the techniques are used correctly, performing the task is less painful. The reduction of inflammation is more variable and may take one or two days to be noticeable to the patient, depending upon the activities eliminated and the amount of stress reduced in the joint. When patients are taught how to monitor the signs and symptoms of inflammation, they are able to appreciate the benefits of joint protection methods. This provides positive reinforcement that is invaluable for encouraging patients to continue to use joint protection methods.

PATIENT INSTRUCTION

A wide range of methods for teaching joint protection instruction has been developed; in fact almost every clinic has developed its own system. Most programs instruct patients in the principles (and specific techniques) of joint protection as defined by Joy Cordery, OTR, in her original article on the topic and often include a list of dos and don'ts based on these principles for the patient to memorize.[1] While the Cordery principles form the conceptual framework for the joint protection process, the methods used for incorporating these principles in daily activities are different for each patient.[1] The instructions given need to be specific to each patient's pattern of arthritis.[1] A standard list of dos and don'ts given to all patients negates the importance of individualizing the process for each patient; and if each recommendation requires a behavior change, the list may pose an overwhelming responsibility for the patient, a factor that contributes to noncompliance.

Janet Sliwa, OTR, has developed guidelines for instructing patients with systemic polyarthritis in joint protection methods.[2] These guidelines capitalize on the value of individualized instruction and on teaching concepts rather than rules. Both factors encourage patient participation and problem solving in the joint protection process. A modified version of these guidelines is included here to demonstrate how these teaching principles can be incorporated into a joint protection program and to encourage therapists to critically analyze their own teaching methods in relation to these concepts. Sliwa's guidelines for instruction include the following:[2]

1. Explain the rationale and value of joint protection, based on the inflammatory process.
2. Teach the patient how to recognize and monitor the signs and symptoms of inflammation, i.e., pain, warmth, and swelling.
3. Encourage the patient to evaluate disease activity level through recognition of inflammatory signs.
4. Stimulate awareness for the need to modify activities based on disease activity level.
5. Identify activity pacing as the process of balancing activities with rest periods.
6. Explain to the patient that pursuing activities despite pain may cause joint damage and that ignoring the symptoms of fatigue may precipitate an exacerbation of disease.
7. Have the patient describe alternative methods for pacing activities.
8. Identify the consequences of static positioning at rest and dynamic forces during activity.
9. Explain and demonstrate proper and improper joint alignment and the consequences of prolonged malalignment.
10. Have the patient practice correct alignment and methods for reducing stress and pain in activities selected by the patient.
11. During the instruction have the patient identify appropriate principles and their application.
12. Throughout the instruction provide verbal, written, or demonstrative reinforcement when the patient expresses or demonstrates joint protection concepts correctly.
13. All written handouts or home programs should be designed for the patient's level of understanding.
14. Have the patient describe the relevance and importance of the instruction to his or her overall medical and rehabilitative program.

Additional information on developing patient education programs can be found in Chapter 2.

PRINCIPLES OF JOINT PROTECTION: RATIONALE AND TREATMENT IMPLICATIONS

Respect for Pain

Fear of joint pain can lead to unnecessary inactivity while total disregard for joint pain can lead to unnecessary joint damage and increased pain. Patients need to respect pain, that is, to understand the source of joint pain and how to monitor activity appropriately.

Clients should carry out activities and exercise only up to the point of fatigue or discomfort, before pain occurs. Time or effort spent on an activity should be reduced if pain does occur and lasts *more than one hour* after the client discontinues the activity. It is important that the client distinguish between usual arthritic discomfort and pain resulting from excessive stress to a joint. His or her understanding of the two can be facilitated through discussion. Occasionally a patient (not on steroid medication) will have a high pain tolerance or may not perceive the pain because of psychological denial. These processes should be considered when a patient with active synovitis reports doing strenuous activity without a proportional amount of pain. For these patients monitoring swelling and warmth is a more effective guideline than pain is for participating in activity; these patients should not do stressful activity using swollen joints.

For the client who is experiencing pain with activities, it is essential to review activities that are commonly overdone and discuss how to lessen them. For example, if a client does a moderate amount of housework in a two bedroom home and his or her knees hurt for the following two days, instruction in work simplification to minimize ambulation and knee stress is indicated.

Rest and Work Balance

The efficient and appropriate use of rest during the day's activities is probably the most effective weapon a person with arthritis can use against the demands of the disease. It is also the most difficult to incorporate into the patient's daily life.

Rest is prescribed for three reasons:

1. To help restorative processes in the body combat systemic disease.
2. To improve a person's overall endurance for activity.
3. To enhance the endurance of specific muscle groups.

Chronic pain and systemic diseases such as rheumatoid arthritis and systemic lupus erythematosus put a tremendous drain on a client's physical and psychological resources, thus resulting in excessive fatigue. Clients with systemic diseases need greater amounts of rest and sleep. *How much?* The consensus of rheumatologists is *10 to 12 hours* per 24-hour period, including a *1 to 2 hour nap* in the afternoon. It is crucial that each client understand the physiologic basis for resting and that suggestions regarding rest are specific to him or her as an individual.

The most effective method to increase functional endurance is *rest before becoming exhausted*. Taking a short 5 to 10 minute rest during activities is difficult but can significantly increase overall functional endurance. The concept of *resting for 10 minutes in the middle of vacuuming* is totally foreign for the majority of housewives. This practice implies lengthening the total time spent doing housework, and the desire to get housework over with is usually a strong one. Resting is also effective during activities such as shopping; sitting for only a few minutes *before* one becomes tired will greatly expand the total endurance for the activity. However, rest breaks during work not only increase endurance but also allow the client more energy later on for the activities he or she enjoys.

The practice of resting before one becomes tired or exhausted is so effective that it should be the number one priority in energy conservation instruction. Once a person employs this practice the benefits are usually self evident. With encouragement and some self discipline the patient (or therapist) can use this process to advantage.

Maintenance of Muscle Strength and Joint Range of Motion (ROM)

See Chapter 28, Functional Activities, and range of motion and muscle strength sections of Chapter 29, Exercise Treatment.

Reduction of Effort

Reducing the effort required in activities is recommended for people with arthritis because reduced effort produces less stress and therefore less pain to involved joints. In addition, it improves total endurance and allows clients more energy for activities they enjoy.

Principles of work reduction include (1) avoidance of excessive loads and heavy equipment by incorporating adaptive methods or assistive equipment[1] and (2) incorporation of basic energy conservation principles. The latter are not included here because they are discussed thoroughly in other resources.[3,4,5,6]

The following list of questions (compiled by Ceis Wilden, OTR) has been valuable for training patients to analyze their own activities. The list is not comprehensive, but its simplicity and directness facilitates patient use. It teaches patients an *approach* for questioning and analyzing their daily activities. After using it once patients often identify additional factors not included on the list and this patient participation reinforces the learning process.

Work Simplication: Task Analysis

Questions

1. How many trips were made between any two points?
2. Could the number of trips be reduced?
3. Could the order of performing different parts of the job be reduced?
4. Are materials and needed equipment within easy reach?
5. Do storage areas contain only the needed materials or are they cluttered with seldom used things?
6. Can any part of this be omitted or changed and still produce the desired results?

7. Are good body mechanics used in posture, sitting, standing, lifting? How can they be improved?
8. Are two hands used to the best advantage?
9. Would the use of wheels be helpful?
10. Are sitting facilities comfortable and of the proper height?
11. Are the materials pre-positioned and ready for use?
12. Is the rate of work too fast?
13. Should someone else do part of the task?

Avoidance of Positions of Deformity

The patient should avoid external pressure and internal joint stresses that facilitate common deformities.[1] The exact pressures and stresses to avoid depend on the joints involved and the disease entity being treated. This is especially important in cases of (1) MCP joint synovitis, when strong grasp and pressure against the MCP joints can play a significant role in deformity;[1,7] (2) knee involvement, when sleeping with the knees flexed can lead to contracture; and (3) ankylosing spondylitis, when characteristic deformities of neck flexion and hip flexion can be prevented.

Posture during work, leisure (particularly watching TV and reading), and bed rest are important considerations.

Use of Stronger/Larger Joints

Any given amount of stress is better tolerated by the larger joints.[1]

Use of stronger and larger joints includes use of feet to close low drawers and hips to push open doors; lifting packages with forearm and trunk; and use of palms rather than fingers to lift or push.

Proper body mechanics in lifting and daily activities should be observed (decribed in this chapter under back protection). However, back protection methods may require modification for patients with hip or knee pain.

Use of Each Joint in Its Most Stable Anatomic and Functional Plane

The patient should learn to use each joint in its most stable anatomic and functional plane.[1] This is especially important in protecting knees, wrists, MCP joints, and back. Using this procedure minimizes excessive stretch on joint ligaments and allows muscle power to be used to the greatest advantage.

When rising from a sitting position the client should avoid leaning to either side, since rotational forces may stress knee ligaments, thereby increasing instability.

Avoidance of Staying in One Position

Muscles become fatigued in a static position, and thereby transmit positional stress to the underlying ligaments and related structures. Additionally, prolonged positioning promotes stiffness. Sustained joint compression can cause pressure on damaged articular surfaces. Therefore the patient should avoid staying in one position for a prolonged period of time.[1]

A client should move frequently enough to avoid stiffness and the pain associated with prolonged static positioning. *It is recommended that clients change position* or stretch about every 20 minutes. This amount varies for each client. Some can tolerate 30 minutes without stiffness, while others can tolerate only 10 minutes without getting stiff.

Avoidance of Activities that Cannot be Stopped

Activities must be stopped immediately if they become too stressful.[1] Continuing a task in the presence of sudden or severe pain is likely to cause joint damage. Therefore, the client should be taught to avoid activities that cannot be stopped immediately upon stress, e.g., standing while showering, walking down a long hallway, or carrying a package a long distance. These tasks should be attempted only if there is a way to take a rest break as needed.

Use of Assistive Equipment and Splinting

This includes any assistive device or adaptive equipment, ranging from functional wrist splints and electric can openers to furniture adaptations. Many medical articles recommend that assistive devices should be issued only as a last resort, when the patient cannot perform the activity in any manner. This is valid in some instances, e.g., if stretching to reach the toes is good for a person, then a long shoe horn or sock donner may in fact be detrimental. But when working with arthritis patients it is also important to consider the use of equipment to protect joints prior to the presence of deformity and not only as a compensation for loss of function. (For further discussion of the use of splints and equipment to protect joints, see Chapter 25, Splinting for Arthritis of the Hand, and Chapter 27, Assistive Equipment.)

APPLICATION OF JOINT PROTECTION PRINCIPLES TO SPECIFIC JOINT INVOLVEMENT

All of the general principles of joint protection at the beginning of this chapter apply to each joint. The following specific principles are suggested in addition.

Fingers with Inflammatory Joint Disease

As mentioned earlier, the patient must avoid activities or positions that enhance deformities particular to his or her disease. (See Chapter 21, Hand Pathodynamics and Assessment, for the dynamics of deformities and Part II, Major Rheumatic Diseases, for deformities unique to each disease.) Children with polyarthritis develop a pattern of deformity that is different from adults. Typically they develop flexion contractures of the MCP, PIP, and DIP joints.[8] Ulnar drift of the MCP joints is uncommon; in fact, radial drift is seen more frequently.[8] Joint protection instruction needs to be individually designed to meet the needs of each child.

MCP INVOLVEMENT

MCP Volar Subluxation and Ulnar Drift

These deformities develop during the active phases of synovitis, when the joint capsule and ligaments not only are weakened by the inflammatory process but also are on stretch as a result of *intra-articular swelling*.[7] Almost all normal functional hand patterns, such as power grasp, hook grasp, palmar pinch, and strong lateral pinch, produce stress on the MCP joints that foster subluxation and drift.[7] The work of Smith and associates provides the theoretical basis for this joint protection concept.[7] (See Figure 37 in Chapter 25.)

Avoidance of hand usage that fosters drift and subluxation is most important during periods of active synovitis. This is difficult because most hand activities facilitate deformity. The most practical way of protecting the joint structures during active synovitis is by splinting the hand to minimize the influence of the long finger flexors during functional activities[7] and to teach clients to substitute bilateral prehension and to use their palms instead of fingers during activities. Splints for this purpose are described in Splinting for Arthritis of the Hand, Chapter 25. When considering splinting for this purpose it is important to keep in mind that immobilization or restriction of the MCP joints *may* cause additional stress to the PIP joints. See Hand Pathodynamics and Assessment, Chapter 21, for a detailed discussion of the role of flexor tendons in MCP joint deformity.

During periods of remission the value of joint protection techniques to prevent or forestall MCP subluxation and drift is highly questionable. However, joint protection techniques for the hands during remission are of value in reducing stress to the joints and thus reducing pain and improving functional hand strength. (Strength is enhanced by minimizing the pain inhibition factor.)

Methods suggested during periods of synovitis to reduce pain and improve functional strength include the following (Figs. 96, 97, and 98):

1. Use of the palm, heel of the hand, and lateral edge of the palm whenever possible. These are the strongest, most stable parts of the hand and the least vulnerable to

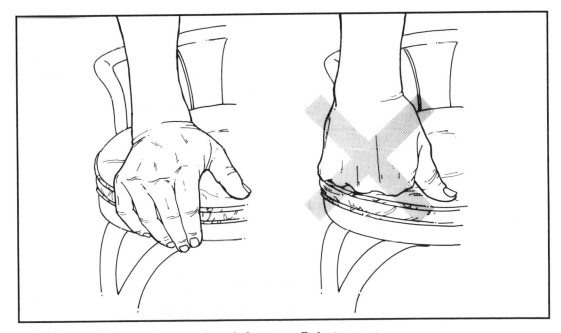

FIGURE 96. Pushing off from a chair: *Left*, correct; *Right*, incorrect.

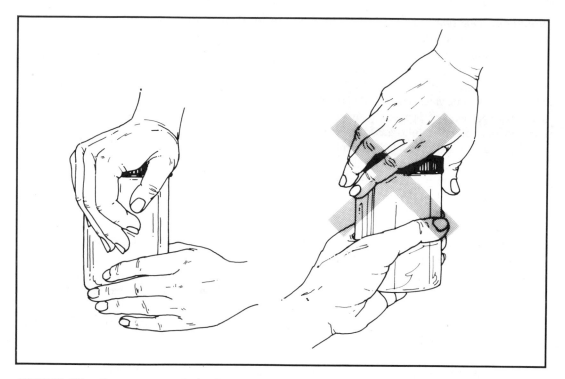

FIGURE 97. Opening a jar: *Left*, Correct, using heel of hand and avoiding metacarpophalangeal pressure; *Right*, incorrect.

stress. This method applies to lifting, pushing, opening jars, transferring, and manipulating switches and equipment. In addition, this practice serves to strengthen the finger extensors, since the fingers must actively extend to allow palmar contact.

2. Use of two hands instead of one when lifting (bilateral prehension).[1]
3. Use of the forearm for lifting and pulling, whenever possible. For car door and home appliance handles that are difficult for patients with weak hands to open, minimize stress by attaching a strap loop through the handle so the patient can open the door (or drawer) with the forearm (or palm of the hand) by slipping it through the loop.

Swan Neck Deformities

When swan neck deformities are due in part to intrinsic muscle tightness, the following is advisable:

1. Avoidance of prolonged intrinsic plus positions (see Fig. 44, Chapter 21) such as holding a book while reading, resting the chin on the dorsum of fingers, and resting or watching television with the MCP joints flexed and PIP joints extended and activities such as crocheting, knitting, and hand sewing. (See section on crocheting and

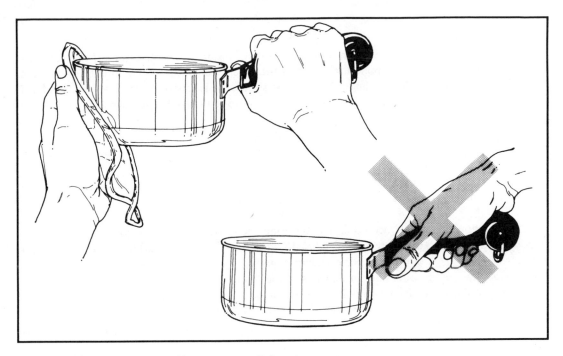

FIGURE 98. Lifting a pan: *Above*, correct; *Below*, incorrect.

knitting in Functional Activities. Chapter 28, for adaptive methods for performing these crafts.)

2. Hand activities or exercises that encourage full PIP flexion while the MCP joints are in extension (intrinsic muscle stretching exercises).
3. Splinting to keep the MCP joints in full extension and encourage PIP flexion. Splints may be used for positioning during stretching exercises, or they may be used during functional activities or all night. (See Chapter 25, Splinting for Arthritis of the Hand.)

PIP INVOLVEMENT

Boutonniere or Flexion Deformities

The three principles of treatment for these deformities are (1) avoidance of keeping fingers in a flexed position at rest; (2) daily ROM exercises; and (3) antideformity exercises, i.e., active DIP flexion with the PIP joint stabilized in full extension. It is desirable to maintain joint mobility with these deformities in order to facilitate personal hygiene and the application of gloves.

Splinting for boutonniere deformities needs further investigation. Several therapists have told me of cases in which early splinting has caused a reduction of the boutonniere. Personal experience with splinting moderate boutonniere deformities has not been successful. (Resources on splinting boutonniere deformities are at the end of Chapter 25, Splinting for Arthritis of the Hand.)

Wrists

Methods suggested for pain reduction and improvement of functional strength in MCP joint involvement of the hands also minimize stress to the wrist. Activities or positions that enhance volar subluxation and radial deviation of the wrist should be avoided. (See Chapter 21, Hand Pathodynamics and Assessment, for discussion of pathodynamics.) The following should be avoided:

1. Activities that involve wrist flexion and rotation, such as stirring with the utensil diagonal to the palm (Fig. 99).
2. Heavy lifting and traction, such as carrying suitcases and purses with hands forming a hook grasp (Fig. 100).

Reduction of stress is accomplished by using the wrist in straight alignment as much as possible and by using the forearm and trunk to lift items whenever possible. Wrist stabilization splints should be used during periods of active synovitis or when pain interferes with hand function. (See Chapter 25, Splinting for Arthritis of the Hand.)

One of the most effective methods for reducing stress to the wrist is the use of commercial elastic-vinyl gauntlet support splints. These splints allow approximately 50 degrees of flexion and extension, but they prevent circumduction, thus reducing considerably rotational stress

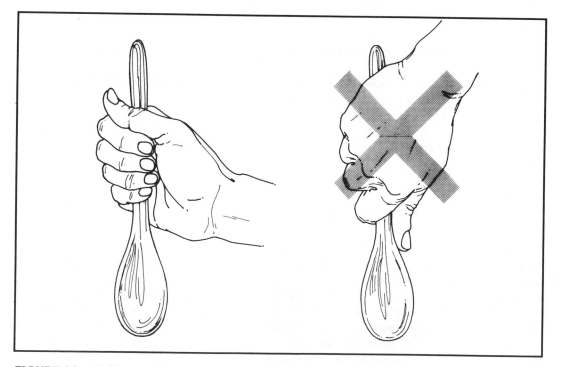

FIGURE 99. Holding a spoon for stirring: *Left*, correct with wrist in straight alignment; *Right*, incorrect.

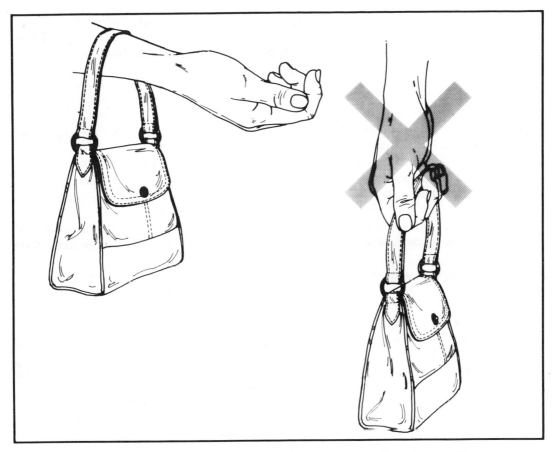

FIGURE 100. Carrying a purse: *Left*, correct, avoiding metacarpophalangeal stress; *Right*, incorrect.

to the wrist. These splints require the patient to use his or her wrists in a neutral, stable alignment during functional activities. These splints have a removable metal reinforcement. This reinforcement provides greater support for inflamed wrists, but for some patients it is too restrictive for daily use. The splint can be effective for joint protection even with the metal support removed.

Knees and Hips

Trauma to osteoporotic vertebra and hips can be reduced if the patient does not plop down when sitting into low seats. Stress to knees may be lessened by using seats of an appropriate height with arm rests. (See Chapter 27, Assistive Equipment.) Rising from a seat is also less painful and easier if the person moves to the edge of the seat prior to rising.

Facilitation of quadricep strength may be achieved prior to standing by having the patient (1) do a quad set, (2) straighten the knee completely once, or (3) flex and extend the knee two to three times in midrange. The choice of facilitation method depends upon which causes the least amount of discomfort since pain inhibits muscle strength.

For patients who are overweight, weight reduction is the most valuable method of joint protection. All overweight patients should receive dietary counseling and encouragement to participate in a weight reduction program. For patients with DJD of the knees, weight reduction alone can often eliminate symptoms.[9]

Feet

Patients with early foot involvement should be instructed in foot and toe ROM exercises to prevent insidious contractures secondary to digital muscle spasm.

Appropriate shoes are extremely important. They should be firm and lightweight with a resilient sole, provide good support for the longitudinal arch, have a soft upper with adequate width to accommodate splayfoot and hallux valgus deformity, give adequate depth (client should be able to curl toes inside the shoe), and have a firm heel counter.

The patient who reports that he or she can wear only soft shoes such as slippers should have a medical foot examination to determine if he or she would benefit from shoe adaptations or orthotics.

The following adaptations and orthotics have proven valuable for arthritic foot problems.

1. *Plastazote (¼-inch thick) shoe liners.* Easily cut from sheet Plastazote, these liners help to distribute pressure evenly over the foot and reduce pressure over the MTP heads. These are most effective in the course of the disease before subluxation takes place. These are often fitted in OT.
2. *Plastazote foot orthotics.* These are custom-made and designed to support the longitudinal arch and provide an MTP bar to reduce stress to the MTP joints by shifting the pressure of weight bearing proximal to the painful metatarsal heads. These orthotics can also be designed to provide accommodation of abnormal valgus. These orthotics are worn inside regular shoes. They are more effective than MTP bars fixed to the sole of the shoe.
3. *Polyprophylene or rigid plastic orthotics (similar to runner's orthotics) with an MTP bar.* These can be made with a heel cup, to reduce inversion and eversion and thereby reduce stress to the subtalar joint, and with a post to stabilize or reduce ankle valgus.
4. *Commercial extra-depth shoes.* These are most effective when the liner is removed and replaced with a Plastazote liner or orthotic.
5. *Custom-made soft leather sandals and shoes.* These are most frequently made to reduce pain that prevents ambulation in patients with severe deformity. The inside conforms to the deformity, distributing pressure over the entire sole of the foot and has a built-in MTP pad. These shoes can also be made with a heel cup to stabilize or reduce hindfoot subluxation.

Back

Avoidance of strain to lower back may be attained by observing proper body mechanics while sitting, driving, transferring, and working. (See end of this chapter for specific back protection methods.) Note: Proper or standard body mechanics for back protection may not be possible if there is knee or hip involvement. Individualization of instruction is essential. There are several publications on this topic. [12,13,14,15,16]

Neck

Stress may be avoided by keeping neck and back aligned as straight as possible during activity. (See later in this chapter for specific neck protection methods.) A support pillow may be used behind the head to keep proper alignment while reading or watching television. When doing desk work (reading or writing), methods such as elevating the work on a platform (e.g., on a portable bed tray) and using a book rack can facilitate appropriate neck alignment. [17,18]

A soft or semi-rigid (Plastazote) collar should be used when indicated, especially during activities with a high risk of neck injury, such as driving, and repetitive motion should be avoided. (For patients with limited hand or shoulder involvement it is helpful if the collar can be adapted with a side opening.)

The therapist should use a mirror to instruct the patient in proper neck alignment during activities. This is particularly effective because there are no visual body cues regarding neck position when the head is in straight posture alignment.

Shoulders and Elbows

Stress to these joints may be reduced by using long, sweeping, circular motions in activities, instead of abrupt back and forth motions, e.g., in cleaning tasks, such as wiping a table or washing a car. Clothing that is simple to get arms into should be used.

Women should use lightweight handbags that can be carried on the forearm for shoulder involvement or with a shoulder strap for elbow or hand involvement.

BACK PROTECTION INSTRUCTION

The following list of instructions has been prepared to use as a guide for client education and training. The instructions are written as directives for the purpose of clarity rather than to be used as a handout for patients.

A current, and probably the most successful, method of instruction is to teach the client the *two basic principles* of minimizing stress to the back—namely *reducing the lordotic curve* and *keeping the spine straight*—followed by demonstrations of specific home or work situations that require the client to work out how to incorporate these principles. This approach makes a list of methods or rules unnecessary and allows individualization of treatment.

The use of back protection methods for low back pain syndromes are most effective when used in conjunction with an exercise program in physical therapy to (1) strengthen the abdominal and back musculature, and (2) strengthen the quadricep and arm musculature (to accomplish lifting tasks.)

The basic principles of back protection are

1. *To reduce the lordotic curve.* Both the natural and exaggerated lordotic curves of the lumbar spine increase pressure on the posterior portion of the intervertebral disc. (This principle is true for most patients. However, occasionally, reduction of the lor-

dotic curve causes increased pain for a patient. These patients should be instructed in the postures that relieve pain.)

2. *To keep the spine as straight as possible during sitting and lifting activities.* Slouching, forward bending, or rotation of the lumbar spine increases pressure on the intervertebral discs.

Therapists who instruct patients in back protection techniques should be knowledgeable about the patient's specific pain syndrome and the total conservative management of low back pain. Information on low back pain is available in several texts.[14,15]

Specific Suggestions for Incorporating the Basic Principles

SITTING

1. Use straight back chairs with arms rather than over-stuffed chairs. Rocking chairs that support the lower back are helpful since they allow motion to ease back tension. (Principle 1)
2. Sit with buttocks as far back into the seat as possible.
3. Keep back as straight as possible when sitting or rising. When rising, pivot to the edge of the chair, lean forward at the hips, and use leg strength to rise. (Principle 2)
4. When sitting, keep the knees bent and higher than the hips by using a foot prop or crossing one leg over the other (Principle 1)
5. Avoid sitting for prolonged periods.

DESK OR TABLE WORK

1. All the general rules for sitting apply during desk work; a foot prop under the desk or table helps to keep one or both knees above the hips.
2. The type of desk and seating, working, and lighting arrangements should foster proper posture. If they do not, adaptations are necessary.
3. Always directly face the task; e.g., if sitting and facing the desk, do not reach to the side to pick up the phone directory. Turn your whole body toward the directory and pick it up using the arm muscles, not the back muscles. A stable swivel chair facilitates repetitious turning. (Note: People typically lift moderately heavy desk items with their back muscles and need to be taught how to lift using only the arm muscles.)

DRIVING

1. Get into the car by sitting on the side of the seat and pivoting into the car, keeping the knees together. (Principle 2)
2. Keep the seat as close to the pedals as possible to increase hip and knee flexion. (Principle 1)
3. Use a seat-back support. There are two kinds: one that provides a rigid or firm surface and one that provides contoured support for the back.
4. For severe back problems, a brace-corset may be indicated during distance driving.

5. Use seat belts and shoulder harnesses to minimize danger in the event of sudden stops.

STANDING AND WALKING

1. Women and men should wear sturdy low-heeled shoes.
2. During prolonged standing, shift weight from one foot to the other. Flatten the lower back by tightening the abdominal muscles and by tucking the buttocks under. Also keep knees slightly flexed. Avoid locking the knees in extension.
3. Avoid prolonged standing when possible.
4. Open doors wide enough to walk through comfortably. Avoid crowded conditions, sports events, and theaters, which often necessitate turning sideways while walking through areas, or at least be conscious about back alignment in such situations. The safest solution is to wear a corset in these situations.

LIFTING AND TRANSPORTING OBJECTS

1. When lifting items below waist height, e.g., on a low shelf or on the floor, face the object with feet about 12 inches apart and one foot forward and squat down, keeping the back straight (as if doing a deep knee bend). Place hands underneath the object if possible. Then, keeping the back straight, tighten the stomach and back muscles. Raise your body and the object using only the leg (quadricep) muscles. This is the only recommended method of lifting. Lifting with the back by keeping the legs straight and bending at the waist is contraindicated because the mechanical stress to the third to fifth lumbar vertebrae is excessive and approximately 150 percent greater than with the leg-lift method. (Note: the recommended method of lifting with the legs is included in all body mechanics literature; however, a person needs strong quadricep muscles and good knee joints to carry out this advice. Professional furniture movers and truck drivers with low back problems probably would have no trouble, but the average housewife or sedentary worker will probably need quadricep strengthening to benefit from this method. Clients often need quite a bit of practice to incorporate this method spontaneously.)
2. Assistance should be sought to lift any items that cannot be lifted in the recommended manner.
3. Heavy items *should not* be lifted overhead. When removing lightweight items from a high shelf: (1) use a stepstool whenever possible, (2) place one foot on a sturdy step to ease low back muscle tension, or (3) place one foot forward and reach for the object with body weight on the forward foot and transfer weight to the back foot as you bring the object down, keeping the back as straight as possible. Reverse the process for placing an object on the shelf. (Do not keep feet even or parallel when reaching high.)
4. Carry objects as close to the body as possible because stress to the spine increases proportionately to the distance of the carrying lever arm.
5. Avoid carrying heavy objects that necessitate leaning backwards for balance, since back hyperextension increases the lordotic curve. (Principle 1)

6. Slide objects instead of lifting whenever possible, keeping the back straight. (Principle 2)
7. Avoid carrying unbalanced loads, e.g., one heavy suitcase with one arm and nothing with the other. (Principle 2)
8. When pushing an object keep one foot forward with knees bent, tighten the back muscles to keep the spine straight, and then use the leg (quadricep) muscles to move the object.

COUNTERWORK

1. Keep frequently used items within easy reach or at counter level. (Principle 2)
2. Use a high stool with back support and footrest or footbar to keep one or both knees flexed. (Principle 1)
3. When standing for a prolonged period, keep one foot on a stepstool or an opened lower drawer to ease back muscle tension. (Principle 1)

HOUSE AND YARD CARE

1. Alternate tasks and incorporate short rest periods to avoid fatigue.
2. Use adaptive equipment to avoid bending, e.g., extended handles, dusters, bathbrushes, toilet brushes, and dustpans.
3. Eliminate unnecessary motions and tasks.

MOPPING, VACUUMING, SWEEPING, AND RAKING

1. Use equipment with handles long enough to avoid stooping. (You may adapt handles with extensions.)
2. Face the material or area being cleaned. Do the work in front, not to the side, to minimize twisting. Keeping the knees slightly bent while working also helps reduce the tendency to twist.

FIREPLACE LIGHTING

Kneel or light fire from a low stool, using long fireplace matches.

WASHING OF CAR, WALL, OR WINDOWS

1. For portions above head level, keep one foot on a stepstool or use a stepladder keeping feet at different levels. Reach with one arm at a time. (Principle 1)
2. For lower portion, kneel (as described for lifting), keeping the back straight.
3. Keep water bucket or cleansing materials on a chair or stool to avoid bending.

TUB CLEANING

1. Kneel and use an extended handle toilet brush for cleaning.
2. After bathing, put a strong washing detergent in the water to reduce or prevent tub ring, thereby reducing the necessity for scrubbing.

CLOTHES WASHING

1. A front loading washer is preferred over a top loading because it allows loading from a kneeling or squatting position or from a low stool. The top loader necessitates bending. (Principle 2)
2. Wash frequently rather than once a week or every two weeks.
3. Transfer multiple small loads rather than single large ones.
4. Lower clothesline to shoulder height. Elevate wash basket on a chair. (Principle 2)

BEDMAKING

1. Raise the bed 3 to 4 inches on blocks to miminize back stress. If this is not sufficient or possible, an alternate method is making the bed while on one's knees. (Principle 2)
2. Straightening the covers while in bed before arising will minimize this daily chore.
3. Have bed away from wall or on coasters for easy moving.

INFANT-CHILD CARE

1. Always use arm or leg muscles rather than back muscles when lifting an infant.
2. Have the child stand on a chair or stepstool while you are dressing or performing facial hygiene for small children. (Principle 2)
3. Kneel while washing a child in the tub. (Principle 2)
4. Wash, change, and dress the infant at counter height. (Principle 2)

DRESSING AND HYGIENE ACTIVITIES

1. Lower extremity dressing (including shoes) should be done from a sitting position, bending the knees (one at a time) instead of the back. If dressing in this manner is not possible, devices such as long-handled shoehorns, dressing sticks, and stocking aids are helpful. (Principle 2)
2. Comfortable garments with front openings should be used to minimize the need for twisting during upper extremity dressing. (Principle 2)
3. During bathing or showering a cloth backscrubber (one pulled from side to side) is preferable over a long-handled brush for back washing. The long-handled backbrush, however, is helpful for lower extremity washing.
4. Hair washing is best done in the shower.
5. Bending over the sink for washing the face, brushing the teeth, and shaving can be

accomplished by bending the knees and hips and keeping the back straight (instead of bending at the back).

6. An electric shaver is preferable over a safety razor for men since it does not require bending to use the sink. (Principle 2)

BED REST

1. Recommended sleeping positions* for reducing the lordotic curve are:
   a. Sidelying with knees and hips flexed (fetal position).
   b. Supine with pillow under knees.
2. Lying prone is not recommended. If, for some reason, it is essential, a small pillow should be placed under the pelvis to reduce the lordotic curve.
3. When lying in bed, do not reach overhead or rest both arms behind your head since this increases the lordotic curve.
4. When rising from a lying position, roll to the side and move to the edge of the bed, keeping the back straight and the hips and knees bent. Use the arms to push up to a sitting position while lowering the feet to the floor.
5. A mattress on top of firm box springs should be used. A bed board (3/4-inch plywood) should be used only as a last resort when it is not possible to purchase a firm bed.
6. The value of a water bed for back pain is uncertain and appears to depend on the individual. The supportive effect depends a great deal on how much it is filled. An air-filled or padded bumper facilitates transfer in and out of bed. Water beds have been reported to enhance the maintenance of a stationary position, thereby reducing the need to change positions.
7. Electric blankets are often helpful since they provide consistent warmth and are lightweight and easy to manage.

SEXUAL POSITIONING

The recommended positions are those that allow hip and knee flexion, e.g., the lower position in the traditional missionary position or various sidelying positions. Many if not most patients are able to alter their positioning to accommodate back pain without any advice. However, there are many patients who use only the traditional position and may need to hear advice from an authoritative medical person to consider alternative methods.

NECK PROTECTION INSTRUCTION

The one objective of all neck protection methods is *to keep the neck in neutral alignment during activities.* Another way to conceptualize this principle is *to keep the back and neck in as straight a line as possible.*

Motions or positions that should be avoided include neck extension (hyperextension), *prolonged* forward and lateral flexion or rotation, and repetitive motion in any direction.

---

*These positions are contraindicated for people with arthritis of the hips or knees.

A soft neck collar can be an excellent training aid for instructing patients in neck protection techniques. A soft neck collar maintains the neck in neutral alignment. If a patient practices the daily activities below while wearing a soft collar, he or she learns how to position work, reading, and so forth, to accommodate the restriction of the collar. This is the positioning and alignment the patient should use without the collar. After learning proper body mechanics the patient can discontinue using the collar or save it for specific activities during which it may be too difficult to maintain alignment without an aid.

Generally a soft collar needs to be ordered by a physician. Using a collar only as a teaching aid versus having the patient wear one all the time needs to be cleared with the referring physician.

Specific Suggestions for Incorporating the Basic Principles

SITTING AND DESK WORK

1. Chair type and desk height should facilitate proper posture. When sitting erect in a chair, the desk should be at a height that supports the elbows, with the elbows touching the body or two inches away. If the desk is too short, it becomes necessary to slouch to support the elbows. Also the lower the table is the more neck flexion is required to perform desk work.
2. Prolonged writing should be done on an angle, e.g., at a drafting table, with a tilted desk top, or through the use of a clip board propped up on an angle. This reduces the neck flexion necessary for horizontal work.

READING

1. Prolonged reading should be done with the book at eye level on an angle with the desk or table. This can be accomplished through the use of an inexpensive book rack propped up on a stack of books or on a file tray.
2. Reading in bed or slumped in a chair is contraindicated since this can require prolonged forward flexion of the neck.
3. Bifocals that require neck hyperextension in order to use the reading portion are not recommended. Reading glasses or bifocals with a large lower portion are preferred.

SECRETARIAL WORK

1. Typing: Ideally, the copy draft should be placed at eye level directly above the typewriter.* This eliminates the need for repetitive neck rotation and flexion which is necessary when the draft lies flat and to the side of the typewriter.
2. Telephone use: Frequent or prolonged use of a telephone can put a severe stress on the neck muscles. The most efficient method for eliminating this stress is to use a device* (designed like a drafting light) that maintains the receiver at an ear level posi-

---

*A draft holder and telephone holder designed for these purposes are produced by Luxo Lamp Corporation, Monument Park, Pt. Chester, NY 10573. Available through most distributors.

tion, without the use of hands or neck muscles to position it. Another alternative is to use a light weight headphone.

DRIVING

1. Place the seat as close to the wheel as possible to facilitate proper spine alignment.
2. Add or adjust mirrors to minimize neck motion. A side mirror on the right side of the car and a bubble mirror attached to the side mirrors can be helpful in reducing the need for turning to see blind spots (a task not possible if the neck muscles are in spasm).
3. Headrests positioned so they do not necessitate neck hyperextension are recommended. Permanent headrests that are set too far back should be built up with foam padding or exchanged for a different type of pad.

LIFTING AND TRANSPORTING OBJECTS

Lifting methods described in the back protection section also apply to neck protection, because bending the back to pick up something instead of squatting necessitates neck hyperextension. Likewise, reaching for objects overhead instead of using a stepstool requires neck hyperextension.

BED REST

1. Sleeping in a sidelying or supine position is recommended; sleeping in a prone position is contraindicated because it maintains the neck in a prolonged rotated position.
2. A firm mattress and springs should be used with a bed board as indicated.
3. A round, tubular pillow designed for cervical pain syndromes (Cervipillo) is an important adjunct to neck protection because it maintains optimal neck alignment in both the supine and side-lying positions. These pillows are available at major rehabilitation equipment distributors and have high patient acceptance. Thick multiple pillows are contraindicated since they cause excessive neck flexion. Patients with respiratory difficulty who need head elevation should raise the head of the bed 4 to 8 inches on blocks.

SELF-CARE ACTIVITIES

In general, commonly used items should be placed within easy reach.

Dressing. Avoid pullover garments that require neck extension.

Hair Care. Shampoo hair in the shower since this is the only means of maintaining proper neck alignment during hair care.

Facial Hygiene. Use a wash cloth while maintaining the neck in good alignment. Rinsing the face without a cloth or brushing the teeth over the sink can put the neck into severe extension. If bending over the sink is necessary it should be done with the chin tucked in. For men, an electric shaver requires less hyperextension than a safety razor.

Drinking. Drinking from bottles, small glasses, or cans should be avoided. Wide mouth glasses and cups or straws are recommended.

REFERENCES

1. Cordery, J. C.: *Joint Protection: A responsiblility of the occupational therapist.* Am. J. Occup. Ther. 19:285, 1965.
2. Silwa, J.: *Performance objectives for joint protection instruction.* AHP Newsletter, Arthritis Foundation, Vol. 12, No. 4, Winter, 1978-79.
3. Gilbert, D.: *Energy expenditures for the disabled homemaker: Review of studies.* Am. J. Occup. Ther. 19:321, 1965.
4. Fish, H. U.: *Take it easy, Nos. 1,2 and 3.* American Heart Association, New York. (Pamphlets on work simplification methods for the homemaker.) Also in the *Heart in the Home* booklet.
5. Rusk, H. A., et al: *A Manual for Training the Disabled Homemaker.* Rehabilitation Monograph VIII, ed. 2. Institute of Rehabilitation Medicine, New York University Medical Center, New York, 1961. (Excellent section on work simplification.)
6. Zee, E., Feit, L., Jallo, L., Stewart, J., Warner, K., and Wood, B.: *Manual on Motion Economy.* Occupational Therapy Department, City of Hope Medical Center, 1500 East Duarte Road, Duarte, Calif. 91010. (In English or Spanish)
7. Smith, E. M., Juvinall, R., Bender, L., and Pearson, J.: *Role of the finger flexors in rheumatoid deformities of the metacarpophalangeal joints.* Arthritis Rheum. 7:467, 1964.
8. Chaplin, D., Pulkki, T., Saarimaa, A., and Vainio, K.: *Wrist and finger deformities in juvenile rheumatoid arthritis.* Acta Rheum. Scand. 15:206, 1969.
9. Templeton, C. L., et al: *Weight control group approach for arthritis clients.* J. Nutrition Educ. Vol. 10, Jan-Mar, 1978.
10. Wood, B.: *The Painful Foot.* In Kelley, W. M., et al. (eds.): *Textbook of Rheumatology.* W. B. Saunders, Philadelphia, 1981.
11. Ishmael, W. K., and Shrobe, H. B.: *Care of Your Feet.* J. B. Lippincott, Philadelphia, 1967.
12. Berland, T., and Addison, R. G.: *Living with Your Bad Back.* Bantam Books, New York, 1972.
13. Ishmael, W. K., and Shrobe, H. B.: *Care of Your Back.* J. B. Lippincott, Philadelphia,
14. Macnab, I.: *Backache.* Baltimore, Williams & Wilkins, 1977.
15. Finneson, B. E.: *Low Back Pain.* J. B. Lippincott, Philadelphia, 1973.
16. Preston, G. M.: *Advice on housework for patients with low back pain.* Occup. Ther. (Br.) March, 1976, p. 24.
17. Jackson, R.: *The Cervical Syndrome,* ed. 4. Charles C Thomas, Springfield, Ill., 1977.
18. Ishmael, W. K., and Shrobe, H. B.: *Care of Your Neck.* J. B. Lippincott, Philadelphia, 1966.

ADDITIONAL SOURCES

Adler-Korbel, M.: *A Joint Effort.* The Western Washington Chapter, Arthritis Foundation, Dexter Horton Building, Seattle, Washington 98104.

Brattstrom, M.: *Principles of Joint Protection in Chronic Rheumatic Disease.* Yearbook Medical Publishers, Chicago, 1975.

Haviland, N., Kamil-Miller, L., and Sliwa, J.: *A Workbook for Consumers with Rheumatoid Arthritis.* American Occupational Therapy Association, Distribution Center, 1383 Piccard Drive, Rockville, Md. 20850.

Johnson, E. W., and Wolfe, C. V.: *Bifocal spectacles in the etiology of cervical radiculopathy.* Arch. Phys. Med. Rehab. 53:201, 1972.

Joint Protection and Energy Conservation for the Early Rheumatoid Arthritis Patient. A slide-tape presentation with a patient teaching booklet. Graphic Plus Associates, 214 Boulevard of the Allies, Pittsburgh, Pa. 15222.

Work Simplification. (A patient instruction booklet.) Bellin Memorial Hospital, 744 South Webster Avenue, P.O. Box 1700, Green Bay, Wisconsin 54305 ($2.50)

27

ASSISTIVE EQUIPMENT

This chapter is limited to the specific considerations needed in assistive equipment when working with arthritis patients. Equipment or adaptive methods are used as a treatment modality to achieve the following goals:

1. *Reduce pain* and preserve joint integrity by minimizing extraneous stress.
2. *Increase the patient's independence* in a task that otherwise could not be performed because of a physical limitation.

FACTORS TO CONSIDER WHEN EVALUATING AND ORDERING EQUIPMENT

The evaluation of the patient's equipment needs is part of the Activities of Daily Living (ADL) assessment. When selecting or designing equipment for patients with arthritis, it is important to keep the following considerations in mind:

1. *The patient's equipment needs in the morning may differ from those in the afternoon; they may also differ during periods of exacerbation and remission.*

Example: Many patients are dependent the first two to four hours in the morning but independent in the afternoon as their morning stiffness wears off. A portable raised toilet seat would allow easy removal by the patient when it is not needed in contrast to a permanent seat which cannot be easily removed.

2. *The equipment may affect other joints of the body.*

Example 1: One of the most common situations is the issuance of a cane, crutch, walker-aid, or wheelchair to protect the lower extremities without consideration of the deforming stresses that the ambulation aid can cause to the wrist, hand, or shoulder.

Example 2: Equipment ordered for shoulder or elbow range limitations frequently have long lever arms and can cause severe stress to the hands, e.g., extended handle brushes or reachers.

3. *Activities and equipment involving strong grasp are contraindicated for patients with metacarpophalangeal involvement.*

Solution: For patients with active MCP synovitis, MCP subluxation, or tight intrinsic muscles, provide a splint to maintain MCP extension during the activity. When this is not feasible, adapt the handle to keep the MCP joints in extension. This should also include adaptation of cane, crutch, and walker-aid handles. Adapted handles to keep the MCP in extension can be of three shapes: rectangular, cone, and elliptical cone. (Note: Patients with protective ulnar drift splints frequently need handles built up to facilitate grip.)

4. *Some patients with wrist or hand involvement are unable to grip standard transfer assist equipment.*

Solution: Order grab bars or transfer bars that attach to the edge of the tub or floor-to-ceiling poles so the patient can hook his or her forearm around the bar for leverage. Bars may need to be padded. Also, patients with thumb CMC adduction contractures may not have sufficient motion to grasp transfer bars or ambulation aids adequately. For these patients a narrow or thinner bar may be needed to allow functional grasp.

5. *Convenience appliances are not always convenient for patients with arthritis.*

Example: Many electrical appliances such as electric can openers, knives, and toothbrushes operate with buttons that are too difficult for patients with hand involvement to use or they can be too heavy for a patient to hold long enough to complete the task required. Therefore, it is imperative that the therapist be familiar with the strength and dexterity required to operate an appliance before ordering it for a patient.

6. *A change in ambulation aids requires instruction in ADL.*

Example: If there is a decrease in ambulation status and the patient needs to use a crutch, walker, or wheelchair, it is important that he or she receive retraining as to how to do work with the required aids.

COMMON FUNCTIONAL LIMITATIONS AND POSSIBLE SOLUTIONS

The following list will familiarize therapists with *some* of the equipment or methods used for certain physical limitations. Not all the physical problems are included nor is the solution list exhaustive. It is designed to stimulate thinking and to acquaint therapists, new to arthritis patient care, with some of the equipment available. The Arthritis Health Professions Section of the Arthritis Foundation has recently revised and updated a self-help manual that includes a comprehensive review of assistive equipment for arthritis patients. (See resources at end of chapter.)

Hand Involvement

Joint protection for hands (see Chapter 26)
Adapted, built-up handles
Nonslip pads or plastic sheets, e.g., Dycem mats (to reduce stress required to stabilize items)
Faucet turners
House or car key adaptations
Lamp switch extenders
Soaped runners on kitchen drawers for easier sliding
Light weight kitchen utensils
Electric can opener
Jar opener
Tea kettle tipper

Bowl holders
Saucepan stabilizers
Spring loaded clipping scissors
Suction bottle/glass brushes
Electric scissors
Strap loops for forearm (for oven doors, drawers, sliding doors) (allows operation with forearm)
Shoulder strap for handbags, suitcases, shopping bags
Blanket cradles or ribbon handles on blankets (to make blanket manipulation easier)
Electric blankets (to minimize bulk)
Sheet tucker (small wooden paddle)
Universal cuff to hold brushes, silverware, pencils
Book racks
Writing devices
Electric shaver or cup holders
Buttonhooks
Soap on a rope (for shower or tub)
Car door openers
Aerosol can dispenser
Luggage carrier (can also be used around the house)

Shoulder Involvement

Extended handles with enlarged grip on hairbrushes, combs, toothbrushes, tableware, backbrushes
Long cloth back scrubbers (preferred over backbrushes)
Extended drinking straws
Coat holders
Reachers
Dressing sticks
Front-opening clothes
Sponges and dustpans with extended handles for floor care
One-handed hair rollers

Neck Involvement

Typing draft holder
Adjustable book holders
Cervical contour pillows (available from medical distributors)
Telephone receiver holders

Knee Involvement

Elevated chairs in the living room, kitchen, at work (and in the clinic)
High kitchen stool
Raised toilet seat

Arm bars for toilet
Shower bench
Tub grab bars
Walking aids
"Half step" or short steps
Tea cart for transporting dishes, etc.
Shopping carts

Hip, Back, or Elbow Involvement (which limits hand to foot or floor range)

Reachers
Sock dressers
Elastic shoe strings
Dressing sticks
Pants dressing poles
Extended shoehorns
Double-faced carpet tape on the end of a stick (to pick up small items like pills or broken glass)

Lack of Hip Flexion (extension contractures)

Specially adapted chairs and toilet seats that allow the patient to sit upright with the hips in less than 90 degrees of flexion.

EQUIPMENT RESOURCES

Equipment is described in more detail (with purchasing or construction information) in the following publications.

Aids and Adaptations. Compiled by the Occupational Therapy Department, Canadian Arthritis and Rheumatism Society, British Columbia Division, Vancouver, Canada. (Contains designs and instructions for fabrication.) Available from C.A.R.S, 45 Charles St. E., Toronto, Ontario, Canada. Cost $2.50.

Davis, W.: *Aids to Make You Able,* ed. 3. 120 pp. Available from Fred Sammons Inc., Box 32, Brookfield, Ill. 60513.

Hodgeman, K., and Warpeha, E.: *Adaptations and Techniques for the Disabled Homemaker.* Rehab. Publ. No. 710, 1973. Sister Kenny Institution, 1800 Chicago Avenue, Minneapolis, Minn. 55404. Cost $1.75.

Lowman, E. W., and Klinger, J. L.: *Aids to Independent Living.* McGraw-Hill Book Co., New York, 1969.

Professional Self Help Aids Catalog. Fred Sammons Inc., Box 32, Brookfield, Ill. 60513. No charge.

The Independence Factory: Self Help Device Catalogs, Vols. 1, 2, 3. The Independence Factory, P. O. Box 597, Middletown, Ohio 45042. (Manufactures and/or provides fabrication plans.)

Self-Help Manual, ed. 2. Arthritis Health Professions Association, Arthritis Foundation, 3400 Peachtree Road, N.E., Atlanta, Ga. 30326, 1980. (Cost: $4.95; excellent resource.)

ADDITIONAL SOURCES

Bare, C., Boetke, E., and Waggoner, N.: *Self Help Clothing for Handicapped Children.* 1962 National Easter Seal Society for Crippled Children and Adults, 75¢.

Casamassimo, P.: *Toothbrushing and Flossing: A Manual of Home Dental Care for Persons Who Are Handicapped.* (Covers techniques, aids, and adaptations.) $1.50. Also, *Helping Handicapped Persons Clean Their Teeth.* 15¢ National Easter Seal Society for Crippled Children and Adults, 2023 West Ogden Avenue, Chicago, Ill. 60612.

Chamberlain, M. A.: *Aids and equipment for the arthritic.* Practioner 224(1339):65, January, 1980.

Chamberlain, M. A., Thornby, G., and Wright, V.: *Evaluation of aids and equipment for bath and toilet.* Rheum. Rehab. (Br.) 17(3):187, August, 1978.

Clothing Designs for the Handicapped. Accent Special Publications, Box 700, Bloomington, Ill. 61701. Designs for men, women, and children. Section on aids, directions for altering clothing and patterns. $15.00.

Fastow, K.: *Adapted knife for rheumatoid arthritis.* Am. J. Occup. Ther. 32(2):112, 1978.

Flaherty, P. T., and Jurkovich, S. J.: *Transfer for Patients with Acute and Chronic Conditions.* Rehab. Publ. No. 702, 1970. Sister Kenny Institution, Minneapolis, Minn.

Ford, J. R., and Duckworth, B.: *Physical Management for the Quadriplegic Patient.* F.A. Davis, Philadelphia, 1974.

Hale, G.: *The Source Book for the Disabled.* Paddington Press Ltd., London, 1979.

Klinger, J. L.: *Mealtime Manual for People with Disabilities and the Aging.* Available by writing to Mealtime Manual, Box 38, Ronks, Pa. 17572 or from Fred Sammons Inc.

Kaufman, M.: *Fare and feeding for patients with arthritis.* Am. J. Occup. Ther. 19(5):281, 1965.

May, E., Wagonner, and Hotte, E.: *Independent Living for the Handicapped and Elderly.* Houghton Mifflin, Boston, 1974.

McCullough, H. E., and Farnham, M. B.: *Kitchens for Women in Wheelchairs.* Illinois University Extension Service, Circular 841, 1961.

Moore, J. W.: *Adapted knife for rheumatoid arthritis.* Am. J. Occup. Ther. 33(2):112, 1978.

Ober, B.: *Clothing for the Aging Women.* Available from the Center for Studies in Aging Resources, North Texas State University, P.O. Box 13438, Denton, Texas 76203. $2.50.

Rusk, H. A., and Lowman, E. W.: *Self Help Devices.* Rehabilitation Monograph, XXI. Institute of Rehabilitation Medicine, New York University Medical Center, New York, 1965.

Sorenson, L., and Ulrich, P. G.: *Ambulation Guide for Nurses.* Rehab. Publ. No. 707, Sister Kenny Institution, Minneapolis, Minn., 1974.

Kitchen Conversions for Arthritis Patients. Columbia Hospital, Rheumatic Disease Program, 2025 East Newport Ave., Milwaukee, Wisconsin 53211.

Wright, V., and Moll, J. M. H.: *Seronegative Polyarthritis.* Elsevier, North-Holland Press, Amsterdam, 1976, pp. 411–415. (Includes a section on aids for patients with fused necks. Describes a unique right angle mirror for driving that allows patients to see traffic approaching from the side.)

28

FUNCTIONAL ACTIVITIES

Functional activities refers to crafts, games, and activities of daily living so structured as to achieve a specific therapeutic goal, such as increasing range of motion (ROM), strength, or dexterity. When these activities are performed with rheumatic disease patients, the following points are important to keep in mind.

1. When the activity is designed for treatment of a specific area, e.g., strengthening elbow musculature, it is important to be aware of the effect of the activity on other body parts. The severity of synovitis can vary from joint to joint. An activity effective for strengthening the elbow may aggravate the shoulder or wrist.
2. Home carry-over is a crucial factor in the treatment of chronic conditions. Selection of activities should be relevant to the follow-up home program. For example, floor loom weaving may be effective for maintaining a patient's upper extremity strength during hospitalization, but it is not as effective for insuring home follow-through as, perhaps, frame weaving or caring for house plants.
3. Joint protection principles should be applied to activities. For example, a patient with MCP synovitis should not perform activities involving strong grip or pinch (handles should be built up or splints worn as indicated), and the patient prone to joint stiffness should stand up or stretch during prolonged sitting activities. (For additional joint protection methods, see Joint Protection and Energy Conservation Instruction, Chapter 26.)
4. The basic treatment principles in using functional activities for restoration of ROM or strength are the same as those used for exercise (see Chapter 29). The functional activity program needs to be coordinated with the physical therapy program to avoid overexertion of specific muscle groups.

THERAPEUTIC CRAFTS AND GAMES

Crafts and games can be used specifically for physical restoration, but in general they play a minor role in rheumatic disease rehabilitation. Even though they can be an effective method for strengthening, increasing ROM, and improving endurance, they frequently are not as efficient as an exercise, and rising medical costs mandate efficient treatment. However, in certain instances, they can be both an effective and efficient modality.

Example 1: For an inpatient on a progressive shoulder-strengthening program, additional strengthening can be achieved in the evening or on the weekend with the use of elevated crafts and weighted arm cuffs. (Weights are not indicated for Grade 2 (poor) muscles as gravity offers sufficient resistance.) For example, frame weaving and macrame used in this manner can play a significant role in physical restoration.

Example 2: For strengthening finger extensors, frame weaving in which the patient packs the weft with the dorsum of the fingers is an effective treatment method. The project should have a loose weave; the amount of resistance is graded by the thickness of the weft.

Example 3: Peg games can be used to encourage motion of the metacarpophalangeal (MCP) joint when the proximal interphalangeal (PIP) joint is immobilized with a temporary splint. This can be a particularly helpful activity following MCP implant arthroplasty.

The efficiency of crafts in rheumatologic rehabilitation is a highly individualized matter. Therapeutic crafts and games effective for one patient may not be helpful for another. The use of crafts for general mental diversion has definite value but is *not* within the realm of current occupational therapy practice in rheumatology except when psychological responses, such as depression, are thwarting the medical regimen. Therapists should keep an open mind toward the use of crafts and games because additional exploration and experimentation are needed in this area.

Crocheting and Knitting

Crocheting and knitting are considered separately from other crafts because of the special role they play as avocations for many individuals confined by disease to a sedentary life. Both crocheting and knitting are unique in that they are traditional crafts which are easily learned, require minimal and available equipment, and are productive, i.e., they produce a usable, functional product. In addition they are crafts that can be performed by patients with severe hand limitations. Many therapists advise patients against performing these activities because of the effects that prolonged static positioning in an intrinsic plus position may have on the joints. However, the psychological benefit of being productive and making something that is useful, stylish, and valued by others is of great importance for rheumatic patients. Careful consideration must be made in advising patients with regard to these activities.

In general the only hand conditions in which knitting and crocheting may cause harm are (1) active MCP synovitis, (2) beginning swan neck deformities caused in part by intrinsic tightness, and (3) degenerative joint disease (DJD) of the carpometacarpal (CMC) joint of the thumb.

These crafts can have an adverse effect for a patient with active MCP synovitis by facilitating ulnar drift and MCP volar subluxation. Crocheting and knitting involve power pinch in a prolonged static intrinsic plus position and place ulnar deviating pressure on the MCP joints. (See Chapter 26, Joint Protection and Energy Conservation Instruction, for detailed discussion.) A patient, however, can perform crocheting and knitting without an adverse effect by wearing a hand splint that prevents the ulnar deviating pressures such as the splint shown in Figure 86 in Chapter 25, Splinting for Arthritis of the Hand.

For the patient with beginning or mild swan neck deformities caused in part by intrinsic muscle tightness, crocheting and knitting may increase the degree of intrinsic tightness by maintaining the fingers in a static intrinsic plus position. Any adverse effects resulting from participation in these crafts can be prevented by (1) wearing a hand splint that keeps the MCP joints in extension (as described above) or (2) performing intrinsic stretching exercises in addition to the crocheting and knitting.

The patient with degenerative joint disease of the thumb will probably find crocheting and knitting painful. However he or she can perform these activities without any adverse effect by using a thumb CMC stabilization splint (described in Chapter 25, Splinting for Arthritis of the Hand).

Generally, a patient with typical degenerative joint disease (in the fingers), progressive systemic sclerosis, or severe chronic inactive rheumatoid arthritis hand deformities would *not* be adversely affected by crocheting and knitting with the exception that prolonged positioning may cause increased joint stiffness when the activity is stopped. This patient usually is aware of this kind of problem and avoids increased stiffness by taking frequent rest breaks or doing the activity for short periods only.

An additional point to consider when advising patients about crocheting and knitting is that the psychological benefit of being productive and making something that is useful, stylish, and valued by others may be of greater importance to the patient than whatever amount of hand function *might* be retained by not doing the craft (or doing the craft without adequate protection).

LEISURE ACTIVITIES

Counseling on leisure activities to help patients develop avocational interests that are within their capabilities can play a valuable role in helping patients cope with disability and the restrictions it places on their lifestyle. This kind of counseling, like other interventions, is not needed by all patients. However, many patients, discouraged by their inability to participate in favorite hobbies or activities, need encouragement and a realistic plan for participating in alternative activities.

Occupational therapists by virtue of their training are in a unique position to provide this service to patients, for they are the only members of the health care team knowledgeable in the areas of rheumatology, kinesiology, and activity analysis. When patients have severe disabilities expertise in all of these areas is needed to develop a viable, successful, avocational program that the patient will enjoy and continue over a period of time.

Resources on leisure activities suitable for patients with arthritis involvement are listed at the end of this chapter. An increasing number of resources are available on gardening, since this is a popular activity for adults and children alike.

ACTIVITIES OF DAILY LIVING

Because the rheumatic diseases are chronic, it is especially important to minimize debilitation that occurs secondary to disuse and bed rest. One method for counteracting this problem is to have the patient perform activities of daily living to tolerance during hospitalization. For a patient with an acute condition this may mean only feeding and facial hygiene, but, for a patient on a rehabilitation service, activities could include making his or her bed, dressing and bathing daily, and attending a dining room for meals.

The use of activities of daily living as a therapeutic medium for patients with rheumatic disease is the same as for patients with other physical disabilities. The main role of these activities in physical restoration is in maintaining muscular tone and improving endurance.

To improve endurance, it is necessary to graduate the length of time the patient is able to participate in selected activities, e.g., cooking or personal hygiene (hair brushing, shaving). The activity selected should incorporate joint protection principles and should allow the patient to stop readily as pain and tolerance dictate.

ADDITIONAL SOURCES

Occupational Therapy and Activities

Barish, H.: *Introduction to Acrylic Painting—An Approach to Encourage Creative Expression in Older Adults.* Potentials Development Inc., 775 Main Street, Buffalo, N.Y. 14203 ($2.95)

Cohen, J.: *Occupational Therapy Following Hand Tendon Surgery.* In Symposium on Tendon Surgery in the Hand. American Academy of Orthopaedic Surgeons. C. V. Mosby, St. Louis, 1975, p. 292.

Cynkin, S.: *Occupational Therapy: Toward Health Through Activities.* Little, Brown, Boston, 1979, 157 pp.

Edwards, B.: *Drawing on the Right Side of the Brain.* (A course in enhancing creativity and artistic confidence.) J. P. Tarcher Inc., Los Angeles, 1979, 204 pp.

English, C., and Nalebuff, E. A.: *Understanding the arthritic hand.* Am. J. Occup. Ther. 25:352, 1971.

Eyler, R.: *Treatment of flexion contractures.* Am. J. Occup. Ther. 19:86, 1965.

Hale, G. (ed.): *The Source Book for the Disabled.* Paddington Press Ltd., New York, 1979, 288 pp. (Includes a chapter on a wide range of leisure and recreational activities and an excellent section on gardening.)

Rosenthal, I.: *The Not-So-Nimble Needlework Book.* Grosset and Dunlap, New York, 1977. (Includes projects and self-help aids and techniques. $5.95.)

Walker, A.: *A treatment program for rheumatoid arthritis.* Am. J. Occup. Ther. 14:207, 1960.

Gardening

Chaplin, M.: *Gardening for the Physically Handicapped and Elderly.* Royal Horticultural Society, London, 1978, 144 pp.

Gardening in Containers. A Sunset Book. Lane Publishing Co., Menlo Park, Calif., 1977. ($2.45)

The Easy Path to Gardening. Available from the Disabled Living Foundation, 346 Kensington High Street, London, W14 8NS.

29

EXERCISE TREATMENT

The occupational therapist applies the principles of exercise through functional activities for physical restoration. However, direct exercise is also an essential part of effective occupational therapy for many specific clinical situations.

EXERCISE FOR RANGE OF MOTION

Range of Motion (ROM) exercises are ones in which the patient or the therapist moves the body part through complete available range of motion. These exercises are utilized to *maintain* joint mobility and, when active or passive stretch is incorporated at the end of range, they can be used to *increase* joint mobility.

When prescribing ROM exercises, five issues need consideration: (1) how joint disease affects range of motion, (2) the type of exercise to use, (3) the minimal number of repetitions necessary to maintain or increase mobility, (4) the time of day the exercises should be done, and (5) follow-through.

How Joint Disease Affects Joint Mobility

Before recommending an exercise program it is critical to evaluate the musculoskeletal involvement and accurately determine the source of joint limitations. Range of motion can be limited by any of the following:

Joint synovitis
Tenosynovitis
Decreased tendon excursion
Muscle spasm (especially in juvenile chronic polyarthritis)
Muscle weakness
Tendon attenuation/rupture
Edema
Soft tissue contractures (fibrosis)
Bone erosions
Bony ankylosis

When inflammation is present, anti-inflammatory measures must be taken in addition to ROM exercise.

When deciding on a program for a particular patient, several factors need to be considered:

1. Synovitis not only weakens the joint capsule and supportive ligaments but also creates intra-articular swelling, placing these structures on stretch.[1] When a joint is swollen, excercise needs to be gentle to avoid addition of trauma.
2. Periarticular or extra-articular swelling causes joint compression and this by itself tends to cause range limitations; hence there is a need to reduce edema.
3. Pain induces spasms in the flexor-adductor muscles surrounding the joint (protective muscular splinting), limiting joint extension.[2]
4. Bed rest or inactivity secondary to pain increases the risk for adhesions, musculotendon shortening, and muscle weakness.

The interrelationship of these factors varies depending on the phase of arthritis present. In the acute and subacute phases, there is a greater risk of losing ROM because of periarticular edema, disuse, and muscular spasm. In the chronic-active phase dynamic forces acting upon weakened and overstretched supporting structures are the major threat to joint integrity. In noninflammatory joint disease ROM is often limited by bony growth (osteophytes).[3]

Types of Exercise: Force or No Force

The philosophy regarding active versus passive exercise for patients with arthritis is one of the most misunderstood concepts in rheumatologic rehabilitation. Physicians, fearful that therapists will apply strenuous exercise, often request active-assistance exercise, believing it is less strenuous than passive exercise. This may not always be the case. A patient can exert more stress on a joint by attempting active motion than he or she would exert during gentle passive motion. When a person has acute synovitis with associated pain and muscle spasm, active exercise increases the tension in the muscle and increases joint compression forces. Often in the presence of active synovitis, greater and less painful mobility can be achieved with gentle passive exercise. In certain joints such as the wrists, elbows, and ankles, active exercises may be the most effective and the easiest to carry out. For the larger joints, such as the shoulders, knees, and hips, passive exercise that incorporates muscle relaxation is often preferable for maintaining mobility during acute or active synovitis. In instances in which there is a lag in motion, e.g., due to tenosynovitis or weakness, passive ROM exercises are the only type recommended.

There are three forms of ROM exercises:

1. *Active ROM:* patient moves body part through full joint range without assistance, using the muscles related to the joint.
2. *Active-Assistance ROM:* active motion through partial range with assistance from an external force to complete range. External forces include:
   a. gravity-assist through positioning
   b. equipment such as deltoid aid and pulleys

c. functional exercises such as finger ladder climbing, cone stacking, and wand exercises
d. water (for ROM in hydrotherapy or in the tub)
e. verbal cues (encouragement) or visual feedback during exercises
f. another person (manual assistance)
g. use of muscles other than those involved in the motion of this act (self ROM)
3. *Passive ROM:* the body part is moved through complete ROM solely by an external force.[4]

The terms used to prescribe ROM exercises, i.e., active or passive, describe how the motion should be done but state nothing about the amount of force that should be used. If you want a patient to perform only active exercise without stretch, the procedure needs to be carefully demonstrated. Many patients become overzealous and think that if a little is good more is better, thus causing joint damage with inappropriate stretching.

The duration of pain is a guide for prescribing exercise. *Pain or discomfort resulting from the exercise should not last for more than one hour following the exercises.* If joint pain lasts for several hours or the patient feels excessive joint discomfort the following day, the exercises were too stressful and should be reduced.[5]

Stretch at the end of ROM is recommended to increase ROM in the chronic-active or chronic-inactive phases. Gentle pressure at the end of ROM may be indicated for the subacute phase to assure that *complete* ROM is being achieved. However, *stretch is not recommended in the acute phase.* This is primarily because it induces pain facilitating protective muscle spasm and puts additional stress on structures already on maximal stretch due to intra-articular swelling. Trauma at this point can cause additional scarring.[6]

How Much? How Often?

There is no hard and fast rule regarding the number of repetitions necessary to maintain or increase mobility. Some patients, e.g., those with stable, chronic conditions, may need to perform *only one complete ROM daily* for maintenance, while patients in an acute or subacute phase (when there is more periarticular swelling and less physical activity) *may* need to perform *two complete ROMs per day.*[7] Although this sounds simple, keep in mind that it may take two to five warm-up reaches for a person to achieve a complete ROM.[8]

To increase joint mobility, positioning of the joint to allow gentle-sustained passive stretch is the most effective method. This procedure takes advantage of muscle relaxation and lengthening of both the agonists and antagonist muscles.[9] For fixed contractures sustained stretch requires the use of progressive or serial splinting or casting.

When Exercises Should Be Done

Exercises should be done at the best time of the day for a patient, when he or she feels the most limber and following adequate analgesic medication. For some patients doing the exercises in or following a warm shower or bath is the ideal time. For other patients specific application of heat or cold prior to exercising may be indicated.[8]

Follow-Through

The self-ranging maintenance program of the patient is a major treatment concern because most forms of arthritis are chronic. I believe it is essential that all home programs be written out for the patient. If there is questionable comprehension or if there are follow-through problems, the exercise emphasis should be placed on the one or two joints most crucial to functional independence.

I have found it effective to start instruction of the home ROM program on the first day of treatment for inpatients, usually completing instruction by the third session. Subsequent ROM treatment during hospitalization consists of having the patient perform his or her ROM program under observation (patient is allowed to refer to the written program). This method does not guarantee follow-through, but it at least guarantees that the patient *can* perform his or her program independently at the time of discharge. It also allows time to modify the program.

The other instructional method I have found particularly effective is to use exercises that provide visual feedback of progression or regression for the patient. Treatment is directed towards having the patient monitor and alter his or her treatment as indicated between follow-up appointments.

1. *Shoulder and elbow ROM:* instead of having the patient reach as high as possible, have him or her face a wall, stand as close as possible, then reach as high as comfortably possible with each arm, and mark the wall at that point. A maintenance ROM exercise for shoulder flexion and elbow extension would be to touch each mark once a day with each hand.
2. *Finger hyperextension range:* have the patient place palms together, keep MCP joints touching, and hyperextend the fingers. While fingers are separated, patient can hold them to a ruler and measure opening span to monitor progression. (Maintenance of hyperextension ROM is not critical to function; however, it is the first motion lost in the presence of MCP joint involvement. This exercise helps maintain the extensibility of the volar structures.)
3. *Thumb web space:* with hand flat on a paper and thumb extended, have patient trace web space. Subsequent tracings can be done in a different color to mark improvement or maintenance.
4. *Finger abduction:* this can also be monitored with tracings of the hand while the hand is palm down on paper.
5. *Temporomandibular excursion:* have patient measure aperture between upper and lower teeth (with a ruler or marked index card in front of a mirror). This is especially important for progressive systemic sclerosis patients. It allows them to monitor jaw range and increase their exercises as needed.

EXERCISE FOR MUSCLE STRENGTH AND ENDURANCE

Basic Principles

When strengthening exercises are being employed for rheumatic disease clients, the following factors need consideration:

1. Does the client have a systemic disease? If so, the client's total daily activity regimen must be considered to avoid overexertion.
2. What is the extent of joint involvement in individual joints: acute, subacute, chronic active, and chronic inactive? The degree of inflammatory involvement can change from day to day. It is important to be aware of the effect a specific exercise may have on adjacent joints or body parts, e.g., exercise to strengthen the external rotators of the shoulder may aggravate elbow involvement.
3. Is the joint painful? When pain is a factor, all exercises should be done with the joint or body part positioned in the least painful position. All efforts should be made to minimize discomfort during treatment.
4. What is the goal of strengthening: Grade 5, Grade 4, or Grade 3 strength; Grade 5 or Grade 4 strength may be impossible for muscles associated with a damaged or inflamed joint. (See grading system defined on page 292.)
5. How will the goal be determined? By muscle test, a plateau of strength gains, functional ability? Having a definite program that gives the client visible feedback of progress can be a significant motivation factor.
6. How will strength be maintained once the goal is obtained? A definite program for maintaining achieved strength is essential.
7. The muscle groups treated should demonstrate some fatigue at the end of treatment, but not overfatigue. If pain brought on by exercise persists for over an hour after the activity is stopped or limits function, the amount of exercise should be decreased the following day.

Type of Exercise

Exercise for strengthening muscles takes two forms: isometric and isotonic. The method of choice for clients with joint disease is the method that induces the least amount of pain since pain inhibits strength.[10] Isometric exercises are usually the least painful for clients with joint disease since they eliminate motion, which is frequently a direct source of pain in damaged joints.

Isometric exercise can be as effective or more effective than isotonic resistive exercise for both maintaining and improving muscle strength and endurance in clients with rheumatoid arthritis.[11,12] Resistive isotonic exercise had been hailed as the superior strengthening method in the past, because it is the most efficient technique for increasing muscle bulk.[11] However, there is *no direct positive correlation between muscle bulk and muscle strength.*[10] A muscle can have severe atrophy and the patient can still demonstrate Grade 4 or 5 strength. This is a common phenomenon in rheumatoid arthritis, particularly in the intrinsic musculature of the hand. (Disuse weakness is not the same as disuse atrophy.) Specifically, because of this phenomenon, strengthening exercises should be directed toward the recovery of function rather than normal muscle structure or form.

Although isometric exercise is preferred when pain is a factor, isotonic exercise has a definite place in rheumatologic rehabilitation and is of particular value when motor function is being relearned, e.g., in tendon transplants and other postoperative treatment.

Amount of Exercise

The amount of exercise needed depends upon the specific treatment goal.

TO COUNTERACT DISUSE WEAKNESS

The amount of exercise for this goal is based on studies that demonstrate that (1) the strength of a normal muscle decreases at a rate of 3 to 5 percent per day during inactivity, and (2) a single daily contraction at 50 percent maximal strength is sufficient to maintain normal muscle strength.[13] A reasonable exercise protocol to maintain strength or counteract disuse weakness for clients with physical dysfunction and normal muscle innervation would be a single maximal strength contraction per day for each muscle group.

In addition to exercise, an important adjunct to combating disuse weakness and maintaining general conditioning is to have the client perform activities of daily living to tolerance.

TO IMPROVE MUSCLE STRENGTH AND ENDURANCE

One exercise program is needed to improve both strength and endurance. Clinically it has been shown that clients on exercise programs to improve endurance (i.e., low resistance-high repetition) demonstrate gains in strength, and clients on programs to increase strength (i.e., high resistance-low repetition) demonstrate gains in endurance.[11,14,15]

Several studies that evaluate strengthening techniques have been conducted for both normal subjects and people with rheumatoid arthritis.[11,12,13,16] In these studies, it has been demonstrated clinically that as little as six isometric contractions per day can significantly increase muscle strength. Two to four isometric exercises per day could constitute a strengthening program for the severely weak patient, while the client with Grade 4 or 5 strength may need more repetitions to improve strength and endurance. Again, there is no hard and fast rule regarding the number needed. Probably the best guide is the number of repetitions necessary to bring on just fatigue (not pain).

TO MAINTAIN STRENGTH GAINED IN TREATMENT

The optimal maintenance program is highly dependent upon the client's total daily regimen once maximal or the desired amount of strength is achieved. Sedentary patients may need to do a daily isometric exercise program, while more active clients may only need to do specific strengthening exercises once a week for maintenance. It has been demonstrated in normal subjects that maximal strength can be maintained with exercise as seldom as once every two weeks.[13]

Methods of Strengthening

ISOMETRIC EXERCISE

Definition

Maximal muscle contraction without joint motion. Often called muscle setting.

Positioning

The muscle or muscles being strengthened should be positioned slightly shorter than their resting length[17] (the point of maximal muscle tension during contraction). When it is not possible to stabilize the joint in this position, position the muscle at its shortest length. If this position causes pain, the joint should be positioned in a manner that produces the least amount of discomfort.[10]

Procedure

Have the client contract the muscle as tightly as possible without moving the joint and hold for six seconds (count of eight), or the desired amount of time, and then relax for six seconds. Repeat procedure for the prescribed number of repetitions. Studies in Poland have demonstrated that exercises done with a consistent rhythm are more effective than those done in a haphazard manner.[14]

PROGRESSIVE RESISTIVE EXERCISES (PRE)

Definition

A strengthening technique using isotonic exercise and definite grading of resistance. The type of resistance can vary from very gentle manual pressure to the application of heavy weights.

Indications

Indications for PRE are:

1. Postsurgical treatment when retraining of the motor unit and strengthening of the maximal number of muscle fibers is desired, e.g., tendon transfers.
2. To specifically increase muscle bulk.
3. In general, when joint pain is not a factor.

Precautions

Muscles need to be able to hold against slight resistance or more (Grade 3.5 strength) to use this method.

Procedure

The following procedures are suggested:

1. Assess the client's maximal resistance level. This is determined by trial and error. It is the maximal amount of resistance the client can move steadily and smoothly through active range of motion and return to resting. If the client trembles, starts fast, uses momentum, or releases fast, it is too much weight.

2. Begin the strengthening program with less than the maximal resistance tolerated. The right amount is that which causes slight muscle fatigue but does not overfatigue the muscle or cause pain that lasts for longer than one hour after the end of exercise.
3. The starting position is with the muscle lengthened. Have the client move the resistance smoothly and steadily through available range of motion.
4. The number of repetitions depends upon the treatment goal. Two to six repetitions per muscle group a day are sufficient to increase strength.

ACTIVE-ASSISTIVE EXERCISE USING A DELTOID AID

Definition

Treatment involving isotonic exercise through active range of motion with assistance from a counterbalance weight mechanism to complete range of motion.

Indications

To strengthen shoulder flexors and abductors with Grade 2 strength. (Note: equipment also provides resistive exercise to shoulder extensors and adductors.) This method can be incorporated during self-care activities, such as feeding, or with therapeutic crafts.

Procedure

Establish the minimum assistive weight, that is, the minimum amount of weight necessary to assist the arm through the desired amount of abduction or flexion. Begin the program with *more than* the minimum amount of weight necessary, reducing the assistance as strength improves.

MUSCLE RE-EDUCATION

Definition

Therapeutic exercise during the period of initial return of voluntary motor control.

Indications

Primarily for postoperative cases (e.g., tendon transplants, arthroplasties), neuropathies, and peripheral nerve injuries.

Procedure

Positioning is the same as for individual muscle testing. Directions for this are given in *Muscle Testing: Techniques of Manual Examination* by Daniels and Worthingham.[18]

    Restoring mental awareness of motor function is accomplished by demonstrating passive motion (visual), giving verbal description of motion and action (auditory), and stroking point of insertion of prime muscles (tactile). Robert Bennett gives an in-depth discussion of muscle re-education in Chapter 10 in Licht's book, *Principles of Therapeutic Exercise.* [19]

Developing muscle function:

1. The therapist manually assists the part through full available range while requesting maximum active contraction from the client. Palpate and decrease assistance as patient gains control of motion.

2. The patient should not use substitute muscles. If this occurs (especially if the patient is trying too hard), eliminate those muscles by increasing the amount of assistance.

3. It is important to establish good patterns of motion (control) before decreasing assistance.

4. Cutaneous stimulation techniques such as tapping, vibration, and brushing can be utilized to facilitate motor response.

REFERENCES

1. *Understanding Inflammation—A Giant Step.* A reprint from the 1969 Arthritis Foundation Annual Report. (Available from the Arthritis Foundation, 475 Riverside Dr., New York, N.Y. 10027.)
2. Swezey, R. L., and Fiegenberg, D. S.: *Inappropriate intrinsic muscle action in the rheumatoid hand.* Ann. Rheum. Dis. 30:619, 1971.
3. *Arthritis Manual for Allied Health Professionals.* Arthritis Foundation, New York, 1973, Chap. 2 (Available, no charge.)
4. Toohey, P., and Larson, C. W.: *Range of Motion Exercise: Key to Joint Mobility.* Rehab. Publ. 703. Sister Kenney Institute, Minneapolis, MN, 1968. (Resource for how to do passive ROM.)
5. Kendall, P. H.: *Exercise for arthritis.* In Licht, S. (ed.): *Therapeutic Exercise,* ed. 2., Elizabeth Licht Publications, New Haven, CT, 1965, pp. 702-720.
6. Flatt, A.: *Care of the Rheumatoid Hand.* C. V. Mosby, St. Louis, 1974, p. 37.
7. Mead, S., and Knott, M.: *Ice therapy in joint restriction, spasticity and certain types of pain.* Gen. Prac. 1961, p. 16.
8. Swezey, R. L.: *Essentials of physical medicine and rehabilitation in arthritis.* Semin. Arthritis Rheum. 3:352, 1974.
9. Flatt: *Care of the Rheumatoid Hand,* p. 44.
10. Kendall: *Exercise for arthritis,* pp. 715-718.
11. Liberson, W. B., and Asa, M. M.: *Further studies of brief isometric exercises.* Arch. Phys. Med. Rehabil. 40:330, 1959.
12. Machover, S., and Sapecky, A. J.: *Effect of isometric exercise on the quadriceps muscle in patients with rheumatoid arthritis.* Arch. Phys. Med. Rehabil. 47:737, 1966.
13. Muller, E. A.: *Influence of training and inactivity on muscle strength.* Arch. Phys. Med. Rehabil. 51:449, 1970.
14. Personal communication from M. Musar, Ph.D., RPT, Department of Rehabilitation, Rheumatological Institute, Warsaw, Poland.
15. DeLateur, B. J., Lehmann, J. F., and Fordyce, W. E.: *A test of the DeLorme axion.* Arch. Phys. Med. Rehabil. 49:245, 1968.
16. Rose, D. L., Radzyminski, S. F., and Beatty, R. R.: *Effect of brief maximal exercise on the strength of the quadriceps femoris.* Arch. Phys. Med. Rehabil. 38:157, 1957.
17. Darling, R. C.: *Physiology of exercise and fatigue.* In Licht, S. (ed.): *Therapeutic Exercise,* ed. 2. Elizabeth Licht Publications, New Haven, CT, 1965, p. 33.
18. Daniels, L., and Worthingham, C.: *Muscle Testing: Techniques of Manual Examination.* W. B. Saunders, Philadelphia, 1972.
19. Bennett, R.: *Principles of therapeutic exercise.* In Licht, S. (ed.): *Therapeutic Exercise,* ed. 2. Elizabeth Licht Publications, New Haven, CT, 1965, pp. 472-485.

30

POSITIONING
AND LYING PRONE

In a rehabilitation hospital with a rheumatic disease unit, bed positioning and prone positioning will probably be carried out by nursing personnel. However, in hospitals without a specific arthritis rehabilitation section, it is usually up to therapists to instruct the patient, family, and staff nurses in the proper positioning procedure for specific rheumatic diseases.

POSITIONING

Positioning for joint disease involves standard positioning procedures to achieve natural anatomic alignment and the addition of some specific splints. With joint disease, however, positioning is a primary treatment. The speed with which contractures can develop and the severity of the contractures necessitate efficient preventive care.

The Bed

AT NIGHT

The bed should be flat. Patients who have difficulty with reflux esophagitis or hiatus hernia should have the entire head of the bed, not just the mattress, raised 8 inches on blocks to aid esophageal motility and peristalsis, without encouraging hip flexion contractures.

DURING THE DAY

Head of bed raised only. *Knee gatch should not be raised* if there is active hip or knee involvement.

For patients with chronic arthritis, knee flexion in bed is permissible as long as it is alternated with periods of knee extension and as long as ROM is maintained.

It is common practice in hospitals to raise the knee portion of the bed slightly (technically called the semi-Fowler position) when the patient is sitting up, so the patient will not slide in bed. Ideally a footboard should be used that can be moved towards the center of the bed, so the patient can sit up in bed with knees straight and feet against the board.

Head and Neck

The first objective of cervical positioning is to support the cervical muscles, thereby allowing complete relaxation, and consequently reducing muscle spasm, pain, and stiffness; the second objective is to maintain the normal lordotic curve of the cervical spine.

The method selected should be comfortable, and the occipital bone, or back of the head, should be touching or close to the mattress. Sleeping with a regular pillow or without a pillow causes flexion of the spine and flattening of the lordotic curve and tension on the cervical ligaments and joints.

To determine the depth of the lordotic curve of the neck, have the patient stand with his or her back against a wall, head level, and occipital bone touching the wall. The distance between the back of the neck and the wall indicates the depth of the curve (providing the patient does not have marked thoracic kyphosis). A proper cervical support will fill this space and maintain this alignment.

The objectives of cervical support can be achieved by several methods: a cervical pillow; a soft, thin down pillow that can be shaped around the neck; or a soft towel or foam roll. The method does not matter as long as the objectives are achieved.

For people with ankylosing spondyloarthritis proper neck positioning is critical and can prevent deformity. They should use a soft neck roll or adapted cervical pillow that supports and maintains the normal lordotic curve of the neck but that allows the occipital skull to touch the mattress. (See Chapter 8, Ankylosing Spondylitis.)

Spine

Position as straight as possible. A small pillow under the low back may help maintain normal lordotic curve for patients *without* low back involvement.

Elbows

A volar positioning splint or bivalved cast may be the only solution for progressing elbow contractures or isolated elbow involvement. Care must be taken to maintain both flexion and extension range of motion (ROM).

Splint straps over the olecranon should be padded with fleece to avoid pressure over the ulnar nerve, which is more vulnerable when the elbow is flexed. The fleece padding also helps to keep the strap in place.

Patients with elbow nodules, sensitive skin, or ulnar nerve sensitivity often find hospital sheets or synthetic sheets irritating to the dorsum of the elbow. Slip-on elbow protectors, the type with a foam pad inside a knit sleeve, can greatly improve comfort during bed rest. These are particularly helpful to patients who rely on their elbows for mobility in bed. Currently there are two different brands of elbow protectors on the market. Both are excellent but have different qualities. The Heelbo has a stronger, more durable knit sleeve. It works well for children and patients with thin arms, because it fits more snugly and is less bulky. However, the snug fit makes it difficult for patients with painful hand involvement to pull on. Heelbo works well for people who need protection during the day, while they are working, since it is less bulky, fits under clothing, and has a less obtrusive appearance.

Another brand, Diamond, is less expensive and has more padding and greater bulk; however, its loose knit sleeve allows independent donning by most people with arthritis. It is helpful to have both brands available to meet the needs of all patients.

The lamb's wool elbow protectors are not recommended, because they are difficult to keep on and because their construction encourages elbow flexion contractures. The inexpensive thin foam protectors available in bulk are simply ineffective.

Hands and Wrists

In the hand the only adequate means of positioning joints with acute synovitis is with hand splints: full hand resting splint, wrist stabilization splint, or protective ulnar drift splint.

The wrist should be maintained in slight dorsiflexion (about 30 degrees) and slight (10 degree) ulnar deviation with the thumb in palmar abduction and opposition. Exceptions to this are (1) if there is wrist flexor tenosynovitis or median nerve compression, the wrist is kept in 10 degrees of extension; and (2) if there is a possibility of bilateral ankylosis, the nondominant wrist should be in neutral and the dominant or preferred hand in 20 degrees of extension. The degree of desirable finger flexion depends upon the joints involved. (See instructions for use of specific hand splints in Chapter 25, Splinting for Arthritis of the Hand.)

Hips

Neutral (full extension, zero rotation) is the desired position. Hip rotation can be controlled either by towel or blanket rolls placed on the lateral side of the hip, knees, and ankles or by a splint for the ankle with a rotation stop bar.

Knees

Full extension is the desired position, since knee flexion contractures are a serious threat to ambulation. Orthoplast, plaster, or aluminum full-length leg-resting splints should be considered for beginning or progressing contractures.

It is highly recommended that children with chronic knee inflammation wear Orthoplast full leg-foot splints at night. Incorporating the foot in the splint usually increases wearing comfort and avoids pressure areas around the ankle. If the patient complains of pressure from the top (proximal) edge of the splint, it usually means the splint is too short and needs to have a longer thigh protion.

Ankles

The ankles should be kept in 90 degrees of dorsiflexion. There are several methods for maintaining this position. The most effective is a posterior, short-leg, ankle-resting splint or bivalved cast (with or without a rotation stop bar). These splints allow the patient the most freedom to move in bed.

A footboard is essential for holding up the bedcovers so they do not rest on the feet, thus pulling them down into plantar flexion. The footboard is also helpful in teaching the patient daily ankle ROM, because the patient can press against the board until both the heel and ball of the foot touch the board. However, a footboard is not recommended as the only means of prevention of footdrop because a footboard becomes ineffective if the patient moves at all.

Whenever an occupational therapist fits a patient with an ankle splint, it is recommended that skin status and ankle ROM be carefully documented in the medical chart at the time of application. Frequently, patients develop pressure sores or flexion contractures that have gone unnoticed or undocumented prior to the splint application. These conditions may later be unjustly blamed on the splint and the occupational therapist who applied it.

Lamb's wool or knit sleeve protector pads (described above for elbows) can help reduce the risk of pressure sores on the base of the heel.

Another method of positioning that can be used with patients who do not have active ankle synovitis is to position a pillow under the entire lower leg (but not under the knee or heel). This method allows gravity to assist knee extension, and it elevates the foot to reduce edema and eliminates pressure on the heel. This method is commonly used following knee surgery.

Prone Positioning

Prone positioning is a specific therapeutic procedure for stretching the hip into full extension. The hip is a large joint with a strong capsular structure. Hip flexion contractures are the most common sequela to arthritis of the hip. Several factors contribute to hip flexion contractures. Hip flexion and external rotation is the position that relaxes the joint and reduces intra-articular pressure, so it is the position the patient assumes when there is hip pain. Most patients with hip pain sit as much as possible. All sitting and most sleeping postures maintain the hip in flexion. For many patients their hips are maintained in a flexed position 24 hours a day. For some patients hip pain causes spasm of the associated hip flexors and adductors, further reducing active motion. There is a strong Y-shaped ligament along the anterior capsule that can become contracted in the presence of chronic flexion positioning.

Patients with hip involvement should be encouraged to develop a routine for lying prone every day.

There is no hard and fast rule to the length of time spent lying prone. Some major rehabilitation centers advocate a goal of 90 minutes per day. Some patients can start right off with 3 sessions of half an hour each, while others can start with only 10 minutes per day and then build up tolerance.

PROCEDURES

Have the patient lie prone on a firm bed *with feet hanging over the edge* (to prevent pressure into plantar flexion). Small pillows should be used under the shoulders to increase comfort, straighten shoulders, and make breathing easier. Any amount of pillows can be used to improve comfort as long as they do not interfere with hip extension.

CAUTION: REGARDING PATIENTS WITH LOW BACK PAIN

Lying prone and lying supine with knees straight frequently aggravates low back pain by increasing the lordotic spinal curve. These positions are usually contraindicated or impossible for the patient with low back pain.

In fact, a patient with low back pain is advised to sleep with pillows under his or her knees or to sleep side-lying with knees bent. Obviously, this is a problem for the patient with concomitant knee or hip arthritis. This particular patient needs to be diligent in ROM exercise programs to prevent hip and knee contractures. The preferred hip ROM method for these patients is by stretching one hip at a time with the ipsilateral knee bent and the contralateral hip slightly flexed.

Range of motion and positioning programs need to be individually tailored for these patients.

ADDITIONAL SOURCES

Bergstrom, D., and Coles, C. H.: *Basic Positioning Procedures.* Rehab. Publ. No. 701. Sister Kenny Institute, 1800 Chicago Ave., Minneapolis, Minnesota 55404, 1971.

Jackson, R.: *The Cervical Syndrome,* ed. 4. Charles C Thomas, Springfield, Ill., 1978.

Nursing Care of the Skin, revised ed. Rehab. Publ. No. 711. Sister Kenny Institute, 1800 Chicago Ave., Minneapolis, Minnesota 55404, 1975.

Welles, C.: *Body mechanics of the bed patient as related to occupational therapy.* Am. J. Occup. Ther. 1952. (Excellent resource.)

APPENDICES

DIAGNOSTIC CRITERIA FOR RHEUMATOID ARTHRITIS

Classic Rheumatoid Arthritis

This diagnosis requires seven of the following criteria. (In criteria 1 through 5, the joint signs or symptoms must be continuous for at least 6 weeks. Any one of the features listed under Exclusions will exclude a patient from this and all other categories.)

1. Morning stiffness.
2. Pain on motion or tenderness in at least one joint (observed by a physician).
3. Swelling (soft tissue thickening or fluid, not bony overgrowth alone) in at least one joint (observed by a physician).
4. Swelling (observed by a physician) of at least one other joint (any interval free of joint symptoms between the two joint involvements may not be more than 3 months).
5. Symmetrical joint swelling (observed by a physician) with simultaneous involvement of the same joint on both sides of the body. (Bilateral involvement of proximal interphalangeal, metacarpophalangeal, or metatarsophalangeal joints is acceptable without absolute symmetry.) Terminal phalangeal joint involvement will not satisfy this criterion.
6. Subcutaneous nodules (observed by a physician) over bony prominences on extensor surfaces or in juxta-articular regions.
7. Roentgenographic changes typical of rheumatoid arthritis (which must include at least bony decalcification localized to or most marked adjacent to the involved joints and not just degenerative changes). Degenerative changes do not exclude patients from any group classified as rheumatoid arthritis.
8. Positive agglutination test—demonstration of the rheumatoid factor by any method which, in two laboratories, has been positive in not over 5 percent of normal controls.
9. Poor mucin precipitate from synovial fluid (with shreds and cloudy solution).
10. Characteristic histologic changes in synovium with three or more of the following: marked villous hypertrophy, proliferation of superficial synovial cells often with palisading, marked infiltration of chronic inflammatory cells (lymphocytes or plasma

cells predominating) with tendency to form lymphoid nodules, deposition of compact fibrin either on surface or interstitially, or foci of necrosis.

11. Characteristic histologic changes in nodules showing granulomatous foci with central zones of cell necrosis, surrounded by a palisade of proliferated macrophages, and peripheral fibrosis and chronic inflammatory cell infiltration, predominantly perivascular.

Definite Rheumatoid Arthritis

This diagnosis requires five of the above criteria. In criteria 1 through 5 the joint signs or symptoms must be continuous for at least 6 weeks.

Probable Rheumatoid Arthritis

This diagnosis requires three of the above criteria. In at least one of criteria 1 through 5 the joint signs or symptoms must be continuous for at least 6 weeks.

Possible Rheumatoid Arthritis

This diagnosis requires two of the following criteria and total duration of joint symptoms must be at least 3 weeks.

1. Morning stiffness
2. Tenderness or pain on motion (observed by a physician) with history of recurrence or persistence for 3 weeks.
3. History or observation of joint swelling.
4. Subcutaneous nodules (observed by a physician).
5. Elevated sedimentation rate or C-reactive protein.
6. Iritis (of dubious value as a criterion except in the case of juvenile rheumatoid arthritis).

Exclusions

1. The typical rash of systemic lupus erythematosus.
2. High concentration of lupus erythematosus cells.
3. Histologic evidence of periarteritis nodosa.
4. Weakness of neck, trunk, and pharyngeal muscles, persistent muscle swelling, or dermatomyositis.
5. A clinical picture characteristic of rheumatic fever.
6. A clinical picture characteristic of gouty arthritis.
7. A clinical picture characteristic of acute infectious arthritis.
8. Tubercule bacilli in the joints or histologic evidence of joint tuberculosis.
9. A clinical picture characteristic of Reiter's syndrome.
10. A clinical picture of the shoulder-hand syndrome.
11. A clinical picture characteristic of hypertrophic osteoarthropathy with clubbing of fingers and/or hypertrophic periostitis along the shafts of the long bones, especially if an intrapulmonary lesion (or other appropriate underlying disorder) is present.

12. A clinical picture characteristic of neuroarthropathy with condensation and destruction of bones of involved joints and with associated neurologic findings.

13. Homogentisic acid in the urine, detectable grossly with alkalinization.

14. Histologic evidence of sarcoid or positive Kveim test.

15. Multiple myeloma as evidenced by marked increase in plasma cells in the bone marrow or Bence-Jones protein in the urine.

16. Characteristic skin lesions of erythema nodosum.

17. Leukemia or lymphoma with characteristic cells in peripheral blood, bone marrow, or tissues.

18. Agammaglobulinemia.

It should be noted that these criteria were developed prior to the new classification of rheumatic diseases adopted by the American Rheumatism Association in 1963, in which ankylosing spondylitis, psoriatic arthritis, and arthritis associated with ulcerative colitis and regional enteritis are listed as distinct from rheumatoid arthritis.

REFERENCES

1. Rodman, G. P. (ed.): *Primer on the Rheumatic Diseases.* Prepared by a Committee of The American Rheumatism Association Section of the Arthritis Foundation, 1973.

2. Ropes, M. W., et al.: *1958 Revision of diagnostic criteria for rheumatoid arthritis.* Bull. Rheum. Dis. 9:175, 1958.

3. Blumberg, B., et al.: *ARA nomenclature and classification of arthritis and rheumatism.* Arthritis Rheum. 7:93, 1964.

CLASSIFICATION OF PROGRESSION OF RHEUMATOID ARTHRITIS

Stage I, Early

*1. No destructive changes on roentgenographic examination.
2. Roentgenologic evidence of osteoporosis may be present.

Stage II, Moderate

*1. Roentgenologic evidence of osteoporosis, with or without slight subchondral bone destruction; slight cartilage destruction may be present.
*2. No joint deformities, although limitation of joint mobility may be present.
3. Adjacent muscle atrophy.
4. Extra-articular soft tissue lesions such as nodules and tenosynovitis may be present.

Stage III, Severe

*1. Roentgenologic evidence of cartilage and bone destruction in addition to osteoporosis.
*2. Joint deformity, such as subluxation, ulnar deviation, or hyperextension, without fibrous or bony ankylosis.
3. Extensive muscle atrophy.
4. Extra-articular soft tissue lesions such as nodules and tenosynovitis may be present.

Stage IV, Terminal

*1. Fibrous or bony ankylosis.
2. Criteria of Stage III.

---

*The criteria that must be present to permit classification of a patient in any particular stage or grade.

REFERENCES

1. Rodman, G. P. (ed.): *Primer on the Rheumatic Diseases*. Prepared by a Committee of The American Rheumatism Association Section of the Arthritis Foundation, 1973.
2. Steinbrocker, O., Traeger, C. G., and Batterman, R. C.: *Therapeutic criteria in rheumatoid arthritis*. J.A.M.A. 140:659, 1949.

3

POLYETHYLENE GAUNTLET SPLINT (MANUAL FABRICATION METHOD)

Important—Read the entire directions before beginning splint.

MATERIALS AND EQUIPMENT

1. Polyethylene (low density) $\frac{1}{8}''$ or $\frac{3}{32}''$ thick. Can be purchased from most wholesale plastic distributors. It is very inexpensive compared with other thermoplastics.
2. Positive mold of the forearm (distal half) and hand with the thumb in palmar abduction, but mold only needs to extend to the end of the palm and middle of the thumb proximal phalanx. When making the negative mold be sure to form in the transverse arch. A rod should extend and should be centered in the shaft of the mold and extend out the proximal end for positioning in the vise. If a regular vise is used a wood stick $\frac{3}{4}''$ by $\frac{3}{4}''$ thick can be used. The stick should be positioned so the sides coincide with the anterior dorsal planes. If necessary use padding or additional plaster to build up the ulnar styloid or other bony prominences on the mold so the finished splint will form a bubble over those areas.
3. Oven 325°.
4. Piece of nylon tricot, 18″ by 18″.
5. A flat cookie sheet, Teflon coated.
6. Stockinette, cotton.
7. 8″ long, $\frac{3}{4}''$ stay (as used in corsets).
8. Two asbestos oven mitts.
9. Electric grinder/sander that is shaped to fit inside curved edges, or a Dremel type hand grinder/sander.
10. Hack saw or other fine tooth saw.

METHOD

1. Preparation of the mold:
   a. With a hack saw cut a slit along the dorsum of the mold where the dorsal opening of the splint will be.

b. Cover mold with stockinette.

c. Pound or press the plastic stay into the dorsal slit (on top of the stockinette). This provides a guide for the final cutting.

2. Cut the polyethylene. Size: Length of the mold by 4″ wider than the needed circumference. (This does not have to be precise as the material stretches and the excess can be cut off.)

3. Place mold rod in a vise so the wrist is horizontal with the volar aspect on top and the distal end towards the therapist. (Mold should be near oven if possible.)

4. Preparation of the polyethylene:

a. Place the polyethylene on the nylon tricot on the cookie sheet. (The polyethylene becomes fluid and hot to handle. The tricot should be large enough so you can pick up the plastic, using the tricot, i.e., about 1 and ½″ wider on the top and bottom, and 3″ wider on the sides.) The tricot produces a flat finish on the outside of the splint; for a shiny finish, use a piece of Teflon cloth.

b. Heat the material for 10 min. at 325° or until it just turns clear.

5. Making the splint (this is tricky and takes practice):

a. When the plastic is ready remove cookie sheet from oven and place near mold. (You have to work fast as the material cools rapidly.)

b. Lift the plastic using only the tricot and bring it over the mold. Flip it upside down and wrap and stretch it around the mold, pressing the edges along the stay and together. (It is okay if they seal together because you cut it later.) In other words, you seal up the mold (including the thumb area), but not the proximal and distal ends. Be sure to get a nice tight fit along the dorsal edge.

c. Take off the tricot.

d. Let the material cool slightly about 5 minutes, wrap with an Ace wrap, and let sit overnight. This allows the plastic to cool evenly.

e. Next day, take off Ace wrap. Position splint in the vise, dorsum of wrist up. Using a sharp mat knife, cut along the stay to make the dorsal opening of the splint. Cut the distal end as desired (see Chapter 18 regarding distal length of wrist stabilization splints). Cut thumb opening out, be careful not to cut it too large about a ½″ radial to the thenar crease. (You can always cut back later if necessary.)

6. Finishing. Take the splint off. Smooth down the edges with a Dremel type tool felt grinder attachment. With a drill make holes in a random pattern for ventilation (smooth hole edges).

7. Sew or rivet two to three Velcro closures, as desired.

GLOSSARY

This glossary defines specific terms used within this text and clinical rheumatologic terms that are not defined in standard medical dictionaries.

Abduction pillow. Large triangular pillow used to position the legs in abduction following hip surgery.

Acromegaly. Enlargement of the hands, feet, and face, secondary to a pituitary gland tumor; may be associated with DJD and back deformity.

Acrosclerosis. Scleroderma and Raynaud's phenomenon confined to the hands.

Adhesive capsulitis (of the shoulder). Frozen shoulder, development of adhesions in the shoulder joint and in surrounding soft tissue.

Agglutination test, sheep cell. Method of testing for RA factor; less commonly used than the latex fixation test.

Air compression sleeves. Plastic sleeves that fit around the hand or arm and are intermittently filled with air to compress the enclosed body part; used to reduce edema

Alopecia. Loss of hair; baldness.

Amyloidosis. Disease in which amyloid is deposited in tissues or in joints causing an arthritis; one of the causes of the carpal tunnel syndrome.

ANA. Antinuclear antibodies. Antibodies that react with nuclear antigens; found in the serum of nearly all patients with systemic lupus erythematosus and 20 percent of patients with rheumatoid arthritis, progressive systemic sclerosis, or polymyositis.

Analgesic. Medication or modality used to relieve pain.

Anaphylactoid purpura. Henoch-Schönlein purpura. (See Chapter 7.)

Anastomosis. A communication between two formerly separate structures.

Angiitis. Inflammation of blood vessels, including both arteries and veins.

Ankylosing spondylitis. Chronic bone and joint disease in which the inflammatory process has a predilection for the sacroiliac, spinal apophyseal, and sternal joints.

Ankylosis. Bony or fibrous fixation of a joint. (See Chapter 21.)

Anorexia. Lack or loss of appetite.

Anserine bursitis. Inflammation of the bursa beneath the distal aspect of the sartorius, gracilis, and semi-tendinosus muscles on the medial aspect of the proximal tibia.

Antinuclear antibodies. Antibodies that react with nuclear antigens; found in the serum of nearly all patients with systemic lupus erythematosus and 20 percent of patients with rheumatoid arthritis, progressive systemic sclerosis, or polymyositis.

Aortic arch arteritis. Arteritis of the large muscular arteries arising from the aortic arch. (See Chapter 7.)

Architectural barriers (mobility barriers). Architectural structures (such as narrow doors, curbs, or telephones placed too high) that limit a person's ambulation, wheelchair mobility, or functional independence.

Arteritis. Inflammation of the arteries.

Arthralgia. Pain in a joint.

Arthrodesis. Surgical procedure designed to produce fusion of a joint.

Arthropathy. Disease affecting a joint.

Arthroplasty. Any surgical procedure that reconstructs a joint; may or may not involve prosthetic replacement.

Arthroscope. Instrument for examining joint interiors. (The examination is called an arthroscopy.)

Arthrotomy. Surgical incision into a joint.

Articular. Of or pertaining to a joint.

Avascular necrosis. Necrosis of part of a bone secondary to ischemia; most commonly seen in the femoral or humeral head. Currently referred to as osteonecrosis.

Baker's cyst. Cystic swelling behind the knee in the popliteal space causing accumulation of fluid in various bursae.

Ballottement. A method for determining joint effusions by tapping or pressing on a joint; usually elicited in the knee by pressing on the patella.

Bamboo spine. Descriptive term for the radiographic appearance of the spine in ankylosing spondylitis.

Behçet's syndrome. Systemic disease of unknown etiologic factors that presents with recurrent painful oral and genital ulcers and iritis; an inflammatory arthritis is present in most patients.

Bennett double ring splint. Slip-on metal finger splint to limit proximal interphalangeal joint hyperextension.

Blanching. Changing to white.

Bony spurs. A pointed projection of bone. (Syn: osteophyte)

Bouchard's nodes. Osteophyte formation around the proximal interphalangeal joint typical of degenerative joint disease; similar to Heberden's nodes.

Boutonniere deformity. Finger deformity with flexion of the proximal interphalangeal joint and hyperextension of the distal interphalangeal joint.

Broach. Technique of preparing the intramedullary canal of a bone with a cutting instrument, usually for prosthetic replacement.

Buck's traction. Lower extremity traction unit, with adhesive skin attachment to the lower part of the leg.

Bunion. Hallux valgus with a painful bursitis over the medial aspect of the first metatarsophalangeal joint.

Burned out phase. Chronic inactive phase of rheumatoid arthritis or other inflammatory joint disease.

Bursa. Closed sac, filled with fluid and lined with a synovial-like membrane; serves to facilitate motion between two structures.

Bursitis. Inflammation of a bursa which can be due to frictional forces, trauma, or rheumatic diseases.

Calcific tendinitis. Inflammatory involvement of a tendon associated with calcium deposits; commonly affects the supraspinatus and biceps tendons in the shoulder.

Calcinosis. Pathological calcification of the soft tissues; occurs in a wide variety of systemic diseases.

Calcinosis circumscripta. Subcutaneous calcifications.

Capsulotomy. Incision through the joint capsule.

Carpal tunnel syndrome. Compression of the median nerve in the carpal flexor space; commonly seen in patients with flexor tenosynovitis. Initial symptoms are usually pain and tingling in the fingers, especially at night. Prolonged entrapment can lead to sensory loss and atrophy of the thenar muscles.

CARS. Canadian Arthritis and Rheumatism Society.

Causalgia. Burning pain accompanied by trophic skin lesions due to nerve injury.

C bar. Curved part of a hand splint that maintains the thumb web space.

Charcot's joint. See Neuropathic joint.

Chondrocalcinosis. Calcification of joint cartilage or menisci; may be seen in pseudogout, hyperparathyroidism, ochronosis, and other conditions.

Claudication, intermittent. Pain, tension, and weakness upon walking (not at rest) due to occlusive arterial disease.

Cock-up toe. Deformity with dorsiflexion of the metatarsophalangeal joint and flexion of the interphalangeal/distal interphalangeal joints.

Collagen. Protein molecule that provides the basic support for all connective tissue including fibrous tissue, cartilage, and bone.

Compression gloves. Any type of stretch glove designed to reduce edema such as Futuro Cotton-Stretch Glove and Jobst Custom Elastic Gloves.

Connective tissue. General term used to describe tissue that connects one part of the body to another; includes fibrous tissue, bone, cartilage, synovium, blood vessels, ligaments, tendons, and parts of muscle.

Cor pulmonale. Failure of the right side of the heart secondary to pulmonary disease.

Crepitation. A grating, crunching, or popping sensation (or sound) that occurs during joint or tendon motion.

CRST syndrome. Tetrad of symptoms consisting of calcinosis, Raynaud's phenomenon, sclerodactyly, and telangiectasia.

Cup (mold) arthroplasty. Arthroplasty that interposes a metal cup between the head of the femur and the acetabulum.

Cushingoid features. Characteristic physical changes with alterations in fat metabolism and the deposition of sucutaneous fat (1) in the face, producing moon facies or (2) at the dorsum of the neck called buffalo hump. Other features include obesity, purpura, and striae. This is a common side effect of long-term steroidal therapy.

Cyanosis. Bluish discoloration of the skin; used to describe the color of the hands in Raynaud's phenomenon or in other types of vascular insufficiencies.

Darrach procedure. Resection of the distal end of the ulna.

Degenerative joint disease. Noninflammatory slowly progressive disorder of joints caused by deterioration of articular cartilage with secondary bone formation.

Dermatomyositis. Variety of skin rashes that may accompany polymyositis.

de Quervain's disease. Stenosing tenosynovitis of the first dorsal compartment of the wrist involving the abductor pollicis longus and extensor pollicis brevis.

Diarthrodial joints. Synovial lined joints.

Diathermy. A method of producing deep therapeutic heat by passing electronic or sound waves through tissue.

Discoid lupus. A disease of the skin presenting with well-demarcated erythematous scaly plaques. In later stages the skin becomes atrophic and scarred; although usually confined to the face, neck, ears, and scalp it may occur on the extremities. About 10 percent of patients will develop systemic lupus erythematosus.

Discogenic. A problem or symptom caused by derangement of an intervertebral disc.

Dislocation. Disruption of a joint characterized by lack of contact between articular surfaces.

Dolorimeter. A device for quantitating the amount of external pressure a person can tolerate over a joint; used as an indicator of pain tolerance.

Dupuytren's contracture. Joint contracture secondary to shortening, thickening, and fibrosis of the palmar fascia; typically involves the fourth or fifth digits.

Dysphagia. Difficulty in swallowing. Frequently seen in progressive systemic sclerosis as a result of esophageal fibrosis and in polymyositis because of esophageal muscle weakness.

Edema. Perceptible accumulation of excess fluid in the tissues.

Effusion. Excess fluid in the joint indicating irritation or inflammation of the synovium.

Erythema. Redness.

Erythema nodosum. Inflammatory rheumatic disease involving painful subcutaneous nodules in the legs; many patients have a self-limited arthritis.

Exacerbation. Increase of disease process either systemically or localized to a single joint; a flare up.

Extension contracture. Fixed limitation of joint flexion.

Exostosis. Ossification of muscular or ligamentous attachments.

Felty's syndrome. A combination of rheumatoid arthritis, splenomegaly, anemia, and leukopenia.

Fibrosis. Deposition of fibrous tissue.

Fibrositis. Syndrome of pain, tenderness, and stiffness in deep tissue, such as muscle.

Finger ladder. Notched board positioned on a wall so that a person can "walk" each increment with the fingertips in a manner that increases shoulder flexion or abduction; it is an active-assisted exercise.

Flexion contracture. Fixed limitation of joint extension.

Fusiform swelling. Fusiform means spindle shaped and refers to the shape of the joint when there is synovitis. It is indicative of the inflammation being confined to the joint capsule.

GC. Gonorrhea (gonococci); can produce a secondary arthritis.

Ganglion. A cystic mass usually containing thick gelatinous material arising from or in close proximity to synovial lined joints or tendon sheaths. Most commonly found over the dorsal and radiovolar aspects of the wrist

Genu. The knee. Genu valgum: valgus deformity (knock knee); genu varum: varus deformity (bowleg).

Girdlestone procedure. Excisional arthroplasty of the femoral head and neck.

Gold therapy. Use of gold compound injections for treatment of rheumatoid arthritis.

Gout. Disease characterized by acute episodes of arthritis with the presence of sodium urate crystals in the synovial fluid or deposits of urate crystals in or about the joints and other tissues.

Hallux valgus. Valgus deformity (lateral deviation) at the first metatarsophalangeal joint.

Hashimoto's thyroiditis. Inflammatory disease of the thyroid that eventually leads to hypothyroidism; may be seen in association with systemic lupus erythematosus.

Heberden's nodes. Bony overgrowth or enlargement at the margin of the distal interphalangeal joint; characteristic of primary degenerative joint disease.

Henoch-Schönlein purpura. Self-limiting vasculitis that affects the small vessels of the skin, genitourinary tract, synovium, and kidneys.

HLA-B27. A genetically determined antigen associated with ankylosing spondylitis.

Honeycomb lung. Radiologic appearance of the lung in pulmonary fibrosis.

Housemaid's knee. Prepatellar bursitis; a swelling between the skin and lower patella or patellar tendon that may result from frequent kneeling.

Hydrarthrosis. Noninflammatory effusion of a synovial lined joint.

Hypersensitivity angiitis. A general term referring to inflammation of small vessels resulting from drug reactions, serum sickness, or other inciting factors.

Hypertrophic arthritis. Another term for degenerative joint disease.

Intrinsic minus position. Extension or hyperextension of metacarpophalangeal joints with flexion of proximal and distal interphalangeal joints (claw deformity).

Intrinsic plus position. Flexion of the metacarpophalangeal joints and extension of the proximal and distal interphalangeal joints.

Iritis. Inflammation of the iris and certain adjacent structures, typically seen in juvenile rheumatoid arthritis and the rheumatoid

variants; can cause scarring and lead to visual loss.

Isometric exercise. Exercises involving maximal muscle contraction without joint motion.

Isotonic exercise. Exercises involving muscle contraction with joint motion.

Jaccoud's deformity. Development of metacarpophalangeal ulnar drift and proximal interphalangeal hyperextension without joint inflammation following rheumatic fever. (Syn: Jaccoud's polyarthritis, postrheumatic fever arthritis)

Jog of motion. Minimal joint motion, usually less than 10 degrees excursion in any plane.

Joint mice (loose bodies). Small detached pieces of cartilage and bone found free in the joint which may be symptomatic if they get trapped between the joint surfaces; found in degenerative joint disease and Charcot's joint.

Knuckle bender splint. Dynamic hand splint that flexes the metacarpophalangeal joints and is commonly used to correct metacarpophalangeal extension contractures.

Kyphosis. Forward curvature of the spine; e.g., humpback in the thoracic spine.

Lag. Difference between active and passive range of motion.

Latex fixation. Method of testing for rheumatoid arthritis factor; person may be described as Latex positive if factor is present and negative if it is absent.

L.E. Prep (preparation). Serological study to identify the lupus erythematous cell; one method of measuring antibodies to systemic lupus erythematosus nuclei seen in systemic lupus erythematosus.

Littler intrinsic release procedure. Excision of the oblique fibers of the extensor mechanism to overcome an intrinsic contracture.

Loose bodies. See Joint mice.

Lupus hair. Broken disorderly hairs about the forehead; seen in systemic lupus erythematosus patients.

Malabsorption. Inability to absorb foods; seen in progressive systemic sclerosis with severe intestinal fibrosis.

Malaise. Feeling of general discomfort or uneasiness; an out-of-sorts feeling.

Mallet finger deformity. Deformity involving only flexion of the distal interphalangeal joint; secondary to disruption of the insertion of the extensor tendon into the base of the distal phalanx.

Metatarsal bar. Ridge on the sole of the shoe to relieve metatarsal pressure and pain.

Metatarsal pad. Pad placed inside the shoe proximal to the metatarsal heads to relieve metatarsal pressure and pain.

Metatarsalgia. Pain over the metatarsal heads on the plantar aspect of the foot.

Moon facies. A rounding of the face due to fat deposition; a side effect of long-term steroid therapy.

Morning stiffness. This term describes the prolonged generalized stiffness that occurs in association with the inflammatory polyarthritides (especially RA and AS) upon awakening. The stiffness tends to be generalized and is indicative of systemic involvement. The duration of the stiffness correlates with the activity of the disease. This generalized stiffness is in contrast to the localized stiffness seen in DJD which results from inactivity.

Morphea. Localized scleroderma that may be a small circumscribed area or large diffuse patches; involves only the skin and subcutis.

Morton's neuroma. A neuroma of the plantar digital nerve caused by trauma to the nerve as it passes between the metatarsal heads; results in burning, numbness, tingling, or cramplike pain of the forefoot. May be due to wearing shoes with narrow toe width.

Muscle setting. Isometric exercise; usually used in reference to strengthening the quadriceps muscles (quad sets).

Muscular splinting. Protective reflex muscle spasm.

Mutilans deformity. Severe bony destruction and resorption in a diarthrodial joint. In the fingers it results in a telescoping shortening (opera glass hand).

Myalgia. Muscle pain.

Myositis. Inflammatory disease of striated muscle.

Myositis ossificans (Heterotopic ossification). Ossification of muscles, soft tissues, fascia, and tendons; may be due to musculoskeletal trauma or repeated joint manipulations. The elbow is especially prone to this condition.

Neuropathic joint. Joint with severe destruction and disorganization caused by a disturbance of joint innervation; commonly seen in the knee with syphilitic tabes dorsalis, in the ankle with diabetic neuropathy, and in the shoulder with syringomyelia. (Syn: Charcot's joint)

Oligoarticular. Involvement of a few joints, usually three or less.

Orthosis. Any medical device applied to the body to provide support or increase function; includes splinting, bracing, and corsets.

Osteoarthritis. The most common term used for degenerative joint disease.

Osteonecrosis. This refers to the death of bone cells. It can be due to trauma to the blood supply (avascular osteonecrosis), or it can be idiopathic (aseptic necrosis). Osteonecrosis commonly occurs in the femoral and humeral heads. It can occur in other bones, including the carpal bones.

Osteophyte. Focal bone growth at joint margins occurring in response to joint destruction. (Syn: bony spurs)

Osteoporosis. Condition characterized by a loss of bone cells. It can be a primary condition or associated with other diseases, drug therapies (steroids), or disuse; can be improved or minimized with active motion and exercise.

Osteotomy. Surgical cutting of a bone.

Pannus. Excessive proliferation of synovial and granulation tissue that invades the joint surfaces.

Palindromic rheumatism. Condition in which patient develops, within minutes, attacks of acute arthritis that last from several hours to several days without systemic signs or residual joint damage.

Pauciarticular. Involvement of a few joints.

Periarteritis nodosa. Same as polyarteritis.

Periarticular swelling. Diffuse swelling of the soft tissues surrounding the joint (extra-articular swelling).

Pes planus. Deformity of the foot characterized by loss of the longitudinal arch. (Syn: flatfoot)

Photosensitivity. Sensitivity to light, especially ultraviolet rays.

Polymyalgia rheumatica. Condition characterized by stiffness and pain of the shoulder muscles without weakness; affects older women and sometimes is accompanied by temporal arteritis.

Polyarteritis nodosa. Inflammatory disease of the medium-sized arteries producing diffuse musculoskeletal and neurologic symptoms.

Polymyositis. Diffuse inflammatory disease of striated muscle that leads to muscle destruction and symmetrical proximal muscle weakness.

Positive mold. In splinting it is the plaster replicate of the body part, e.g., of the wrist. A negative mold is the outer shell used to cast the positive mold.

Pott's disease. Tuberculosis of the spine.

Primary disease. A disease of unknown etiologic factors.

Prodrome. Early symptom of a disease.

Prosthesis, joint. An artificial substitution for part or all of a joint. Examples are:

Austin-Moore. Metal femoral head and neck replacement.

Charnly-Mueller. Total hip replacement with a metal femoral component and plastic acetabular component.

Geometric. Total knee replacement with a metal femoral component and plastic tibial component.

MacIntosh. Metallic tibial plateau replacements.

Nibauer. Silastic finger implants covered with a Dacron mesh.

Swanson finger prosthesis. Silastic implants for the metacarpophalangeal and proximal interphalangeal joints.

Protrusio acetabulae. Condition in which the head of the femur pushes the acetabulum into the pelvic cavity.

Pseudogout (Articular chondrocalcinosis). Similar to gout clinically but a condition in which the synovitis is due to deposits of calcium pyrophosphate dehydrate crystals (instead of urate crystals).

Pulmonary osteoarthropathy (hypertrophic osteoarthropathy). Condition with clubbing of the distal interphalangeal joints, arthralgias, and effusion of other joints (knees, ankles, elbows, and metacarpophalangeal joints) as manifestations of various diseases, especially carcinoma of the lung.

Purpura. Condition characterized by hemorrhage into the skin.

Raynaud's disease. Symptoms of digital paroxysmal vasospasm without an associated disease.

Raynaud's phenomenon. Paroxysmal vasospasm of the fingers in association with a disease; occurs in 90 percent of people with progressive systemic sclerosis and 50 percent with systemic lupus erythematosus. Vasospasm results in blanching, erythema, and cyanosis of the hands.

Reduction. Passive correction or realignment of a joint deformity or fracture.

Reefing. Surgical procedure for taking up the slack in an attenuated structure by folding the attenuated area back on itself and suturing it in place; e.g., radial side reefing of the extensor mechanism in the rheumatoid hand.

Reflex dystrophy (Sudeck's atrophy). Abnormal reflex sympathetic nerve involvement secondary to trauma, resulting in severe pain, edema, vasomotor instability, and atrophy of the bone, muscle, and skin.

Reflux esophagitis. Inflammation of the lower portion of the esophagus as a result of regurgitation of acid from the stomach.

Reiter's syndrome. Currently refers to arthritis associated with nongonococcal urethritis or dysentery; in classic cases conjunctivitis and skin lesions are also present. Typically the arthritis is limited to a single episode but it can become chronic.

Reposition. To replace or realign.

Resection arthroplasty. Removal of the articular ends of one or both bones forming a joint, e.g., Darrach procedure and girdlestone procedure.

Rheumatism. Lay term used to refer to any type of muscle or joint pain or ache.

Rheumatoid arthritis. A systemic disease characterized by chronic inflammation of the synovium.

Rheumatoid factor (RA factor). A substance found in the blood of a high percentage of people with classic or definite rheumatoid arthritis. Alone, it does not indicate RA, but, with other RA features, can help lead to a diagnosis of RA. It may also occur in other diseases such as cirrhosis and tuberculosis. A person may be described as seronegative or positive. A latex fixation or sheep cell agglutination test is used to determine if the factor is present.

Rheumatoid-like arthritis. A symmetric small-joint polyarticular arthritis that resembles rheumatoid arthritis but usually is not as severe. Typical of the arthritis found in systemic lupus erythematosus, polymyositis, and progressive systemic sclerosis.

Rheumatoid variants. A group of diseases

characterized by (1) inflammatory joint disease of the spine and sacroiliac joints, (2) asymmetric peripheral arthritis, (3) iritis, and (4) presence of HLA-B27 antigen in a high percentage of patients. This disease classification includes ankylosing spondylitis, psoriatic arthritis, Reiter's syndrome, and the arthritis seen with ulcerative colitis or regional enteritis.

Rocker sole. Shoe sole, curved at the toe to facilitate push off for limited ankle motion.

SI joint. Sacroiliac joint.

Sarcoidosis. Systemic disease of unknown etiologic factors characterized by a reaction of neoplastic granulation tissue. It can affect almost any tissue; therefore symptoms depend on the site. Associated arthropathy may include mild periarticular involvement, acute or chronic synovitis, or destruction of bone.

Sclerodactyly. Sclerosis and tapering of the fingers in progressive systemic sclerosis.

Sciatica. Vague term commonly used to refer to low back pain syndromes with involvement of the sciatic nerve.

Secondary disease. A disease in which the causal factor is known.

Sedimentation rate. The rate at which red blood cells sediment in serum; elevated in any inflammatory disease such as rheumatoid arthritis.

Shoulder-hand syndrome. Condition associated with reflex sympathetic dystrophy of the shoulder and hand secondary to pathology in the shoulder; pain, vasomotor disturbance, and diffuse swelling can lead to severe hand contractures and atrophy of tissues.

Sicca syndrome. A combination of lacrimal gland atrophy, resulting in insufficient tear production (keratoconjunctivitis sicca) and corneal changes, and salivary gland atrophy (xerostomia), resulting in a dry mouth. When associated with a rheumatic disease the triad is known as Sjögren's syndrome.

Sjögren's syndrome. Disease of the lacrimal and parotid glands, resulting in dry eyes and mouth; frequently occurs with rheumatoid arthritis, systemic lupus erythematosus, and systemic sclerosis.

Splayfoot. Transverse spreading of the forefoot.

Spondylitis. Inflammation of the spine involving the apophyseal (interfacet) and costoverterbral joints. Osteitis of the vertebral bodies, paravertebral ligaments, and muscles may be associated with spondylitis.

Spondylosis. Term applied nonspecifically to any lesion of the spine of a degenerative nature; reactive changes in the vertebral bodies about the interspace usually associated with discopathy.

Steinmann pin. A traction or fixation pin.

Still's disease. A variety of juvenile rheumatoid arthritis with severe systemic involvement and high spiking fevers.

Subluxation. Incomplete dislocation.

Swan neck deformity. Finger deformity involving hyperextension of the proximal interphalangeal joint and flexion of the distal interphalangeal joint.

Symptom. Pathology that is felt or experienced. (A *sign* refers to pathology that is observable.)

Syncope. Fainting.

Synovectomy. Surgical procedure to remove the synovial lining of joints or tendon sheaths.

Synovium. Lining tissue in diarthrodial joints, tendon sheaths, and bursa. In the joint it produces fluid to lubricate the joint and is the part of the joint that becomes inflamed in inflammatory joint disease.

Synovitis. Inflammation of the synovium.

Systemic. A condition that affects the body as a whole.

Systemic lupus erythematosus. Systemic inflammatory disease characterized by small vessel vasculitis and a diverse clinical picture.

Tabes dorsalis. Tertiary form of syphilis characterized by neurologic symptoms such as absent position and vibratory senses.

Telangiectasis. Chronic dilation of capillaries and small arterial branches which produces small reddish spots in the skin.

Tendinitis. Tendon inflammation.

Tendon ruptures. Sudden discontinuity in a tendon.

Tenosynovitis. Inflammation of the synovial lining of tendon sheaths.

Thermography. Method of photography that demonstrates the heat distribution in a body part.

Thrombocytopenia. Condition in which there is a reduced number of platelets in the circulating blood.

Tinnitus. Persistent ringing or buzzing sensations in the ear, used as an indicator of aspirin toxicity (aspirin levels are maintained just below the dosage that causes tinnitus).

Tophi. Deposits of uric acid crystals around the joints or in ear cartilage.

Trigger finger (triggering). Inconsistent limitation of finger flexion or extension often caused by a nodule on a flexor tendon or stenosis of the tendon sheath.

UC-BL shoe insert. Plastic custom-molded shoe insert used for ankle or foot support.

Ulnar drift. Abnormal ulnar deviation of the fingers at the metacarpophalangeal joints.

Uveitus. Same as iritis.

Venostasis. Pooling of blood in the lower legs because of poor circulation.

Wall walking. Walking the fingertips up a wall in a manner that increases shoulder flexion or abduction; method used in place of the finger ladder.

Weaver's bottom. Ischial bursitis, inflammation of the bursa separating the gluteus maximus from the underlying ischial tuberosity; usually resulting from prolonged sitting on hard surfaces. This can also occur with bicycling.

Wegener's granulomatosis. A destructive arteritis of the upper respiratory tract, lungs, and kidneys. It may have an associated joint pain.

Zig-zag effect. Ulnar drift at the metacarpophalangeal joints associated with radial deviation of the wrist.

INDEX

A *t* following a page number indicates a table.

Bed
    position of
        in joint disease, 393
Benemid
    for treatment of gout, 105
Bouchard's nodes, 201–202
Boutonniere deformity, 221
    chronic synovitis in, 221–222
    joint protection principles for, 359
    surgery for, 129–130
Bufferin
    for treatment of rheumatic disease, 96t, 99t
Bursectomy
    shoulder, 160–161
Bursitis
    shoulder, 159–160
Butazolidin alka
    for treatment of rheumatic disease, 97t

CALCINOSIS
    in systemic sclerosis, 55–56
Capitello-condylar elbow arthroplasty, 154–155
Cardiac fibrosis
    in systemic sclerosis, 57
Carpal tunnel syndrome (CTS), 120
    at wrist, 248–249
    muscle atrophy and, 226
    surgery for, 119–122
Cation salicylates
    for treatment of rheumatic disease, 99
Chlorambucil
    for treatment of arthritis, 39
Choline salicylate
    for treatment of rheumatic disease, 99
Chronic tophaceous gout, 90
Clinoril
    for treatment of rheumatic disease, 96t
Coban
    for wrapping inflamed joints, 76
Colchicine
    for treatment of gout, 90, 105
Contracture(s)
    extension, 35
    flexion, 35
    in systemic sclerosis, 48
    joint, 209–211
        in dermatomysitis, 62
        in polymyositis, 62
    PIP joint
        in tenosynovitis, 122
    positioning for prevention of, 393–398
Crafts
    therapeutic, 379–381
Crepitation
    in DJD of CMC joint, 204

Crocheting
    as functional activity, 380–381
Cyclophosphamide
    for treatment of arthritis, 39
Cyst(s)
    synovial, 201
Cytoxan
    for treatment of arthritis, 39

DARRACH procedure, 136–138
Deformity(ies)
    hand. See Hand, deformities of.
    positions of
        avoidance of, 355
Degenerative joint disease (DJD), 195–196
    age at onset of, 79
    diagnosis of, 80
    etiologic factors in, 79
    hip involvement in, 82–83
    inflammation in, 7
    neck involvement in, 85–86
    of spine, 80
    osteophytes and, 201–202
    primary, 79
        finger involvement in, 81
        thumb involvement in, 81–82
    prognosis for, 80
    secondary, 79
        ankle involvement in, 83
        back involvement in, 84–85
        elbow involvement in, 84
        knee involvement, 82
        shoulder involvement in, 83–84
        wrist involvement in, 84
    sexes affected by, 79
    symptoms of, 80
Denial
    as response to chronic illness, 13–14
Dependency
    as response to chronic illness, 17
Depression
    as response to chronic illness, 14–16
    identification of, 15–18
de Quervain's tenosynovitis, 118, 236, 240
    vs. DJD of thumb, 203
Dermatomyositis
    age at onset of, 59
    conditions associated with, 63
    diagnosis of, 59
    drug therapy for, 63
    etiologic factors in, 59
    muscle atrophy in, 61
    muscle pain in, 61
    occupational therapy for, 60–61
    prognosis for, 59

Dematomyositis—*Continued*
    sexes affected by, 59
    symptoms of, 60-61
Disability
    patient response to, 13-16
Disalcid, 96*t*, 99
Double crush syndrome, 253
Drug(s)
    experimental
        for treatment of arthritis, 39
    nonsteroidal anti-inflammatory (NSAIDs), 98-100
    remission-inducing (RIDs), 101
        for treatment of arthritis, 38-39

ECOTRIN, 96*t*, 99*t*
Edema
    in systemic sclerosis, 48
Elbow(s)
    fascial arthroplasty in, 155
    involvement of in RA, 35-36
    joint protection principles for, 363
    positioning of
        in joint disease, 394
    range of motion of
        measurement of, 282
    surgery of, 151-152
    synovectomy of, 152-153
    synovitis of
        and hand deformities, 194
    total replacement of, 153-154
        prostheses for, 153
    ulnar nerve entrapment at, 253-254
Energy conservation
    instruction in, 351
    rest/work balance in, 353-354
    work simplification in, 354-355
Equipment. *See* Assistive equipment.
Erythema
    palmar, 246
Exercise(s)
    active-assistive
        with deltoid aid, 390
    amount of, 385
    follow-through on, 386
    for muscle re-education, 390-391
    for muscle strength, 386-391
    for range of motion, 383
    isometric
        for muscle strength, 388-389
    progressive resistive (PRE)
        for muscle strength, 389-390
    timing of, 385
    types of
        for range of motion, 384-385

Extensor communis (EC)
    rupture of, 242
    surgery for, 124-128
Extensor digiti quinti (EDQ)
    rupture of, 242
    surgery for, 124-128
Extensor pollicis longus (EPL)
    rupture of, 243
    surgery for, 124-128

FACE
    in systemic sclerosis, 53-54
Fatigue
    as symptom of rheumatoid arthritis, 37-38
    as symptom of SLE, 42-43
Fenoprofen, 96*t*
Fever
    as symptom of SLE, 42-43
Fibrosis
    cardiac
        in systemic sclerosis, 57
    pulmonary
        in systemic sclerosis, 56-57
Finger(s)
    abduction of
        measurement of, 289
    deformities of. *See under individual names.*
    deviation of
        measurement of, 290
    joint protection principles for, 356
    osteophytes of
        formation of, 201-202
    range of motion of
        measurement of, 283-284, 289
Finkelstein test
    for de Quervain's tenosynovitis, 240-241
Flexion deformity
    joint protection principles for, 359
Flexor digitorum profundus
    rupture of, 244
    surgery for, 124-128
Flexor digitorum superficialis (FDS)
    rupture of, 244
    surgery for, 124-128
Flexor pollicis longus (FPL)
    rupture of, 243
    surgery for, 124-128
Foot
    hallux rigidus in
        correction of, 183
    hallux valgus in
        correction of, 183
    joint protection principles for, 362
    surgery of, 181-182

Hip(s)—*Continued*
    joint protection principles for, 361–362
    positioning of
        in joint disease, 395
    surgery of, 169–170
    total replacement of, 170–173
Hydroxychloroquine
    for treatment of rheumatic disease, 2, 102
Hypersensitivity angiitis, 66

IBUPROFEN
    for treatment of rheumatic disease, 96t
Implant(s). *See under* Prosthesis(es).
Imuran
    in treatment of arthritis, 39
Indocin
    for treatment of rheumatic disease, 97t
Indomethacin
    for treatment of gout, 90
    for treatment of rheumatic disease, 97t
Inflammation
    signs of, 197
Interosseus(i)
    dorsal
        weakness of, 228
    volar
        weakness of, 228
Intrasynovial steroid injection
    for treatment of inflammation, 100–101
Intrinsic plus deformity
    splinting for, 317
Iritis
    as manifestation of AS, 70

JOINT(s)
    ankylosis of, 211–212
    contractures of, 209–211
        in dermatomyositis, 62
        in polymyositis, 62
    carpometacarpal
        arthroplasty of, 143–144
        range of motion of
            measurement of, 287
    distal interphalangeal
        arthrodesis of, 149
        hyperextension of
            measurement of, 286
        range of motion of
            measurement of, 285
    large
        use of
            for joint protection, 355
    metacarpophalangeal
        hyperextension of

measurement of, 286
    implant arthroplasty of, 138–142
    range of motion of
        measurement of, 284
    subluxation in, 206
    synovectomy of, 115–116
    ulnar deviation of
        measurement of, 280–281
metatarsophalangeal
    arthroplasty of, 182
    resection of, 182
proximal interphalangeal, 142–143
    arthrodesis of, 147–149
    hyperextension of
        measurement of, 286
    range of motion of
        measurement of, 285
    synovectomy of, 116–117
radiocarpal
    implant surgery for, 135–136
    prostheses for, 134–135
    subluxation of, 206, 212–213
radioulnar
    replacement of, 136–138
    resection of, 136–138
    subluxation of, 213
stability of, 209
stiffness of
    in ankylosing spondylitis, 69
talonavicular
    arthrodesis of, 183
thumb CMC
    degenerative joint disease of, 204
Joint disease. *See also* Arthritis.
    and joint mobility, 383–384
    forms of, 2
    inflammatory, 3–6
    inflammatory phases of, 2
    noninflammatory, 7
        occupational therapy goals for, 7
        outline of, 5–6
    positioning in, 393
    therapy for
        goals of, 2
        initiation of, 2
        overview of, 1–3
Joint protection
    in swan neck deformity, 358–359
    instruction in, 351
        for neck, 368–369
    patient instruction in, 352–353
    principles of, 353–356
        application of, 356–363
        for back, 364–368
        for neck, 369–371

Prosthesis(es)
finger, 133–134
for total hip replacement, 170
for total knee replacement, 175–177
Neer
for shoulder replacement, 161
nonhinge
for total knee replacement, 178–180
Silastic
for MTP arthroplasty, 182
Protective MCP splint, 332–336
indications for, 335t
Psoriatic arthritis (PA). See Arthritis, psoriatic.
Pulmonary fibrosis
in systemic sclerosis, 56–57
Purpura, types of, 246

RADIAL HEAD
resection of
in elbow, 152–153
Radial nerve entrapment, 254–257
Radial tunnel syndrome (RTS), 257
Radiculopathy
cervical, 247
Range of motion (ROM)
assessment of
methods of, 288–290
composite
measurement of
for fingers, 289
functional
assessment of, 288, 289t
hand
exercises for, 50–51
maintenance of
in systemic sclerosis, 48–49
measurement of, 262
goniometer for, 281–287
method of, 281
Range of motion (ROM) lag
causes of, 204
Rash(es)
erythematous
in SLE, 43–44
evanescent, 245
skin
in dermatomyositis, 62
in drug reactions, 245
in polymyositis, 62
terms used for, 244–245
Raynaud's phenomenon, 246–247
as manifestation of SLE, 44
associated with polymyositis, 63

in systemic sclerosis, 49
treatment of, 51–52
Remission(s)
drug-induced, 2
spontaneous, 1–2
Remission-inducing drugs (RIDs)
for treatment of arthritis, 38–39
for treatment of rheumatic disease, 101
Rheumatic disease. See also Joint disease.
causes of pain in, 4
common medications used for, 104t
concerns of patients with, 18
medical history in
evaluation of, 187
morning stiffness in, 188–189
neurologic involvement in, 247
psychological factors related to, 12–13
symptoms of
evaluation of, 187
Rheumatoid arthritis (RA). See Arthritis, rheumatoid.

SALICYLATES
cation
for treatment of rheumatic disease, 96t, 99
for treatment of rheumatic disease, 96t, 98
Salicylsalicylic acid
for treatment of rheumatic disease, 99
Scleroderma. See Systemic sclerosis.
Shoulder
acromioplasty of, 160–161
bursectomy of, 160–161
in RA, 36
joint protection principles for, 363
Neer prosthesis for, 161
pain in
and hand deformities, 194
range of motion of
measurement of, 281–282
surgery of, 159–160
synovectomy of, 160–161
total replacement of, 161–163
Shoulder-hand syndrome, 194
Silastic implant(s)
for metatarsophalangeal arthroplasty, 182
Sjögren's syndrome
associated with polymyositis, 63
associated with SLE, 45
in systemic sclerosis, 57
Skin
changes in
in rheumatic disease, 244–245
ulcerations of, 245